About the Authors

Bettie Lilley Nosek is a registered nurse, published author, and entrepreneur. Bettie began her career working in the ICU-CCU at Memorial Baptist Hospital in Houston. She then moved to Denver, Colorado, and worked as the Staff Development Coordinator in the operating room at Porter Memorial Hospital.

While in Colorado, she obtained a journalism degree from Loretto Heights College and worked as a copy editor for the *Rocky Mountain Medical Journal*.

After moving to California, she created instructional videos demonstrating infusion pumps and conducted evaluations of infusion pumps at the University of California, San Diego, and Children's Hospital in Los Angeles. She then worked as Director of Surgical Services at Garfield Medical Center in Monterey Park, where she supervised the operating room, recovery room, and central service.

Later, she worked as a Bureau Chief for International Medical News Group, covering medical conventions, and was published in physicians' newspapers and healthcare magazines.

Bettie began her entrepreneurial career by joining her husband in owning a telecommunications company. After running and later selling the company, Bettie started her own consulting firm, helping small businesses develop sales.

She owns several patents, copyrights, and trademarks, and she's a licensed California real estate agent and notary. She lives in Southern California and enjoys playing golf with her husband and being constantly amazed by her granddaughter.

Deborah Trendel-Leader is a registered nurse and freelance medical journalist with a bachelor's degree in nursing. She holds current certifications in critical care, IV therapy, public health nursing, and advanced cardiac life support and has a teaching credential issued by the Board of Vocational Nursing. With her career spanning more than two decades, Deborah has worked in a variety of healthcare facilities, specializing in critical care, and has served as a clinical supervisor/nurse educator in both the hospital and home health settings. She has taught numerous IV therapy certification courses for vocational nursing programs and keeps her IV skills current with continuing education courses specific to the principles, administration, and management of IV therapy. Currently, she is an active member of the Infusion Nurses Society, works per diem in adult critical care, and is a freelance medical journalist for About.com, part of the New York Times Company.

Dedication

From Bettie: I dedicate this book to my wonderful husband and best friend, Jim, who has inspired, helped, tolerated, and believed in me for more than 30 years. His indomitable spirit and unconquerable soul fill me with life's most valuable commodities — love, courage, and hope.

This book is also dedicated to our children, Tamitha, Jason, and Rebecca, who have inspired us with their accomplishments and blessed us with beautiful grandchildren.

I also dedicate this book to my sisters, Dortha and Lynda, who have always been a part of my life and have allowed me to be a part of theirs. I will cherish our love and memories forever.

Finally, I dedicate this book to my lifelong friends, who have grown up with me and shared all of life's passages.

From Deborah: I would like to dedicate this book to my mother, Virginia Trendel, who has been a constant source of support for me throughout my life. I also dedicate this book to my dear friends, Lori Israel and Arlene Wyman, whose inspiration and encouragement have been the backbone of my adult life. Finally, I want to dedicate this book to all of the aspiring nurses and other healthcare professionals who read this book. You're about to embark on one of the most rewarding journeys of your life, and I'm proud to be a part of your journey.

IV Therapy

D

by Bett
Deborah

WILEY

John Wiley & Sons, Inc.

IV Therapy For Dummies®

Published by
John Wiley & Sons, Inc.
111 River St.
Hoboken, NJ 07030-5774
www.wiley.com

Copyright © 2013 by John Wiley & Sons, Inc., Hoboken, New Jersey

Published by John Wiley & Sons, Inc., Hoboken, New Jersey

Published simultaneously in Canada

For general information on our other products and services, please contact our Customer Care Department within the U.S. at 877-762-2974, outside the U.S. at 317-572-3993, or fax 317-572-4002.

For technical support, please visit www.wiley.com/techsupport.

Wiley publishes in a variety of print and electronic formats and by print-on-demand. Some material included with standard print versions of this book may not be included in e-books or in print-on-demand. If this book refers to media such as a CD or DVD that is not included in the version you purchased, you may download this material at http://booksupport.wiley.com. For more information about Wiley products, visit www.wiley.com.

Library of Congress Control Number: 2012949510

ISBN 978-1-118-11644-9 (pbk); ISBN 978-1-118-22445-8 (ebk); ISBN 978-1-118-23766-3 (ebk); ISBN 978-1-118-26256-6 (ebk)

Manufactured in the United States of America

10 9 8 7 6 5 4 3 2 1

WILEY

Authors' Acknowledgments

From Bettie: I would like to thank my agent, Barb Doyen, for giving me the opportunity to write this book and the inspiration needed to see it through to the end. It's been a wonderful journey!

Thanks to the great folks at John Wiley & Sons, Inc., especially Alissa Schwipps, Stacy Kennedy, and Amanda Langferman, who gave me direction and support every step of the way.

Thanks to my coauthor, Deborah Trendel-Leader, for her contributions.

Finally, I'd like to thank the countless hospital patients who knew I was a newbie at starting IVs but held out their arms anyway. Thanks for your vote of confidence and for helping me learn the life-sustaining skill of IV therapy.

From Deborah: This book would not have become a reality for me without the tremendous efforts of my agent, Barb Doyen. She believed in me from the start and served as a constant source of encouragement and support throughout the entire process. I would also like to extend a special thanks to my project editor, Alissa Schwipps, who was always patient and professional in spite of my many time constraints. Additional thanks go out to the great team at John Wiley & Sons, Inc. — my copy editor, Amanda Langferman, technical editors, Jeffrey Bohmer, MD, Kay Coulter, CRNI, and William E. Miller RN, BSN, CRNI, VA-BC, and medical illustrator, Kathryn Born — for their expertise in getting this book ready for print. Finally, I want to express my sincere appreciation to my coauthor, Bettie Lilley Nosek, for her many contributions to the project and for seeing the book with a similar set of eyes.

Publisher's Acknowledgments

We're proud of this book; please send us your comments at http://dummies.custhelp.com. For other comments, please contact our Customer Care Department within the U.S. at 877-762-2974, outside the U.S. at 317-572-3993, or fax 317-572-4002.

Some of the people who helped bring this book to market include the following:

Acquisitions, Editorial, and Vertical Websites

Senior Project Editor: Alissa Schwipps

Acquisitions Editor: Stacy Kennedy

Copy Editor: Amanda M. Langferman

Assistant Editor: David Lutton

Editorial Program Coordinator: Joe Niesen

Technical Editors: Jeffrey H. Bohmer, MD, FACEP; Kay Coulter, CRNI, VA-BC; William E. Miller RN, BSN, CRNI, VA-BC

Editorial Manager: Christine Meloy Beck

Editorial Assistants: Rachelle Amick, Alexa Koschier

Art Coordinator: Alicia B. South

Cover Photo: © iStockphoto.com / Mark Evans

Cartoons: Rich Tennant (www.the5thwave.com)

Composition Services

Project Coordinator: Sheree Montgomery

Layout and Graphics: Carl Byers, Corrie Niehaus

Proofreaders: Rebecca Denoncour, Cynthia Fields

Indexer: BIM Indexing & Proofreading Services

Illustrator: Kathryn Born

Special Help

Caitlin Copple, Jennette ElNaggar, Elizabeth Rea, Danielle Voirol

Publishing and Editorial for Consumer Dummies

Kathleen Nebenhaus, Vice President and Executive Publisher

David Palmer, Associate Publisher

Kristin Ferguson-Wagstaffe, Product Development Director

Publishing for Technology Dummies

Andy Cummings, Vice President and Publisher

Composition Services

Debbie Stailey, Director of Composition Services

Contents at a Glance

Table of Contents

Part II: What's Your Type? Components of IV Therapy ... 69

Chapter 4: Medications Made to Order: Pharmacological IV Therapy 71

Chapter 5: Beefing Up on Blood Component Therapy Basics 93

Introduction

I (Bettie) recently donated blood at a local blood bank, and I have to admit I was a little nervous. I knew that the needle would be a large-bore, 18-gauge needle and the unit of blood would be 500 cc of my own life-sustaining commodity. I worried that the IV nurse would need more than one try to get my vein and that I would feel sick as the blood drained from my body. It's scary for a nurse to be on the *other side* of the needle!

Then the IV therapist said, "Hi, Bettie. My name's Amanda, and I'll be your nurse today. What's your favorite television station?"

With just one sentence, she immediately established rapport and put me at ease for the impending procedure. After that, I experienced a successful one-stick venipuncture and a feeling of confidence that I was in the right hands at the right time.

Lying under a warm blanket, watching my favorite TV news station, with the blood draining from my vein, I thought, "This is the beautiful part of IV therapy nursing — it's not only about providing a life-saving therapy. It's about an opportunity to change a patient's attitude about healthcare and transform a terrifying experience into a show-and-tell moment."

Deborah and I have written *IV Therapy For Dummies* (Wiley) to help IV nurses wrap the knowledge, skills, and techniques we include in this book in a warm blanket of caring and compassion.

About This Book

IV therapy is a broad subject, encompassing many disciplines and subdisciplines within nursing. It's impossible to cover every IV topic in great detail without using a 3-pound textbook, but it *is* possible to provide practical, useful, everyday information in a handy, accessible format.

To provide an easy-to-understand framework, this book answers the following five questions and focuses on the critical how-to information related to each one:

- ✔ Why should you start an IV?
- ✔ When should you start, monitor, and discontinue an IV?
- ✔ Who should start an IV?
- ✔ Where's the best vein for an IV?
- ✔ What equipment should you use for an IV?

In a nutshell, this book gives you an easy-to-understand guide to the most important skills and procedures associated with IV therapy. It also provides something that's unavailable in other books — insider secrets and techniques from frontline nurses who work in the everyday trenches of IV therapy.

Conventions Used in This Book

We use the following conventions throughout the text to make things consistent and easy to understand:

- ✔ All web addresses appear in `monofont`.
- ✔ New terms appear in *italic* and are closely followed by plain English definitions.
- ✔ **Boldface** highlights the action parts of numbered steps and the key words in bulleted lists.
- ✔ On first reference, we spell out a unit of measurement and follow it with the relevant abbreviation to help you become familiar with the abbreviations used in physician's orders. For example, you may see this kind of measurement: 10 milliliters (10 mL).
- ✔ We use generic and brand names for medications. So that you know which is which, we format all drug names on first reference like so: generic name (Brand name); for example, phenytoin (Dilantin).

What You're Not to Read

Although we'd love for you to read this book cover to cover, we understand the demands on your time, so we've clearly marked sections that you don't need to read when your time is limited. When you want the facts and just the facts, feel free to skip the following sections:

- **Text in sidebars:** *Sidebars* are shaded boxes that usually give detailed examples or describe historical perspectives on the topic at hand.

- **Anything marked with a Technical Stuff icon:** This icon indicates information that's interesting but that you can live without. Read these tidbits later when you're not pressed for time.

Foolish Assumptions

We normally don't like making assumptions, but as we wrote this book, the following assumptions helped us direct this book's focus to material that you can use in your everyday nursing practice:

- We assume that you're either a student nurse or a practicing caregiver.

- We assume that you have an understanding of common medical terminology, although we define quite a few of the medical terms we use in this book.

- We assume that you have a general working knowledge of basic nursing skills and that you know how to carry out physician's orders and promote patient safety.

- We assume that you have a passion for caring for others and a desire to help people at their most critical moments.

How This Book Is Organized

To help you navigate this book, we've divided it into six parts. This section provides a breakdown of those six parts and a quick look at what you can find in each one.

Part I: Tapping Into IV Therapy

Part I covers the basics of IV therapy. Chapter 1 kicks things off with a quick overview of the book. Chapter 2 highlights the medical-legal aspects of IV therapy, including federal, state, and institutional standards of care, and explains how you can avoid malpractice problems and keep yourself and your patients safe. Chapter 3 introduces you to the equipment and supplies you need to be familiar with in IV therapy.

Part II: What's Your Type? Components of IV Therapy

Part II walks you through the various types of IV therapy. Chapter 4 reviews the pharmacologic interactions between medications and the human body and explains how drugs work to cure infections and fight disease. Chapter 5 discusses the components and compatibilities of life-saving blood products, while Chapter 6 discusses the pros and cons of another life-saving IV therapy — chemotherapy. Chapter 7 takes you on a journey into the cellular world of fluid and electrolyte balance. Finally, Chapter 8 deals with the increasingly sophisticated regimens of IV nutrition and the important role of parenteral nutrition in restoring health.

Part III: Getting Down to IV Therapy Business

In Part III, you get a glimpse of the overall IV therapy process. Chapter 9 directs your attention to the significance of accurately and completely documenting the IV procedure from start to finish, along with the consequences you can face when you keep inadequate documentation. Chapter 10 reviews some basic math and walks you through a couple of simplified methods for calculating common IV infusion rates and dosages. Chapter 11 lays the groundwork for administering medications by IV push and piggyback and shows you how to put the power of technology to work with infusion pumps, auto-syringe pumps, and patient-controlled anesthesia pumps. Chapter 12 demonstrates how to start, stabilize, monitor, and discontinue peripheral IVs, and Chapter 13 shows you how to do the same with central lines.

Part IV: Administering IV Therapy

Part IV covers all the how-to info you need to know about administering the most common types of IV therapy. In it, you get a rundown on how to assess patients, administer specialty IV substances, and manage adverse IV reactions. In Chapter 14, you find all the details on initiating, monitoring, and discontinuing pharmacological IV therapy (that is, medication infusions), as well as on recognizing and managing adverse drug reactions. Chapter 15 walks you through the steps needed to safely administer blood and blood products. Chapter 16 deals with advanced procedures associated with administering toxic substances like chemotherapy and shows you how to protect yourself and your patient when working with hazardous agents. Chapter 17 discusses the nitty-gritty of replacement therapy with fluids and electrolytes. Finally, Chapter 18 covers the essentials of administering parenteral nutrition.

Part V: Considering Unique Populations

Part V covers the full gamut of IV therapy from pediatrics to geriatrics. Chapter 19 is all about administering IVs to children and overcoming the special challenges you may face as a pediatric IV nurse. Chapter 20 deals with the other end of the age spectrum — elderly patients — and explains the various modifications you need to make to administer IV therapy safely to geriatric patients. Finally, Chapter 21 centers on the growing demand for IV therapy at home and the steps you have to take to create a safe home environment for yourself and your patient.

Part VI: The Part of Tens

Part VI contains ten handy techniques and insider secrets for starting and administering IV therapy. Chapter 22 presents ten take-away tips on the general subject of IV therapy, and Chapter 23 gives you ten how-to tips on starting IVs.

Icons Used in This Book

To make this book easier to use, we include the following icons that can help you find and fathom key ideas and information:

The Tip icon appears whenever the text next to it can save you time or help you promote patient safety when administering IV therapy.

Any time you see this icon, you know the information that follows is important and worth reading more than once.

The Warning icon flags information that highlights dangers to you or your patient's health and safety.

This icon appears next to information that's interesting but not essential to the discussion at hand. When you're in a hurry, skip the paragraphs marked with the Technical Stuff icon and come back to them later.

Where to Go from Here

This book is organized so that you can skip around to find whatever information you need at the time. If you want to know how a chemotherapy drug works, jump to Chapter 6. If you want to find out how to administer chemotherapy, go to Chapter 16. You can use the table of contents to find broad categories of information or the index to look up more specific topics.

If you're not sure where you want to go next, why not start with Chapter 1? It gives you an overview of IV therapy and points you to places where you can find more detailed information.

Part I

Tapping Into IV Therapy

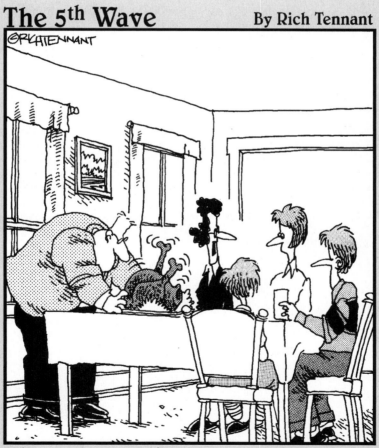

The 5th Wave   By Rich Tennant

"This is what I get for marrying a phlebotomist.
Every Thanksgiving he's got to inject the turkey
with gravy before he'll carve it."

In this part . . .

Part I introduces you to the basics of IV therapy. It starts with a quick overview of IV therapy and the many topics we cover in the rest of the book. It also focuses on the important medical-legal aspects of infusion nursing and the equipment and supplies you may use at one point or another as you work as a nurse in IV therapy.

Chapter 1

Introducing IV Therapy: A Purpose-Driven Practice

In This Chapter

▶ Exploring the types of IVs and the different methods of administration

▶ Figuring out what your role is in IV therapy

▶ Getting familiar with standards of care to protect yourself and your patient

*I*ntravenous (IV) therapy is more than just another medical procedure. It's a universal method of saving lives and restoring health that healthcare facilities all around the world use every day.

In this chapter, you find out how IV medications work to restore vital signs and relieve pain, and you get a glimpse of the various types of IVs used to treat clinical conditions, as well as the assorted methods of administering them. You take a journey through all aspects of IV therapy, including starting, monitoring, and discontinuing IVs, and you explore important methods of promoting patient safety and preventing complications. Finally, you get a closer look at the medical-legal implications of IV therapy and the importance of performing to national standards of care, particularly those set by the Infusion Nurses Society (INS).

What's the Point? The Purpose of IV Therapy

Doctors prescribe IV therapy when they need to deliver fluids and medications quickly, copiously, and frequently. They also use it to administer products like blood, parenteral nutrition, and chemotherapy that can't be delivered any other way.

As a healthcare worker, you use IVs to administer all types of therapies, ranging from a simple normal saline drip to hydrate a depleted marathon runner to a sophisticated thrombolytic drug infusion to dissolve blood clots in a patient who just had a heart attack. Regardless of which type of therapy you use them for, the main purpose of IVs is to save lives.

Administering emergency fluids and medications

During emergencies, you use IV fluids and medications for countless reasons, including the following:

- ✔ To stabilize blood pressure
- ✔ To dilate bronchial tubes in patients with asthma
- ✔ To convert heart arrhythmias back to sinus rhythm
- ✔ To relax vocal cords to facilitate intubation
- ✔ To restore blood volume to prevent circulatory collapse

In short, IV fluids and medications are vital, irreplaceable elements in an emergency response, and they frequently make the difference between life and death. For details on preparing for and administering IV therapy, check out Parts III and IV.

Delivering pharmacological agents

When patients need to receive medications quickly, frequently, or over a long period of time, the intravenous route is the method of choice. The use of IV medications has skyrocketed since the advent of modern IV therapy in World War I. Today, every department of the hospital, from intensive care to medical-surgical units to labor and delivery and beyond, uses IV medications.

Nurses who administer IV medications must know how to administer IV drugs safely, prevent potential complications from both the drug itself and the IV, and monitor the patient's response to therapy. For details on administering IV medications and managing complications, go to Chapter 14. For drug classifications and other IV medication basics, see Chapter 4.

Replacing blood and blood products

Since the first successful human blood transfusion was performed in 1818, blood transfusions have become a mainstay in replacing blood lost through injury, surgery, or disease. Today, more than 5 million people receive blood transfusions each year in the U.S. alone.

Blood transfusions through IV therapy are now routine and relatively safe. In fact, the greatest danger patients face when receiving blood today is having a life-threatening reaction caused by getting the wrong blood type by accident. That's where knowing more about IV therapy becomes essential.

Because nurses administer the vast majority of blood and blood components, they're the last safety net to ensure delivery of compatible blood products. But even with all the safety precautions of initially checking the blood and verifying it again at the bedside, patients still die from blood incompatibilities every year. The biggest key to preventing deaths and other complications related to the administration of whole blood or blood products is a vigilant nurse. To find out more about administering blood components safely and preventing complications, check out Chapters 5 and 15.

Administering chemotherapy medications

Chemotherapy drugs are *cytotoxic* (cell-killing) substances designed to attack and kill cancer cells. Unfortunately, chemotherapy can't distinguish between malignant cells and healthy cells, so it also destroys healthy cells and causes a cascade of debilitating side effects. Yet, even though the side effects may be severe and crippling, millions of cancer patients each year elect to undergo chemotherapy to combat the devastating effects of cancer.

Chemotherapy is a risky business for both the patient and the IV nurse. Patients are at risk for vein destruction and tissue necrosis if the IV becomes infiltrated, and IV nurses are at risk for chemical burns to the eyes, face, or hands when preparing and administering the drugs. In addition, long-term side effects of leukemia and blood abnormalities have been observed in oncology nurses with chronic exposure to chemotherapy agents.

Fortunately, awareness and technology eliminate some of these risks. For instance, nurses use implanted ports to reduce the risk of infiltration and leakage of toxic drugs into surrounding tissues in the patient. Nurses also use high-tech safety gear and protective equipment that shield their face, arms, and hands from the accidental spilling or splashing of toxic chemicals.

Despite the risks, more than 100,000 doses of chemotherapy are given around the world every day, and IV nurses are a critical component in delivering this life-saving therapy. For more on how chemotherapy works, check out Chapter 6. For details on how to administer chemotherapy, turn to Chapter 16.

Maintaining fluid and electrolyte balance

To function properly, the human body must keep fluid in its cells, between its cells, and in the bloodstream. The body maintains a state of equilibrium by keeping a vigilant watch over its fluid and electrolyte levels. When the body's fluids and electrolytes get out of balance, the heart beats irregularly, the kidneys shut down, and the circulatory system collapses. To treat this imbalance, healthcare professionals replace fluids or replenish electrolytes through IV therapy.

During therapy, the IV nurse is responsible for safely administering replacement fluids and electrolytes as prescribed by the physician and monitoring the patient's response to treatment. For the basics on fluid and electrolyte balance, go to Chapter 7. For the lowdown on using IV therapy to administer fluids and electrolytes, turn to Chapter 17.

Providing nutrition

Parenteral nutrition delivers vitamins, minerals, lipids, and other nutritional substances directly into the patient's bloodstream through an IV. This life-sustaining infusion is especially critical for patients who can't absorb nutrients through the digestive tract or can't take foods orally due to injury or surgery. To explore the basics of planning, administering, and monitoring life-saving meals of IV nutrition, check out Chapters 8 and 18.

The Main Ways to Administer IV Therapy

IV therapy isn't a *one-size-fits-all* type of procedure. Doctors use a variety of administration methods from low-tech gravity drips to high-tech smart pumps and everything in between to achieve rapid response to treatment and optimal patient outcome. The most common types of IV administration include the following:

- **Peripheral IVs:** These short-terms vascular access devices (VADs) may be inserted by paramedics, nurses, or physicians. The tip of the device resides in the veins of the upper extremities. You typically use them for short-term rehydration or fluid administrations that last less than one week (see Chapter 12).

✔ **IV push and piggyback:** An *IV push* is when you use a syringe to push a specific dose of a medication through a peripheral or central VAD over a short period of time (usually less than 2 minutes). A *piggyback* is when you attach a secondary bag of fluid or medication to a primary IV set (check out Chapters 3 and 11).

✔ **Central lines:** Central VADs (CVADs) are inserted by physicians, physician assistants (PAs), or specially trained nurses (who may insert only peripherally inserted central catheters, or PICCs). CVADs are placed in the chest, neck, groin, leg, scalp, or arm with the catheter threaded into the veins of the central venous system, such as the superior vena cava or inferior vena cava. You can use them for short- or long-term therapy (turn to Chapter 13 for more info).

✔ **Infusion pumps, syringe pumps, and patient-controlled analgesia (PCA) pumps:** These electronic devices infuse fluids or medications intermittently or continuously with an automatic pump. They can infuse the correct dose at the correct rate for a prescribed amount of time. The *infusion pump* is larger, is usually pole mounted, and has preloaded drug information in its memory. *Syringe pumps* utilize a syringe to give smaller controlled doses of medications over a prescribed duration. *PCA pumps* are like syringe pumps, except they include a hand-held button the patient can use to give himself prescribed amounts of medications when he needs them (see Chapter 11).

✔ **Volume-metered, microdrip, and macrodrip systems:** These types of peripheral IV tubing deliver fluids and medications from their containers to the VAD and into the patient's bloodstream. *Volume-metered tubing* has a small, volume-controlled chamber that sits between the main fluid container and the insertion site; it can deliver a controlled volume of fluid or medication. A *microdrip system* infuses a smaller amount of fluid per hour (less than 100 milliliters per hour), while a *macrodrip system* delivers a large quantity of fluid at a rapid rate (100 milliliters or more per hour). (Skip to Chapters 3 and 11 for details.)

✔ **Intermittent and continuous infusions:** *Intermittent infusions* deliver medications or fluids at specific times and at designated intervals. *Continuous infusions* deliver medications or fluids at a constant rate, one drop at a time, over longer periods (check out Chapter 11).

✔ **Filtered and nonfiltered infusions:** *Filtered infusions* decrease the amounts of undissolved particles or bacteria that enter the patient's bloodstream; they're typically used for infusing blood, blood products, and total parenteral nutrition. *Nonfiltered infusions* are given without a filter (go figure!); they're typically used for maintenance fluids, such as normal saline or lactated Ringer's solution. (See Chapters 5 and 15 for details on administering blood and blood products and Chapters 7 and 17 for details on administering maintenance fluids.)

Understanding the Important Role You Play in IV Therapy

IV therapy is one aspect of nursing that's prevalent in all areas of the health-care spectrum. As an IV nurse, you must have a broad knowledge of pharmacology and technology, including the techniques of starting and monitoring IVs. But you must also be skilled in the art of patient assessment, and you need to be able to deal with a full array of patient populations.

IV therapists are special nurses who relish the challenge of starting IVs in critically ill patients and who reap the rewards of seeing their patients improve with treatment. They understand that their number one role in IV administration is delivering safe, life-sustaining therapies that restore health and extend life.

Getting down to brass tacks: Starting IVs

Whether you're a practicing healthcare professional who wants to brush up on IV techniques or a student nurse who wants to learn all aspects of IV therapy for the first time, one of the most basic and fear-evoking procedures is starting an IV. Practicing on IV mannequins in a safe classroom setting can certainly help prepare you for this task, but facing a real patient in a real-life clinical situation still strikes fear in even the most intrepid nurse.

Chapter 12 gives you a head start on starting peripheral IVs, while Chapter 13 focuses on central lines. Both chapters help you select the appropriate VAD, prepare and assess the insertion site, initiate therapy, and perform proper care and maintenance of the VAD. Chapter 19 takes you on a similar journey, covering IV therapy in children, and Chapter 20 focuses on the other end of the age spectrum with geriatric patients.

Preventing infection

Protecting yourself and your patient from infectious disease is one of your major responsibilities as an IV nurse. This vital role requires vigilance on two important fronts:

- You must protect yourself from blood-borne pathogens, such as Hepatitis B and human immunodeficiency virus (HIV).
- You must protect your patients from infections acquired during their hospital stay, known as *hospital-associated* or *hospital-acquired infections* (HAIs).

Hand washing is the single most important means of preventing the spread of infection and minimizing risk for both healthcare personnel and patients. It's also the first step in building a chain of *aseptic technique* — when every member of the healthcare team adheres to strict guidelines of proper hand washing, appropriate use of sterile gloves and supplies, and prevention of cross-contamination between patients. When any team member fails to maintain a sterile or aseptic environment, the chain of aseptic technique is broken and the patient is at increased risk for infection.

Maintaining a chain of aseptic technique begins with proper hand washing (see the nearby sidebar for a refresher) and continues through the following procedures:

✔ Inspecting sterile supplies and preparing IV medications and fluids

✔ Starting and changing IVs, infusion bags, and tubings

✔ Cleansing insertion sites and changing dressings

✔ Administering medications and discontinuing IVs

In addition to practicing proper hand washing and aseptic techniques, you need to maintain a safe, clean IV environment by following these steps:

✔ Use antiseptic solutions and disinfectants to clean treatment rooms and medication preparation areas.

✔ Frequently disinfect high-touch areas associated with patient care, such as bedrails, bed tables, and faucets.

✔ Ensure that hand sanitizers are available for use by both patients and visitors.

Partnering with your patient is an excellent way to promote infection control. Teach your patient about her role in prevention and ask her to follow these simple techniques to prevent cross-contamination:

✔ Ask visitors to avoid sitting on the bed.

✔ Don't place food, eating utensils, or personal items on the bed.

✔ Request that visitors and healthcare workers wash their hands before and after visiting.

✔ Wash hands before touching the face or mouth.

Talk to the hand: Practicing good hand hygiene

You've probably been using proper hand washing technique for a while now, but because it's such a critical first step in maintaining aseptic technique, we provide a quick refresher here. Follow these steps every time you wash your hands:

✔ Wet your hands with warm or cold water and apply soap.

✔ Rub your hands together to make a lather and scrub them well; be sure to scrub the backs of your hands, between your fingers, and under your nails.

✔ Continue scrubbing your hands for at least 20 seconds. Need a timer? Hum the "Happy Birthday" song from beginning to end twice.

✔ Rinse your hands well under running water.

✔ Dry your hands with a clean towel or allow them to air-dry.

✔ Use a towel or your elbow to turn off the water.

Monitoring infusions and managing complications

Monitoring infusions is an essential part of administering IV therapy, particularly in longer-term IVs. When IVs are in place for long periods of time, the risk for complications greatly increases. Frequent access through injection ports, multiple infusions of different medications, and maintenance flushing procedures increase the patient's risk for complications. The key to combating these complications is carefully assessing, monitoring, and maintaining every infusion from start to finish.

Monitoring and managing peripheral IVs

Peripheral IVs pose a risk for complications because they're placed in extremities that patients use constantly for eating, drinking, and performing other normal activities. Guarding against complications from peripheral IVs requires knowledge of the most common complications, such as phlebitis, infiltration, and clot formation. Vigilant monitoring of the insertion site and peripheral equipment are key elements in preventing these complications. Chapter 12 tells you what you need to know about monitoring peripheral infusions and discusses how you can minimize risk and maximize patient safety during IV therapy in peripheral veins.

As soon as you realize that a complication exists, stop the IV immediately, reassure the patient, and notify the physician. (Turn to Chapter 12 for more details.)

Monitoring and managing central venous lines

Central venous lines are at even greater risk for serious complications than peripheral IVs because they go directly to the patient's central venous system and can expose the patient to a catheter-related bloodstream infection (CRBSI) or *septicemia* (systemic infection).

Whenever you're dealing with a central line, frequently monitor the line to clear any problems that may impede flow and lead to clotting or infection. Also, ensure that the line is stabilized, assess the insertion site, and evaluate the line during routine maintenance procedures, such as flushing and locking. We cover all these procedures and more in Chapter 13.

Supporting your actions by keeping careful records

Keeping careful records through proper documentation is another key role of every IV nurse. In the medical field, documentation provides a clear, concise, permanent record of what you did, what happened when you did it, and what the outcome was after you did what you did. The four primary reasons that complete and accurate documentation is so important in healthcare are

- ✔ It provides continuity of care.
- ✔ It acts as your insurance policy against lawsuits.
- ✔ It tells a story about the steps you took to reach successful patient outcomes.
- ✔ It gives insurance companies a complete picture of your patient and the care you provided so they can issue reimbursement.

Documentation isn't always a nurse's favorite duty, but when done properly, it ensures that you delivered the highest quality of excellence and the greatest level of competence in patient care. Plus, proper documentation is often a nurse's only defense witness in front of a jury in cases of lawsuits. So make sure you document all your nursing actions, including all those related to IV therapy. Turn to Chapter 9 for the lowdown on maintaining proper documentation as an IV nurse.

Familiarizing Yourself with Standards of Care

Whether you like it or not, nursing actions are measured against standards of care and published guidelines, and those standards and guidelines basically determine what a nurse should and shouldn't do. Standards of care measure the degree of excellence and outline the expected level of competence in nursing care.

The nurse's most vital protective strategy in meeting standards of care is being a knowledgeable and safe practitioner of patient care. To do so, you must be aware of nursing standards, published guidelines, legal issues in nursing, scope of nursing practice, and limits of legal liabilities. The following sections touch on these issues; see Chapter 2 for more details.

Understanding the importance of the Infusion Nurses Society

The Infusion Nurses Society (INS) is the global authority on infusion nursing. Founded in 1973 by Ada Plumer and Marguerite Knight, the INS established the first infusion nursing standards of care in 1980 and continues to provide revisions and updates to the standards approximately every five years. The 2011 version, titled *Infusion Nursing Standards of Practice,* consists of 68 standards of care.

INS's standards of care are composed of two sections:

- The first section comprises broad statements applicable to all IV procedures, such as peripheral lines, peripherally inserted central catheters (PICC lines), central venous lines, and central venous ports.

- The second section consists of clinical practice criteria that provide guidance for implementing the standards.

The INS standards cover every IV topic, ranging from infrared light and ultrasound technology used for visualizing veins to catheter stabilization devices and sutureless securement options used to prevent central line infections.

Through these standards, the INS establishes a framework for monitoring nursing care and medical products and provides a structure of reference that distinguishes among malpractice, product failure, and negative patient outcomes. The INS framework also assists in resolving ethical conflicts between infusion nurses and their employers.

In addition to protecting nurses and promoting patient safety, other goals of the INS standards include reducing malpractice and product liability claims and ensuring positive patient outcomes.

Implementing INS standards of care in your daily practice

The best way for you to promote patient safety and avoid malpractice suits is to strictly comply with the current INS standards of care. Familiarize yourself with the standards that apply most frequently to your everyday activities and implement the standards, even when doing so takes a few extra minutes.

Take time to research or refresh your memory of the standards dealing with new procedures and to attend presentations on new infusion equipment. Utilize the chapters in this book to brush up on old skills and check out new ones. Remember that advocating for your patient and using critical-thinking skills are not only your right but also your responsibility.

Avoiding lawsuits by following standards of care

When standards of care are questioned, nurses often find themselves personally involved in lawsuits. The biggest reasons for lawsuits against nurses are

- Communication errors and medication errors
- Failure to assess and monitor or advocate for the patient
- Inappropriate delegation or supervision
- Working while impaired, including excessive fatigue

Nurses are even held accountable by law for not using critical-thinking skills and common-sense judgment when giving patient care. So when a medication order appears unsafe, don't assume that contacting the physician and verifying the order gives you a green light to administer the med. If you administer an unsafe medication and ignore your critical-thinking process, you could find yourself on the wrong side of a lawsuit.

The best defense for the nurse facing a lawsuit is to prove that she performed to the expected level of competence by documenting her actions (refer to the earlier section "Supporting your actions by keeping careful records" and Chapter 9). After all, accurate documentation and thorough charting are the most vital aspects of proving that you've met all nursing standards of care.

Turn to Chapter 2 for more info on keeping within the letter of the law as an IV nurse.

Staying focused on ethical principles

Ethics is an integral part of the foundation of nursing. IV therapy embodies the following ethical principles:

- ✔ Preventing illness by educating patients about the importance of wellness and fitness programs and the benefits of prophylactic activities, such as routine well-patient appointments and immunizations

- ✔ Alleviating physical suffering by administering IV pain relief and minimizing emotional suffering by providing psychological support to the patient and family

- ✔ Restoring health by providing IV medications that fight infection, combat cancer, and extend life

- ✔ Advocating for patients when family members are absent or nonexistent and collaborating with other professionals to provide patients with treatment options and needed resources

- ✔ Maintaining appropriate and safe healthcare environments in both the hospital and home setting and displaying moral self-respect through personal hygiene and professional behavior

- ✔ Maintaining personal accountability for standards of care by regularly attending competency and certification courses and complying with INS standards of care and state regulatory practices

Working within your scope of practice

Scope of practice is usually determined by committees of experts focused on defining educational requirements for nurses working in specific areas of healthcare, such as IV therapy. Scope of practice varies from state to state and is based on the particular state's licensing practices. In some states, such as California, licensed vocational nurses (LVNs) aren't allowed to start IVs unless they've been certified through an approved IV certification course. In other states, LVNs are allowed to start IVs or inject medications into an infusion bag under an RN's supervision.

To identify the educational requirements for IV therapy delivery by RNs, LVNs, or nonlicensed personnel in your state, check with the state licensing board to verify the scope of practice dictated by your license.

Some employers encourage nurses to take IV certification courses to ensure they possess a level of knowledge and competence in the specialty area of IV therapy. Check with your facility, nursing organizations such as INS or the Association for Vascular Access (AVA), or your state board to obtain information about IV certification.

Implementing evidence-based infusion practice

Evidence-based practice is a method of determining the best treatment for improved patient care based on evidence from clinical research studies. It's the opposite of the old method of determining treatment based on experience.

Interest in evidence-based practice emerged in the 1970s and is now accepted as the gold standard in dictating treatment and optimizing patient care. It has been incorporated into professional standards of care and implemented in healthcare fields throughout the world.

Evidence-based infusion practice calls for nurses to select and review research studies and apply relevant findings to patient care. Evidence-based nursing integrates the best research evidence with clinical expertise, patient preferences, and existing resources to enable the physician and infusion nurse to make informed decisions about the healthcare of individual patients.

Documenting informed consent

Documenting that informed consent has been obtained and/or placing the signed consent form in the patient's chart is the responsibility of the nurse. Standards specify that the nurse must be knowledgeable about the proper protocol for obtaining informed consent. Informed consent must be obtained from legally competent adults and children and must be documented in the patient's permanent record. Typically the physician has to obtain this consent.

Complying with your employer's policies and procedures

Employer and facility policies and procedures are institutional guidelines designed to protect the patient, nurse, and institution. They act as a framework to enable healthcare professionals to carry out responsibilities while preventing complications and minimizing patient risk.

Of course, nurses have a duty to comply with their employer's policies and procedures, but they have a greater duty to advocate and promote patient safety. When policies and procedures impair a nurse's ability to provide appropriate patient care, medical ethics and standards of care become issues of concern. To address issues of medical ethics and standards of care, consult your local or national nursing organization, state Nurse Practice Act, or state board of nursing.

Chapter 2

Keeping within the Letter of the Law

. . . .

In This Chapter

▶ Comprehending the legal standard of care

▶ Understanding federal and state regulations pertaining to IV therapy

▶ Figuring out how professional standards fit into your practice

▶ Breaking down the elements of negligence

▶ Protecting yourself from erroneous lawsuits with risk-management strategies

. . . .

Mastering the art of intravenous (IV) therapy often puts nurses and other healthcare professionals between a rock and a hard place. On one hand, the specialty brings enormous professional satisfaction. On the other hand, it increases professional risk and liability. Because the practice of IV therapy has evolved to give healthcare professionals like yourself greater responsibility and accountability, never before has it been more important for you to provide quality patient care that falls within the letter of the law.

Administering IV therapy is one of the most important tasks you'll ever perform. It's also the most legally significant. Unfortunately, along with the growth of the specialty comes an increase in lawsuits filed against nurses and other healthcare professionals who implement IV therapy.

In this chapter, we hope to broaden your awareness of the legal issues that you face when performing IV therapy. We cover the legal standard of care, including how it applies to you and infusion therapy. We look at federal and state regulations governing IV therapy, and we go over professional and institutional standards that you need to be aware of. We talk about what constitutes malpractice in the eyes of the law, and we review the most common areas in IV therapy that can lead to malpractice. Finally, through evidence-based practices, we show you how to keep your practice smarter and safer.

Understanding the Legal Standard of Care

When you provide reasonable, practical patient care that's typical of what's expected of you compared to another nurse or healthcare professional with similar training, you're following the *legal standard of care*. For example, suppose you start an IV with your first attempt or you hang an IV piggyback at the time it was actually ordered. As a nurse (or other healthcare professional licensed to perform IV therapy), you're following the legal standard of care. The legal standard of care exists to protect patients from negligence and to hold nurses and other healthcare professionals accountable for their actions.

In a nutshell, the legal standard of care is evaluated based on patient care that is

- ✔ Typical of the performance of another healthcare professional with similar, specialized training
- ✔ Measured by what another healthcare professional with similar training would do in the same situation
- ✔ Based on the healthcare setting and state in which the care is delivered
- ✔ Based on knowledge that exists within a specific historical time frame

Who is behind the legal standard of care? And to whom must you answer if you fall short? The legal standard of care originates from four sources: federal and state laws and regulations and professional and institutional standards. Here's a quick look at where these laws and standards come from:

- ✔ The American Nurses Association (ANA) regulates the national nursing standard of practice.
- ✔ Laws in each state called *Nurse Practice Acts* (NPAs) define the scope of nursing practice.
- ✔ State boards of nursing, such as the Florida Board of Nursing, oversee the NPAs.
- ✔ Common law is derived from principles or social practices rather than from rules and regulations.

Together, the NPAs and common law define nursing practice. Each state is governed by the ANA, which regulates NPAs, and each state regulates common law. Each facility has its own Policies and Procedures (P&P) based on these laws that regulate nursing in that facility. We discuss all these sources in this chapter.

Making Sense of Federal and State Regulations

Federal and state regulations applicable to healthcare are laws designed to control or govern the conduct of healthcare professionals in all settings. The regulations relevant to infusion therapy are unique to the specialty, and they were created by federal and state agencies to protect patients from harm. It's your responsibility to familiarize yourself with federal and state regulations regarding infusion therapy and to provide patient care that follows the standard of care developed by these agencies.

Regulations set by the American Nurses Association (ANA) and each state's Nurse Practice Act (NPA) are based on basic principles, while the Infusion Nurses Society (INS) has developed IV therapy standards based on evidence-based practices. Each facility should develop its own Policies and Procedures (P&P) based on standards as defined by the ANA, NPAs, and INS to regulate and define a nurse's responsibilities. You can use your facility's P&P as a resource when getting to know legal nursing regulations because it should reflect up-to-date federal and state regulations.

Seeing who's watching your back at the federal level

Federal agencies establish laws that govern the practice of infusion therapy. After Congress passes a bill and the president signs it into law (or Congress overrides the veto), the law becomes a federal statute and is published in the *United States Code*. Federal statutes are then interpreted, implemented, and publicized by various federal agencies, such as the Occupational Safety and Health Administration (OSHA), the Food and Drug Administration (FDA), and the U.S. Department of Health and Human Services (USDHHS).

Not all statutes are relevant to infusion therapy. The most applicable include occupational health and safety, infection prevention and control, safety of medical devices, and federally funded insurance programs such as Medicare and Medicaid.

Promoting job safety: OSHA

In 1970, Congress enacted the *Occupational Safety and Health Act,* out of which OSHA was born. OSHA's primary purpose is to reduce workplace injury, illness, and death by establishing and enforcing standards for workplace health and safety.

OSHA is big on exposure control, and it plays a colossal role in the regulation of blood-borne-pathogen and hazardous-material exposure, not to mention those all-too-familiar Material Safety Data Sheets (MSDSs). The agency is also responsible for broadening the use of personal protective equipment (PPE) to protect employees from hazardous materials.

When you perform IV therapy, you run the risk of being exposed to blood-borne diseases such as Hepatitis B, Hepatitis C, and HIV/AIDS. OSHA's standard of care regarding blood-borne-pathogen exposure states that all body fluids are potentially infectious and that anyone handling them must follow strict guidelines for self-protection.

Administering antineoplastic agents such as chemotherapy and other caustic drugs also places you at risk of exposure to hazardous materials. OSHA has a hand in regulating these types of agents, too, which OSHA recognizes as health hazards.

The advent of special handling, administration, and disposal precautions pertaining to blood-borne pathogens and hazardous materials significantly reduces the risks that healthcare professionals face on a daily basis. OSHA requires that healthcare professionals handling these substances be knowledgeable of and well trained in these special precautions. We talk more about handling antineoplastic agents in Chapter 6 and disposing of blood and blood products in Chapter 15.

Always check the facility policy regarding exposure to blood-borne pathogens or other hazardous materials before implementing IV therapy.

Setting guidelines and making recommendations: The multiple roles of the CDC

The Centers for Disease Control and Prevention (CDC), which operates under the watchful eye of the USDHHS, is a federal agency whose mission is to protect people and their communities by promoting health and the prevention of disease, disability, and injury. The CDC also strives to prepare communities for impending serious health threats. Although the CDC doesn't regulate healthcare, it does make recommendations that federal agencies may later use to establish new healthcare regulations.

The *Guidelines for the Prevention of Intravascular Catheter-Related Infections*, updated in 2011, is just one CDC recommendation that applies to infusion therapy. These guidelines are for healthcare professionals who insert IV catheters and for people responsible for monitoring infection control in hospitals, home care, and outpatient settings. Guidelines such as these help improve patient outcomes and cut costs, two aspects of infusion therapy that often go hand in hand.

To review the *Guidelines for the Prevention of Intravascular Catheter-Related Infections* on the CDC website, visit www.cdc.gov/hicpac/pdf/guide lines/bsi-guidelines-2011.pdf.

Regulating medical devices: The FDA

Originally, the FDA was created to regulate products such as food, cosmetics, and prescription and over-the-counter medications to ensure that they're safe and effective for public consumption. In 1976, its role was expanded to include regulating the safety of medical devices.

Medical devices include IV therapy equipment such as vascular access devices (VADs), IV solution containers, and electronic infusion pumps. The INS guidelines state that before using any medical device for infusion therapy, it's your responsibility as a healthcare professional to inspect it thoroughly and report any problems to the FDA.

Although you should always follow agency protocol for reporting adverse events, the FDA encourages consumers and healthcare professionals alike to report serious adverse events, product quality problems, product use errors, and therapeutic inequivalence/failures to MedWatch at 1-800-332-1088, the FDA safety information and adverse event reporting hotline. You can also fax your report to 1-800-332-0178, report online at www.fda.gov/medwatch/report.htm, or mail your report to MedWatch, Food and Drug Administration, 5600 Fishers Ln., Rockville, MD 20852-9787.

Ensuring quality healthcare: Centers for Medicare and Medicaid Services

The Centers for Medicare and Medicaid Services, commonly referred to as CMS, is a federal agency established in 1977 to oversee the Medicare and Medicaid programs. Because these programs are federally funded, CMS ensures quality healthcare to its beneficiaries from healthcare providers participating in these programs. If you're employed by an agency receiving Medicare or Medicaid reimbursement, you must comply with the standards set forth by CMS.

Looking at oversight of the state

State laws are developed independently within each state's *jurisdiction,* or legally defined geographic location. Although state laws can't override federal laws, a state may pass additional regulations. State statutes that govern the practice of infusion therapy include your state's Nurse Practice Act, nurse licensing requirements, and statements of joint policy.

Protecting the welfare of patients: The Nurse Practice Act

Each state has a Nurse Practice Act that determines the scope of practice and legal responsibilities for practicing registered nurses and licensed vocational nurses. Nurse Practice Acts are designed to protect the public from harm by advising nurses of what they can and can't do within a jurisdiction. For example, in some states, licensed practical nurses (also known as licensed vocational nurses in California and Texas) are prohibited from administering IV medications via IV push or IV piggyback. They're allowed, however, to hang IV fluids that don't contain medications. Nurse Practice Acts determine which tasks fall within a nurse's scope of practice and are specific to each state.

If you're a nurse, you're responsible for reviewing and understanding the Nurse Practice Act of the state in which you're licensed. To find out more about the Nurse Practice Act in your state, contact the Board of Registered Nursing or the Board of Vocational Nursing within your state.

When statutes fall short: Statements of joint policy

Statements of joint policy often fill in where statutes leave off. When an existing statute fails to clearly define the role of the nurse in performing certain procedures, your state's nursing association or other interested parties may issue statements of joint policy. For example, in October 2009, the American Association of Pediatrics issued a joint policy statement that determined guidelines for the care of children in the emergency department. The statement said that nurses and other healthcare professionals who initiate IV therapy on children in the emergency room must have the knowledge, skill, and training to do so.

Complying with state licensing requirements

Each state has specific licensing requirements for healthcare professionals performing IV therapy. As a healthcare professional, you're responsible for keeping your license up-to-date and fulfilling the continuing education requirements necessary for license renewal. Minimum requirements for licensure are established by the appropriate state boards.

Note: Although the terms *licensure* and *certification* are often used interchangeably, they refer to two different concepts. *Certification* is voluntary, is offered through a private organization, and provides public information on the individuals who have successfully completed the certification process. *Licensure* refers to the state's grant of legal authority to practice a profession within a designated scope of practice and prohibits anyone who isn't licensed from practicing the profession, regardless of whether or not the individual has been certified.

Maintaining Professional Standards

As a healthcare professional who performs IV therapy, you're expected to be competent at what you do. Professional standards help establish required levels of competency for healthcare professionals like yourself and are even recognized in courts of law. Several agencies play a part in maintaining professional standards in IV therapy: the American Nurses Association (ANA), The Joint Commission (TJC), the Association for Vascular Access (AVA), and the Infusion Nurses Society (INS). Additionally, each facility has its own set of professional, institutional standards that you're responsible for knowing.

Defining a competent level of care: The American Nurses Association

The American Nurses Association (ANA) defines the level of competency expected of today's registered nurse through its publication *Nursing: Scope and Standards of Practice.* The standards are far reaching; they apply to everything from the most basic of nursing skills, such as taking vital signs, to the more advanced skill of administering IV therapy. The ANA remains the primary resource for general nursing practice and, to date, represents more than 3.1 million American registered nurses.

To find out more about the publication *Nursing: Scope and Standards of Practice*, visit the ANA website at www.nursingworld.org/scopeand standardsofpractice.

Improving the quality of healthcare: The Joint Commission

If you've worked in any kind of clinical setting, chances are you're quite familiar with The Joint Commission (TJC), formerly known as the Joint Commission on Accreditation of Healthcare Organizations, or JCAHO. No other agency generates such a buzz as TJC does, should it decide to survey your facility.

TJC is a private accrediting agency that, contrary to popular belief, has nothing to do with government. It sets the standard for safe, high-quality healthcare for organizations such as hospitals, behavioral health centers, nursing homes, ambulatory care centers, and home-care agencies. Its goal is to improve the quality of healthcare through accreditation while denying accreditation if an organization fails to meet specific standards. Through national patient safety goals, TJC assists accredited organizations in recognizing and addressing areas of concern in patient safety.

Maintaining the standard of care: The Infusion Nurses Society

The year 1980 marked the first time the Infusion Nurses Society (INS) introduced standards of care for the safe practice of infusion therapy that applied in virtually any healthcare setting. The *Infusion Nursing Standards of Practice* are a set of evidence-based statements specifically designed to maintain a high standard of care in the area of infusion practice. The standards are supported by current research and technological advances that are evidence based. You hear a lot more about the INS in the rest of this book.

For more information about the *Infusion Nursing Standards of Practice,* call 1-781-440-9408 or visit www.ins1.org.

Following facility policy

Not only must you be familiar with governmental guidelines and professional standards concerning infusion therapy, but you must also adhere to institutional policies and procedures set forth by the facility in which you work. These facility-specific directives are meticulously detailed in your facility's Policies and Procedures (P&P) manual.

Every healthcare facility has policies and procedures pertaining to IV therapy — the facility must in order to be accredited by TJC or any other agency. Most agencies develop IV therapy policies and procedures based on the *Infusion Nursing Standards of Practice* that we mention in the preceding section. Policies and procedures help protect the patient receiving IV therapy and the healthcare professional administering it.

When Bad Things Happen to Good People: Comprehending Malpractice

When you know who's who in setting high-quality standards for infusion therapy (see the preceding sections), you're ready to understand the downside of infusion practice: the fact that your actions, or lack thereof, can cause harm to patients and get you sued (in a malpractice suit).

Negligence is the most common form of malpractice. Because nurses and other healthcare professionals who perform IV therapy have a higher level of responsibility than ever before, they're often at the forefront of malpractice suits. To have a legitimate malpractice case, the *plaintiff* (the person suing) must prove four elements of medical malpractice. We discuss these elements in the following sections.

Do you owe a duty of care?

To successfully prove a malpractice case, the plaintiff must prove that the *defendant* (the person being sued) owed a duty of care to a patient and ultimately didn't live up to that duty.

When do you owe a duty of care to a patient? The answer to this question is more complicated than it seems. Whenever you assume care of a patient in a clinical setting, you also assume a duty of care to him. It doesn't matter whether you're in an ambulance, a home-care setting, or a hospital; if you're assigned to care for a patient, you owe that patient big time.

To owe a duty of care, you must also be in some way responsible for the patient. Do you owe a duty of care to someone even after he's been discharged from the hospital? You often do. Part of discharging a patient means you're responsible for teaching him how to care for himself when he arrives home. For instance, what if you discharge a patient home with a central vascular access device (CVAD) without setting him up with home healthcare or providing specific discharge instructions on how to manage it? Suppose the patient decides to remove the CVAD himself and bleeds out because he's on high doses of anticoagulants. By not properly educating your patient or arranging home healthcare to follow up with aftercare, you didn't act in a way that was reasonable given the standard. As a result, you'll probably be held responsible for any injuries the patient suffered. If, however, you did follow the standard of care and he still pulled the line and bled out, then you wouldn't be considered negligent because you acted in a manner that was expected of you given the situation.

Whenever you provide discharge instructions to a patient, always document the education you provided as well as the patient's understanding of those instructions. Don't forget to have the patient or the patient's legal or medical representative sign the discharge instructions before he leaves the hospital. This documentation provides solid proof that you acted in a professionally responsible manner.

Has there been a breach of duty?

One of the elements that must be proven in a malpractice case is that there was a *breach of duty* to your patient. In other words, you violated the standard of care. This could be from something you did or something you didn't do.

Suppose you administer 80 milligrams of IV push furosemide (Lasix) in 5 seconds, and the patient's blood pressure drops dramatically, causing the patient to code. Did you breach your duty? Technically, yes. A lawyer could say that the standard of care requires that IV push furosemide be administered slowly, over 1 to 2 minutes, so giving it too rapidly could be considered a breach of duty, especially if the patient suffered negative consequences from your actions.

Not doing something that you're supposed to do is just as significant as doing something that you aren't supposed to do, at least in the eyes of the law. Consider a patient who has been prescribed IV amiodarone (Cordarone) for ventricular tachycardia. Perhaps the doctor writes the order *stat* (to be done immediately), but you get too busy and forget to start the infusion until 2 hours later. In the meantime, the patient's rhythm converts to ventricular fibrillation. Would this act of omission be a breach in duty? It certainly would.

Are there grounds for legal causation?

To prove *legal causation,* the plaintiff must be able to prove that, had the standard of care been followed, no injury would've occurred.

Imagine that the patient you're caring for in the telemetry unit of your hospital becomes disconnected from his telemetry monitor. The monitor technician tries to call you on your phone, but you don't answer because you left your phone at the nurses' station and you're socializing in the break room. The monitor tech tries to call you several times to no avail, and then he forgets about the patient and goes about his day. In the meantime, your patient codes, but no one notices because he's been off his monitor now for more than 2 hours. Finally, you go into your patient's room and notice he's blue. You call a code and begin CPR, but the patient dies. Had you followed the standard of care, which in this case required that you keep your phone with you at all times and check your patient at least hourly, the patient might have lived. If the patient's family decides to sue you, they must prove that, had the standard of care been followed and the duty upheld, the patient would still be alive. In this case, failure to follow the standard of care directly resulted in the patient's death; hence, there are grounds for legal causation.

On the other hand, if the patient is admitted to telemetry, has a heart attack, and dies in spite of the standard of care being followed, the patient's family will have a hard time proving malpractice because no one failed to follow the standard; therefore, there are no grounds for legal causation.

Are the damages legally compensable?

For malpractice to be successfully proven, the damages that the patient incurs must be *legally compensable,* meaning the patient suffered substantial physical, emotional, or financial injury from your actions. If he didn't, he has no case.

What if you give your patient the wrong medication, but after you monitor him for several days, he experiences no adverse effects from it? Your patient is discharged and tells his story to his sister, who believes that he should sue for malpractice because she doesn't believe the nurse should get away with making such a grievous error. When your patient goes to the lawyer, the lawyer asks about the impact of the medication error. The patient says that he's just fine but thinks that anyone who makes a mistake such as this should be sued. Will your patient have a case? Absolutely not.

Understanding Common Areas of Malpractice and Negligence

Certain aspects of patient care are more commonly associated with medical malpractice and negligence than others. To avoid a lawsuit, you need to familiarize yourself with each one.

Improper administration of medications

Improperly administering medications is by far the most common area of patient care pertaining to medical malpractice. What constitutes improper administration of medication? Here are some examples:

- ✔ Being unfamiliar with a medication's potential harmful side effects
- ✔ Giving a medication that the patient is allergic to
- ✔ Failing to give a medication at the ordered intervals

- ✔ Administering medications by the wrong route
- ✔ Failing to follow the healthcare provider's instructions for medication administration
- ✔ Giving a medication that was erroneously ordered by the healthcare provider

You're legally responsible for a medication error if that error leads to patient harm. The best way to prevent a medication error is to follow the five rights of medication administration — the right patient, the right medication, the right dose, the right route, and the right time — which we outline in Chapter 12.

Improper use of equipment

Can you really be sued when medical equipment goes awry? That depends on whether you properly inspected the equipment and monitored the patient.

Suppose you set up a patient-controlled analgesia (PCA) pump and it malfunctions, overdosing and killing the patient. Would you be held responsible for the malfunction of the equipment and the patient's death? If you failed to supervise the operation of the PCA, the answer is yes, it's quite possible. If you can prove that you inspected the equipment and monitored the patient appropriately (through thorough, accurate documentation), then you wouldn't be held responsible for a defect in the equipment; the manufacturer would.

Protecting your patient from equipment hazards is part of your job as a healthcare provider and especially as an infusion specialist. This means that before you initiate IV therapy, you need to inspect every piece of equipment used for the infusion, from the vascular access device and administration set right down to the solution container and infusion pump.

Failing to act in a timely manner

Although most facilities allow for a window of time — generally 30 minutes before and 30 minutes after a dose is due to be administered — for administering a medication, failing to give a medication that's ordered or giving it too late can get you into as much trouble as giving the wrong medication or giving a medication incorrectly. If the delay or complete omission results in injury or death to your patient, you'll likely be held responsible.

Check your patient's chart frequently for new orders.

Not keeping a close enough eye on your patient

Whenever you initiate IV therapy, continuous assessment and monitoring is critical to patient care. Say you administer dopamine hydrochloride (Dopamine), an agent that has vesicant potential, to your patient. You start the infusion and everything goes smoothly, but you get busy and don't check on the patient again for several hours. In the meantime, the IV has infiltrated, and tissue sloughing and necrosis have begun. By the time you notice the problem, substantial damage has been done, and giving phentolamine (Regitine), the antidote, does little to help. By the next day, the patient's arm needs surgery. Are you responsible for this patient's injury? Yes. Failure to monitor the insertion site for complications during the administration of a vesicant means that you didn't follow the standard of care and increases the likelihood that you'll be sued for negligence.

Assess and monitor your patient frequently and document your findings when administering any form of IV therapy, whether or not the solution is a vesicant. (See Chapter 9 for the lowdown on proper documentation.)

Causing or contributing to infection

IV therapy involves venipuncture, an invasive procedure that places patients at higher risk for catheter-related bloodstream infections. What if you start an IV but neglect to prepare the skin according to facility policy, or what if you didn't assess the IV site regularly for complications and your patient develops an infection? If your patient suffers damages and your contribution to the problem can be proven in a court of law, you're likely to be held responsible for your actions and found to be negligent.

Before initiating IV therapy, be aware of and follow your facility's policy and procedure related to preventing infection.

Lack of communication with the ordering doc

Failure to communicate with the ordering healthcare provider is similar in nature to failure to act. Take, for example, a patient who begins to deteriorate on your shift. You notice a dramatic decrease in blood pressure and document your findings in the chart, but you fail to notify the physician of your findings. The next nurse comes on, and an hour into her shift, the patient codes. The physician is baffled and reviews the chart the next day, only to find that she was not notified when the blood pressure dropped far below the patient's normal baseline measurement. In fact, she wasn't notified at all, until it was too late. Because you failed to notify the doctor and the patient died as a result of your negligence, you'll most likely be held responsible for the patient's death.

It's better to be safe than sorry. Always notify the healthcare provider immediately when there's a change in your patient's baseline condition.

Having joint responsibility

Did you know that if the primary care provider is found to be negligent in her duty to the patient, you could be held liable for allowing or aiding in her negligence? For example, if a physician orders a dose of penicillin, forgetting that the patient has an allergy to penicillin, and you administer the medication, you're just as culpable as the doctor is for ordering it.

Just because a physician orders a medication doesn't mean that she's infallible. Human error knows no bounds. Doctors are just as capable as making a mistake as anybody else.

What if you try to call the doctor and are unable to reach her? You figure the doctor knows what she's doing and give the penicillin anyway, and the patient has an anaphylactic reaction. Being unable to reach the doctor is no excuse for making a grave medication error and unfortunately doesn't protect you from liability.

If you have a question about an order from a physician, trust your instincts and don't administer it until you've clarified and verified the order. It's acceptable and legally within your scope of practice to question an order that you feel may be erroneous. You should also document why you held the medication, how many times you attempted to contact the doctor regarding your decision, and what method you used to do so, whether by telephone, pager, or in person.

Reducing Your Risk with Risk-Management Strategies

You can help prevent negligence and keep yourself out of court by following your facility's risk-management protocol. *Risk-management* is a system to identify and analyze trends that may be putting you and your facility at risk; you then implement appropriate strategies to reduce and prevent these risks from occurring in the future.

Additionally, you can be proactive in reducing your professional risk in five important ways: listening to your patient, documenting unusual occurrences per agency policy in a separate incident report, documenting your actions in the medical record, carrying professional liability insurance, and maintaining appropriate patient relations.

Listening to your patient

Listening to your patients is just as important as talking to them. Say you go into your patient's room to hang IV phenytoin sodium (Dilantin). Your patient asks you what you're doing, and you tell him that the doctor has ordered an anticonvulsant to help prevent his seizures. Your patient says he's never had a seizure. Do you give the medication, or do you stop in your tracks and go back and check the order? If you're a cautious nurse, you hold the medication and double-check the order and clarify the order with the ordering physician.

Listen to your patient. If he questions an order, go back and check it. Don't give a medication that the patient is questioning until you have clarification.

Completing an unusual occurrence report

An *unusual occurrence* in healthcare can be anything from a medication error to a patient slipping and falling because of a spill. When an unusual event occurs, it's usually documented in an *unusual occurrence report*. Unusual occurrence reports are a way of keeping track of unusual situations that occur in the workplace (see Figure 2-1 for a sample report). They're often used to improve patient care and facility policies and procedures.

Unusual occurrences are noted in separate reports rather than in the patient's chart because documenting an unusual occurrence in the permanent record is a huge red flag to lawyers, alerting them to the possibility of medical error. Unusual occurrence reports are confidential, internal documents; however, they're admissible in court if evidence in the patient's chart shows that one was filed.

Always check with facility policy about how you're supposed to handle an unusual occurrence; then follow facility protocol in completing an unusual occurrence report.

STATE OF CALIFORNIA - HEALTH AND HUMAN SERVICES AGENCY   CALIFORNIA DEPARTMENT OF SOCIAL SERVICES
COMMUNITY CARE LICENSING DIVISION

UNUSUAL INCIDENT/INJURY REPORT

INSTRUCTIONS : NOTIFY LICENSING AGENCY, PLACEMENT AGENCY AND RESPONSIBLE PERSONS, IF ANY, BY NEXT WORKING DAY.

SUBMIT WRITTEN REPORT WITHIN 7 DAYS OF OCCURRENCE.

RETAIN COPY OF REPORT IN CLIENT'S FILE.

NAME OF FACILITY

FACILITY FILE NUMBER

TELEPHONE NUMBER ( )

ADDRESS

CITY, STATE, ZIP

CLIENTS/RESIDENTS INVOLVED	DATE OCCURRED	AGE	SEX	DATE OF ADMISSION

TYPE OF INCIDENT

☐ Unauthorized Absence	Alleged Client Abuse	☐ Rape	☐ Injury-Accident	☐ Medical Emergency
☐ Aggressive Act/Self	☐ Sexual	☐ Pregnancy	☐ Injury-Unknown Origin	☐ Other Sexual Incident
☐ Aggressive Act/Another Client	☐ Physical	☐ Suicide Attempt	☐ Injury-From another Client	☐ Theft
☐ Aggressive Act/Staff	☐ Psychological	☐ Other	☐ Injury-From behavior episode	☐ Fire
☐ Aggressive Act/Family, Visitors	☐ Financial		☐ Epidemic Outbreak	☐ Property Damage
☐ Alleged Violation of Rights	☐ Neglect		☐ Hospitalization	☐ Other *(explain)*

DESCRIBE EVENT OR INCIDENT (INCLUDE DATE, TIME, LOCATION, PERPETRATOR, NATURE OF INCIDENT, ANY ANTECEDENTS LEADING UP TO INCIDENT AND HOW CLIENTS WERE AFFECTED, INCLUDING ANY INJURIES:

_____

_____

_____

_____

_____

PERSON(S) WHO OBSERVED THE INCIDENT/INJURY:

_____

_____

_____

_____

EXPLAIN WHAT IMMEDIATE ACTION WAS TAKEN (INCLUDE PERSONS CONTACTED):

_____

_____

_____

_____

_____

LIC 624 (4/99)   **OVER**

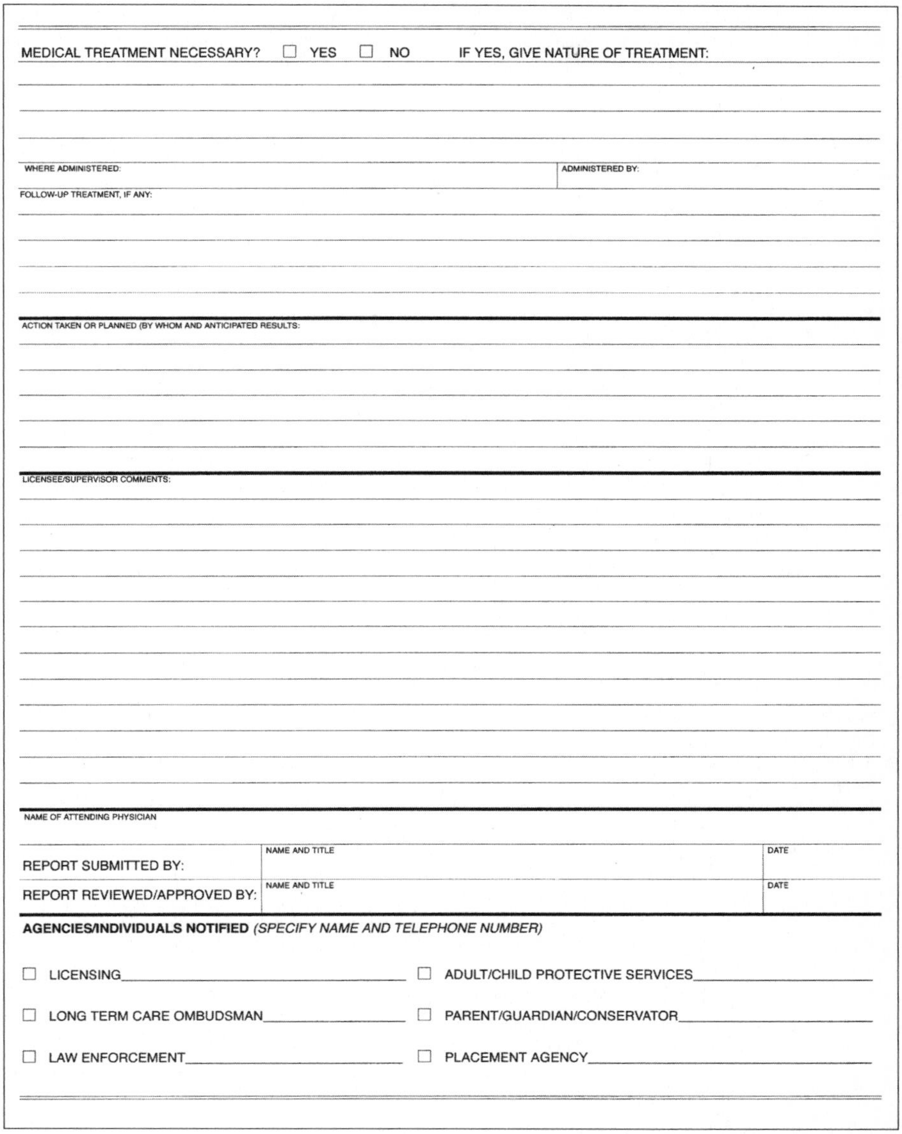

MEDICAL TREATMENT NECESSARY? ☐ YES ☐ NO IF YES, GIVE NATURE OF TREATMENT:

WHERE ADMINISTERED: | ADMINISTERED BY:

FOLLOW-UP TREATMENT, IF ANY:

ACTION TAKEN OR PLANNED (BY WHOM AND ANTICIPATED RESULTS):

LICENSEE/SUPERVISOR COMMENTS:

NAME OF ATTENDING PHYSICIAN

	NAME AND TITLE	DATE
REPORT SUBMITTED BY:		
REPORT REVIEWED/APPROVED BY:	NAME AND TITLE	DATE

AGENCIES/INDIVIDUALS NOTIFIED *(SPECIFY NAME AND TELEPHONE NUMBER)*

☐ LICENSING_____   ☐ ADULT/CHILD PROTECTIVE SERVICES_____

☐ LONG TERM CARE OMBUDSMAN_____   ☐ PARENT/GUARDIAN/CONSERVATOR_____

☐ LAW ENFORCEMENT_____   ☐ PLACEMENT AGENCY_____

Figure 2-1:
An unusual
occurrence
report form.

Illustration courtesy of California Department of Social Services

Documenting accurately

Accurate documentation is the key to avoiding potential lawsuits. If your patient suffers injury or death and your documentation doesn't show that you provided competent patient care that followed the legal standard of care, legal action may be filed against you that could result in the taking of your license, a fine, and even jail time. We talk more about how to document appropriately in Chapter 9.

Carrying professional liability insurance

Carrying your own professional liability insurance is a personal preference, but it's an option you should strongly consider. Having liability insurance means that you transfer your financial risk to a company that insures you. If you get sued for malpractice, the company insuring you agrees to compensate the patient for damages. In return, you sign an insurance policy and pay a monthly premium. Damages awarded to the patient are limited to the terms outlined in the insurance policy.

Although licensed healthcare professionals are responsible for their own actions, many healthcare facilities carry liability insurance for employees who perform negligent acts while on the job, as long as the act is within the employee's scope of practice. Sometimes the amount of the damages exceeds what the employer covers. Inadequate employer coverage can leave you holding the bag with unexpected expenses, so having professional liability insurance can be beneficial.

If you choose to obtain professional liability insurance, do your homework and choose a company with an excellent reputation. How can you determine a company's reputation? Word of mouth is always a great resource for gauging a company's reputation. You can also search the Internet for reviews of the company you're considering and check with the Better Business Bureau in your state to see how many complaints the company has on file.

Maintaining prudent patient relations

Remember the old saying "You attract more bees with honey than with vinegar"? This certainly applies to your relationships with the patients you care for. Who do you think patients are more likely to sue — a mean, crabby nurse who couldn't care less about their welfare or a nurse who's pleasant, friendly, and caring?

Maintaining prudent patient relationships from the minute you meet the patient to the time that he's discharged is paramount to your success as a healthcare professional. If your patient complains, listen to him. Get to the bottom of the complaint if you can, and if you can't, involve your supervisor. If you properly investigate and then resolve patient complaints, you're less likely to be sued for negligence by disgruntled patients and their families.

Chapter 3

Tools of the Trade

*T*o meet the demands of healthcare professionals and patients alike, IV therapy equipment is continuously evolving. In fact, medical technology, in general, always seems to be one step ahead of everything else. No sooner is one innovative piece of new equipment introduced than another one steps in to replace it. In other words, the latest and greatest infusion equipment of today may be outdated by tomorrow.

Even with all these changes, however, one thing that remains constant in IV therapy is the need for the equipment you use to be safe *and* effective. What good would an antimicrobial barrier device be, for example, if it increased the likelihood of catheter-related infections?

IV therapy relies on tools that are designed to protect the patient and the healthcare professional who's using the equipment. Nevertheless, for the equipment to do its job, you must first do yours. This means getting to know your infusion equipment on an intimate level, from its unique design right down to its particular functionality.

In this chapter, we introduce you to some basic tools of the trade that you're likely to see in your everyday practice. We describe the different types of vascular access devices, including which device to use when, and we talk about the advantages and disadvantages of certain solution containers. We discuss the various administration sets out there and their purpose in IV therapy, and we review their major differences. Finally, we talk about adding accessories to the mix.

Vascular Access Devices

A *vascular access device* (VAD) is a thin, flexible, hollow tube (also known as a *catheter*) that's inserted into a vein or an artery for the purpose of injecting or withdrawing fluids. Vascular access devices are categorized based on the vein in which the tip of the device resides. The two types are

✔ **Peripheral vascular access devices:** These devices are inserted by paramedics, nurses, and physicians. The tip of the device resides in the veins of the extremities.

✔ **Central vascular access devices:** These devices are inserted by physicians, physician assistants (PAs), and, on some occasions (for peripherally inserted central catheters or PICCs), specially trained nurses. The tip of the device resides in the veins of the central venous system.

When considering which type of catheter is more appropriate for your patient, keep in mind the following specifics:

✔ The length of time your patient needs therapy

✔ The length of time the device will remain in place

✔ Your patient's age and activity level

✔ The type of solution you're infusing

✔ The condition of your patient's veins

In general, you use peripheral access devices for short-term IV therapy that lasts less than one week, and you use central access devices in situations that require long-term IV therapy. Check with your facility's protocol if you're unsure of which one to use when.

Choosing the best peripheral access device

A peripheral access device or catheter begins and ends in an extremity, such as the arm, hand, leg, or foot, and more uncommonly, the neck. Peripheral IV catheters come in three types: the winged catheter (or *butterfly*), the short peripheral catheter (winged or nonwinged), and the midline catheter (see Figure 3-1).

Access into the external jugular vein is considered peripheral unless the tip of the catheter extends *into* the veins of the chest, such as the subclavian vein.

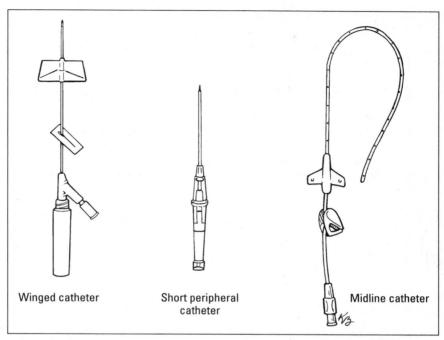

Illustration by Kathryn Born

Figure 3-1:
Comparison
of periph-
eral access
devices.

Winged catheter

Short peripheral
catheter

Midline catheter

Understanding winged devices

As you can see in Figure 3-1, the *winged catheter* is a basic peripheral IV device that has flexible or stiff plastic wings on either side of the catheter hub and sometimes has the extension tubing already attached. You insert a winged catheter into a vein as you would a traditional peripheral IV. To help stabilize the catheter hub, you can apply sterile tape or use a sterile sutureless device to secure the hub to the patient's skin. Many winged catheters have a safety mechanism that easily slides the needle into a protective sheath or applies a metal sheath over the tip for safety and disposal.

A *butterfly* is a type of winged needle with flexible plastic wings that's typically used to draw blood. Extending from the plastic hub is a short piece of tubing with a connector at the end that enables you to attach a syringe or vacuum tube for drawing blood. Although you can use a butterfly needle for an infusion, the Infusion Nurses Society (INS) recommends that you use it only for drawing blood. Because the butterfly needle is difficult to stabilize, it's linked with higher rates of infiltration, a common complication of IV therapy that we discuss in Chapter 12.

Winning the popularity contest: The short peripheral catheter

The *short peripheral catheter* is the catheter of choice when you expect IV therapy to last less than a week. Of all the short peripheral catheters out there, the *over-the-needle catheter,* shown in Figure 3-1, is the most commonly used.

The over-the-needle catheter is a color-coded, soft, plastic device equipped with a hard, plastic hub. A needle with a beveled tip sits inside the catheter and protrudes from its most distal end, allowing for puncture through the skin and vein. The color code on the catheter depends on the needle's gauge and is universal. As soon as the needle hits a vein, a flashback of blood appears in the catheter or chamber behind the hub of the catheter, depending on the manufacturer's preference. When you withdraw the needle, only the catheter remains in the vein.

Many newer-model short peripheral catheters have built-in safety features that retract the needle into a plastic covering or apply a metal sheath over the tip as the catheter advances into the vein and the needle is removed from the catheter. Some of them require that you push a button to retract the needle, while others do it automatically. Check your facility's product guide for details on using short peripheral catheters.

Read the manufacturer's instructions before using any VAD to become more familiar with its unique safety features and the correct way to use it. Change the peripheral IV catheter site every 72 hours or when complications, such as infiltration or phlebitis, occur. If your patient has limited venous access, notify the provider to discuss alternate IV access, such as a midline catheter or central line (see the later section "Keeping it centralized with a central vascular access device" for details).

To meet INS recommendations and to promote proper hemodilution (decreased flow of cells and solids in the blood), choose a short peripheral catheter with the smallest gauge and shortest length possible that still allows for proper administration of the prescribed IV therapy. Unstable patients present an exception to this guideline, as these patients require large volumes of fluid and/or blood products and need a larger-gauge catheter.

Avoid using a short peripheral catheter if the therapy you administer is a *vesicant* (a solution that causes severe tissue damage if leaked into the skin), if the pH of the solution is less than 5 or greater than 9, or if the osmolarity of the solution is greater than 600 mOsm/L. (If you need a quick refresher on pH or osmolarity, turn to Chapter 7.)

Familiarizing yourself with the midline catheter

The *midline catheter* (a type of peripheral catheter) is a longer (8 inches or 20 cm) peripheral access device that's generally inserted into the veins of the arm approximately 2 inches above the antecubital area. These veins include the basilic, cephalic, and median cubital veins. The catheter is then threaded through the veins up the arm to the *axilla* (underarm). Refer to Figure 3-1 for an example of a midline catheter.

In adults, the tip of the midline catheter rests in the upper arm just about 2.5 centimeters or 1 inch below the level of the axilla, which is why the midline catheter is still considered a peripheral device. A physician or certified clinician can insert the midline catheter at the bedside. Because the catheter doesn't reside in a central vein, you don't need to confirm placement of the tip with a chest X-ray.

Midline catheters are recommended when IV therapy will last for longer than one week. The INS states that no established evidence or references specify how long a midline catheter can safely remain in place; however, most manufacturers say you can leave it in for up to 30 days unless complications arise.

Midline catheters are recommended only for intermediate use. You shouldn't use them as a substitute for a central line (see the next section for details).

Similar to the short peripheral catheter, a midline catheter shouldn't be used when the therapy you administer has vesicant potential, when the pH of the solution is less than 5 or greater than 9, or when the osmolarity of the solution is greater than 600 mOsm/L. (For details on pH or osmolarity, turn to Chapter 7.)

Keeping it centralized with a central vascular access device

A *central vascular access device,* also known as a *central line,* is a catheter with the tip located in the superior vena cava near its junction at the right atrium or in the inferior vena cava if the femoral vein is used. The ideal route to the superior vena cava is by way of the subclavian vein, but you can also access it through the internal or external jugular veins or the veins of the arm, including the basilic, brachial, or cephalic veins.

You use a central line in the following situations:

- ✔ When emergency access is required during trauma or surgery
- ✔ When your patient has poor peripheral access
- ✔ When the solution you administer is inappropriate for a peripheral vein
- ✔ When long-term venous access is required

In most situations, you can start using a central line after a chest X-ray has been done and you've verified that the tip is in the correct location. In some facilities, you may need an order stating that the line is ready to use (unless it was placed in an emergency, in which case the doctor will give the okay to use the line until the tip is verified).

Central vascular access devices come in four types. We compare the uses for, advantages and disadvantages of, and the considerations you need to make for these four types in the following list. Figure 3-2 compares their physical features.

- ✔ **Peripherally inserted central catheters (PICCs):** Inserted through the veins of the upper extremities (in adults).

   - **Indications:** When long-term access is needed; when the patient has poor access; when frequent restarts of peripheral lines are needed to complete therapy; with multiple transfusions of blood and blood products, repeated lab draws, multiple radiographic studies, infusion of vesicants irritants, or chemotherapy.

   - **Advantages:** Accommodates transfusions of blood or blood products and long-term infusions of antibiotics or other caustic or vesicant agents; can be inserted at bedside by a physician or PICC-qualified RN (in most states); comes in single, double, or triple lumen; is associated with minimal complications; is well-suited for home use as it permits easy self-care.

   - **Disadvantages:** May lead to thrombophlebitis, arrhythmias (if the tip is in the right atrium), catheter malfunction, and infection.

   - **Considerations:** Insert by using maximum barrier sterile technique; utilize proper disinfection technique when accessing lumens or injection ports; monitor frequently for phlebitis and thrombus formation; flush according to facility policy and manufacturer guidelines with a 10-cc syringe or larger; use aseptic technique when flushing the catheter or doing dressing changes.

- ✔ **Non-tunneled percutaneous central catheters:** Inserted through the skin into the subclavian, jugular, or femoral veins.

   - **Indications:** Recommended for treatment lasting up to two weeks; when the patient needs emergent fluid resuscitation; when the patient has poor access; when frequent restarts of peripheral lines are needed to complete therapy; with multiple transfusions of blood and blood products, repeated lab draws, multiple radiographic studies, infusion of vesicants irritants, or chemotherapy.

   - **Advantages:** Accommodates patients who require multiple infusions; can be inserted at bedside by a physician or trained clinician; accommodates antibiotics, chemotherapy, total parenteral nutrition (TPN), and blood or blood products; aids in central venous pressure monitoring; comes in single or multi lumen.

- **Disadvantages:** Can lead to carotid artery puncture, pneumothorax, infection, and catheter malfunction; has a higher potential for dislodgment; is associated with more serious complications such as cardiac tamponade and major venous air embolism.

- **Considerations:** Insert by using maximum barrier sterile technique; utilize proper disinfection technique when accessing lumens or injection ports; flush according to facility policy and manufacturer guidelines; assess frequently for infection and clot formation; use aseptic technique when flushing the catheter or doing dressing changes.

✔ **Tunneled cuffed catheters:** Inserted surgically by a physician or trained clinician in the chest. The catheter is tunneled under the skin and enters the central vascular system through the jugular or subclavian vein. The tip usually ends in the superior vena cava.

- **Indications:** Appropriate for intermittent therapy or continuous long-term therapy. The Broviac (a smaller-lumen catheter) may be used for pediatric or elderly patients who have smaller central veins. The Groshong (a valved catheter that doesn't require a heparin lock) is indicated for patients with allergies to heparin or patients who are at high risk of thrombocytopenia related to heparin use. The Hickman (a larger-lumen catheter) is ideal for home infusion therapy. All three varieties can have single or multiple lumens. Dialysis catheters are another type of tunneled cuffed catheter.

- **Advantages:** Accommodates antibiotics, chemotherapy, TPN, and blood or blood products; is associated with reduced risk of infection; is well-suited for home use as it permits easy self-care; low potential for dislodgement; is available in single or multi lumen; doesn't always require a dressing when healed.

- **Disadvantages:** Requires surgical insertion and removal; Groshong and Hickman versions may tear and kink easily.

- **Considerations:** Monitor and change the dressing postsurgically; utilize proper disinfection technique when accessing lumens or injection ports; flush according to facility policy and catheter-specific manufacturer guidelines; observe frequently for kinks and tears.

✔ **Implanted ports:** Implanted surgically, typically in the upper chest under the skin, by a physician or trained clinician. The catheter, which is attached to the port, is tunneled under the skin and enters the central vascular system, usually through the jugular or subclavian vein. Ports can also be implanted in areas like the arm, thigh, abdomen, or back.

- **Indications:** When therapy is intermittent and projected for months to years or is needed for longer than three months; is especially beneficial to pediatric and oncology patients because of its portability and "hidden" location under the skin and tissues.

- **Advantages:** Accommodates continuous infusions and vesicant and other caustic medications; requires minimal care, flushing, and dressing changes in between infusions; has minimal effect on self-image.

- **Disadvantages:** Must be removed surgically; is difficult to self-administer IV therapy through if it isn't already accessed.

- **Considerations:** Utilize proper disinfection technique when accessing lumens or injection ports; assess for signs and symptoms of infection postsurgically; access only with a non-coring port access needle to avoid damage to the "resealing" septum; flush with heparin monthly.

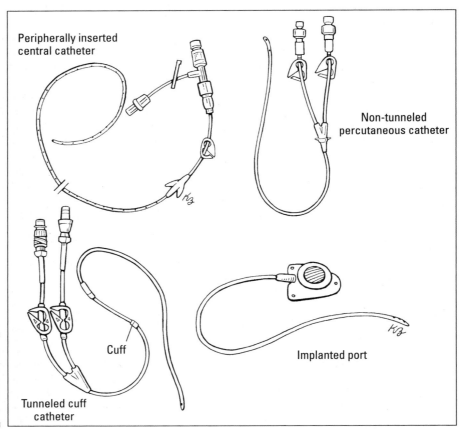

Peripherally inserted central catheter

Non-tunneled percutaneous catheter

Cuff

Tunneled cuff catheter

Implanted port

Figure 3-2: Central vascular access devices.

Illustration by Kathryn Born

Solution Containers

Solution containers are made of glass or plastic and come in a variety of sizes, ranging from bottles or bags that contain between 50 milliliters (mL) and 3 liters (L) of solution to smaller syringes that contain anywhere from 1 to 60 mL of solution. Each container comes with its own set of advantages and disadvantages.

When your infusate can't adapt: Using a glass container

The first solution container used in IV therapy more than 50 years ago was made of glass. You still use glass containers today when you infuse solutions that are incompatible with plastic, such as nitroglycerin or albumin.

Glass containers are vacuum sealed with a solid rubber closure that's held in place with an aluminum band. Graduation marks spaced every 20 to 50 mL are easy to see along the sides of the container. The major disadvantage to glass containers is that they're breakable and more difficult to store.

Unlike plastic containers, glass containers aren't collapsible, so they require a vented administration set to deliver the solution. The vented administration set has a unique spike with a small side channel designed to introduce air into the bottle. Sometimes the air channel is capped, so you have to uncap it before you use the administration set. Figure 3-3 shows a glass container with a vented administration set. If you don't use a vented set with a nonvented bottle, the solution won't flow correctly.

Being aware of the challenges of plastic containers

Plastic containers are easy to use, store, transport, and dispose of — not to mention, they're unbreakable. And because they collapse as fluid flows out, they don't require a vented administration set. Even so, plastic containers do have some disadvantages that you need to be aware of:

- *Sorption* occurs when certain IV medications, like nitroglycerin and insulin, adhere to the surface of the plastic container itself. This can negatively impact the titration of many drugs.

✔ Graduation marks on the outside of the container are difficult to read, particularly when you've already infused a lot of the solution from the container.

Despite these challenges, manufacturers strive to constantly improve the products used in plastic containers. To date, they're the most widely used solution container in IV therapy.

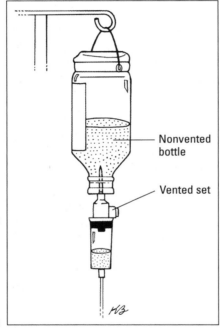

Figure 3-3:
A glass container with a vented administration set.

Nonvented bottle

Vented set

Illustration by Kathryn Born

Knowing your limitations: Alternate solution containers

When it comes to accuracy and ease of use, the syringe makes for an unbeatable alternate solution container. Unlike glass containers, syringes don't break if you drop them. When you put them into a syringe pump, you can easily see the volume infused, as well as the volume remaining. You can put them in your pocket during transport, and they're relatively inexpensive. Available worldwide, syringes can be prefilled or even frozen with virtually any kind of solution or medication.

The major disadvantage to using a syringe is its limitation in volume. Generally, syringes don't contain more than 60 milliliters of solution.

Saving time with ready-to-use drug delivery systems

A *ready-to-use drug delivery system* (DDS) holds a premeasured amount of drug and diluent in two separate compartments. Not only do DDS containers save you time in preparing a drug for administration, but they also work well when the drug you're infusing must be used within a short period of time after it's been diluted.

To use the ready-to-use drug delivery system, rupture the container's diaphragm by firmly squeezing opposing parts of the bag or breaking the seal of the medication vial so that the diluents and medication can mix. Gently invert the bag several times to mix all the medication with the diluent.

One of the problems with ready-to-use drug delivery systems is that the drug doesn't always mix with the diluent. To prevent this issue, rupture the seal and be sure to *thoroughly* mix the drug with the diluent before you start the infusion.

Administration Sets

For the solution to get from the container to your patient, you must use an administration set. The three main types of administration sets used in IV therapy are primary, secondary, and metered-volume chamber, but if you have certain circumstances, you may need to use a specialty set instead. No matter which type of set you use, it's sure to have plenty of features that help make your job easier.

The main event: The primary administration set

Standard *primary administration sets* run between 60 and 110 inches long and are typically used to deliver the primary infusion to the patient. IV fluids used during maintenance or replacement therapy commonly flow through a primary administration set. You can use primary sets continuously or on an intermittent basis, and they may hang by gravity or run through an electronic infusion pump.

As Figure 3-4 shows, a standard primary administration set has a spike to access the solution container, a drip chamber, one or more injection ports, and a device that allows you to control the flow, like a roller clamp or slide clamp. The end of the administration set that's farthest away from the spike is usually equipped with a *Luer-Lok,* a locking device that secures the administration set tubing to the catheter, which helps minimize the risk of disconnection.

You need to replace primary administration sets every 72 to 96 hours for continuous administration, depending on the solution being infused. Always label the administration set tubing with the time and date of the infusion and your initials.

When disconnecting an intermittent primary set from a patient, cover the end of the set with a new, sterile, protective cap. Never loop the tip into another injection port higher up on the administration set. Doing so is considered inappropriate practice and can lead to contamination and infection. Make sure you change intermittent primary administration sets every 24 hours due to the repeated disconnection and risk of contamination.

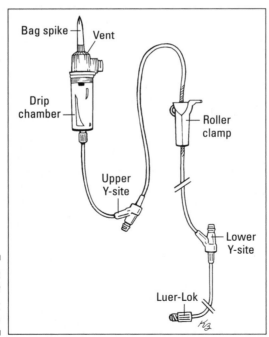

Figure 3-4:
A primary administration set.

Illustration by Kathryn Born

Piggybacking with a secondary administration set

You use a *secondary administration set,* commonly called a *piggyback,* to deliver a wide variety of IV medications, the most common of these being IV antibiotics. Secondary sets generally attach to the primary set through a Luer-Lok (needleless connector) or another type of needle-protected device.

Sharing many of the same characteristics as the primary set, the secondary administration set has a spike, a drip chamber, at least one injection port, and a flow-control device (see the later section), but it's much shorter in length than the primary set, usually about 30 to 36 inches long, as shown in Figure 3-5.

You must replace and label a secondary administration set every 72 to 96 hours for continuous administration, depending on the solution being infused. If you have to disconnect the secondary line after each use, handle it as you do a primary intermittent set by covering the end with a new, sterile, protective cap in between infusions. Also, be sure to change intermittent secondary administration sets every 24 hours due to the repeated disconnection and risk of contamination.

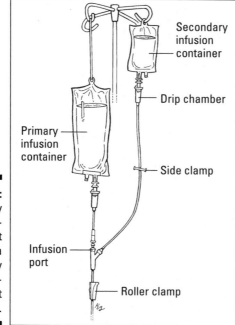

Figure 3-5: A primary administration set (left) with a secondary administration set (right).

Illustration by Kathryn Born

Limiting fluids with a metered-volume chamber set

A *metered-volume chamber set* has a small, volume-controlled chamber that sits between the main fluid container and the actual administration set. It's perfect for the pediatric patient because it delivers precise volume control. Plus, many metered-volume chamber sets have filters built right into the line to keep particles and pathogens from contaminating your patient. Figure 3-6 shows you what one of these sets looks like.

Metered-volume chamber sets allow you to fill the chamber with only 1 to 2 hours worth of fluid volume. Or you can add medication to the injection port at the top of the chamber and mix it right in the chamber, using the primary infusion as a dilutant. Be sure to check your facility's policies on using this type of device for IV administration.

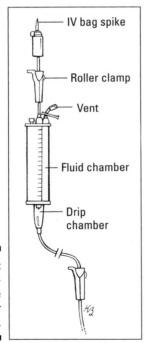

Figure 3-6: A metered-volume chamber set.

Illustration by Kathryn Born

Isn't that special? Considering a specialty set

You may need to use a *specialty administration set* when you infuse medications that require special tubing, such as nitroglycerin, parenteral nutrition, lipids, and blood or blood products. Specialty sets are uniquely designed for the drug or fluid you infuse with them. For example, nitroglycerin administration sets feature non-PVC-type tubing to prevent sorption that may occur with standard, PVC-type tubing. Blood administration sets allow for the uniform flow of blood, despite its viscosity. Whatever their purpose, specialty sets add functionality to your infusion where it may otherwise be lacking.

Generally, if the medication you're infusing requires a specialty set, the packaging in which the drug comes from the pharmacy will say so. An exception to this rule is blood, whereby you use special Y-tubing from your facility supply room.

The *primary Y-set* is a specialized, primary administration set that you typically use when administering blood or blood products. As you can see in Figure 3-7, it has two separate spikes, one drip chamber, and two separate roller clamps. This dual action comes in handy when you're administering blood with normal saline; see Chapter 5 for details.

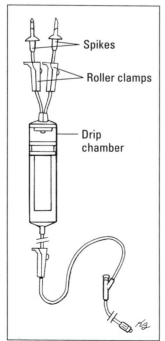

Spikes

Roller clamps

Drip chamber

Figure 3-7:
The primary Y-set.

Illustration by Kathryn Born

Characteristics of administration sets

From drop factors to needleless connectors, administration sets have many unique characteristics built into them that help make your job much easier and a lot safer.

Following the drips with drop factors

Administration sets are available with two different drip systems: macrodrip and microdrip (see Figure 3-8). Which type you use depends on the goal of the treatment.

- A *macrodrip* system is capable of delivering a large quantity of fluid at a rapid rate. It has a *drop factor* (the number of drops in 1 mL) of 10 to 20 drops per mL (gtt/mL). Use a macrodrip system when you infuse at a rate of 100 mL or more per hour.

- A *microdrip* system has a drop factor of 50 to 60 gtt/mL and is an excellent choice for the pediatric or elderly patient who needs a smaller amount of medication or the patient who needs a medication that must be closely regulated. Use a microdrip system when you infuse at a rate of less than 100 mL per hour.

We talk more about the calculation of drop factors in Chapter 10.

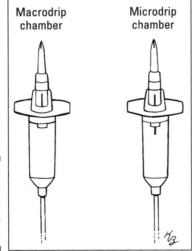

Figure 3-8:
Macrodrip
and
microdrip
systems.

Illustration by Kathryn Born

What's all the fuss about injection ports?

Most primary administration sets feature between one and three injection ports along the tubing so that you can run multiple, compatible infusions at the same time or inject compatible IV push medications into the patient's vein without disconnecting the line.

Injection ports can be needleless, as in the Luer-Lok, or they can require access by a needle. To date, most facilities use needleless injection ports and connection systems (see the later section "Connecting with administration set connectors" for details). Although injection ports requiring needles are still available, the U.S. Occupational Safety and Health Administration (OSHA) currently prohibits using them because of possible needle-stick injuries.

Preventing back flow with the one-way valve

One-way valves are an intrinsic part of many primary administration sets. The *one-way valve* uses a float device to keep the medication flowing in one direction — into the patient — and the blood from flowing back into the line.

One-way valves are particularly important when you infuse a secondary medication. What prevents your primary medication from flowing back into the secondary solution container? You guessed it — the one-way valve. When the secondary infusion is finished, the one-way valve reverses, allowing the primary line to pick up where it left off. Figure 3-9 shows you what a one-way valve looks like.

Hang your secondary solution higher than the primary solution to ensure proper function of the one-way valve and complete delivery of your secondary medication.

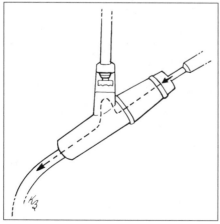

Figure 3-9:
The one-way valve.

Illustration by Kathryn Born

Using administration sets with dial-a-flow regulators

Dial-a-flow administration sets are primary sets with a dial incorporated in the line that you can use to set flow rates from 20 mL to 250 mL an hour without having to count drops. However, you should never use a dial-a-flow system for precise dosages, such as those in the ICU setting.

Connecting with administration set connectors

Every administration set has a connector that plugs directly into the patient's IV extension set or the primary tubing. The two standard needleless administration set connectors are the slip and the Luer-Lok connector. You can also use a combination of the two. Although both types are designed to prevent accidental disconnection, Luer-Loks are threaded — slips are not — which makes the Luer-Lok less likely to leak or accidentally disconnect. Figure 3-10 shows what these two connectors look like.

The purpose behind needleless connectors is obvious: to prevent needle sticks in healthcare workers. Unfortunately, while they have clearly met this goal, mounting evidence suggests that needleless connectors also increase the risk of bloodstream infections in patients. Although technology continuously strives to reduce these risks, they remain an integral part of the clinical setting.

When monitoring your infusion and your IV site, always check your connections. Disconnection of your line is always possible, no matter which type of connector you use. Also whenever you use needleless connectors, be sure to follow your agency's protocol in accessing and changing them.

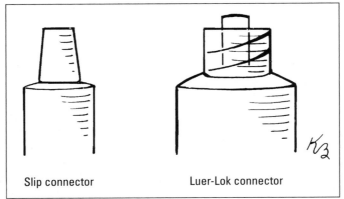

Figure 3-10:
Administration set connectors.

Slip connector   Luer-Lok connector

Illustration by Kathryn Born

Flow-Control Devices

Can you imagine if you had no control over the flow of your IV solution? The results could be disastrous! Flow control is a key part of IV therapy. In general, you can use a manual or an automatic system to control flow. Which type of flow-control system you use for an infusion depends on the patient, the type of therapy you administer, and the healthcare setting in which you practice.

Relying on the manual method: Gravity

Flow-control systems that depend on gravity (often called *gravity-dependent systems*) rely on a pressure gradient that's created by the height of the solution container. To make gravity work in your favor, you must hang the IV solution container 3 or 4 feet above the patient.

Gravity systems are typically the simplest and cheapest systems in use today, and they're supplied with standard IV administration sets. The infusion rate of a gravity system depends on pressure differences across the valve, such as those created by the height of the fluid in relationship to the patient, venous pressure, or obstruction (such as clotting or crimping of the catheter), and on gravity, which provides the infusion pressure.

Some IV solutions (like albumin, which is generally infused rapidly) flow best when you rely on gravity to help out. But for precise rate and volume control, an electronic infusion pump works best (see the later section for details on infusion pumps).

The pressure is on: Adding pressure with a pressure bag

A *pressure bag* is just what it sounds like: a plastic bag that you place directly over a plastic IV solution container and inflate to maintain a specific, constant pressure. Most pressure bags come equipped with a warning label that alerts you to the bag's recommended maximum pressure. Usually, this pressure shouldn't exceed 300 mL of mercury (mmHg) or 6 pounds per square inch (psi).

Generally, you use pressure bags only for serious situations, like critical care, trauma, or surgery. You use them with gravity-dependent infusions that need to be administered very rapidly or when your patient has an arterial line.

Relying on its own power: The mechanical infusion pump

Mechanical infusion pumps require no battery or outside power supply. They rely on their own physical properties of shape and matter to provide a fluid pathway. You can use mechanical pumps to provide continuous intravenous, subcutaneous, or epidural administration of drugs. You throw them away after you use them.

One example of a mechanical pump is the elastomeric balloon pump, shown in Figure 3-11. Medication is delivered to the patient as the elastomeric "balloon" inside the ball consistently deflates and gently pushes solution through the IV tubing and into the catheter or port. It offers duration infusion times from 30 minutes to 5 hours and can deliver multiple medications such as antibiotics and antiviral medications.

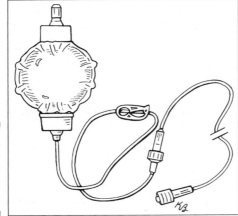

Figure 3-11:
The elastomeric balloon pump.

Illustration by Kathryn Born

Pumping up the volume: The electronic infusion pump

The *electronic infusion pump* uses positive pressure to deliver IV fluids. When you need better control over your infusion, the electronic infusion pump is the way to go.

The two types of electronic infusion pumps available are volumetric pumps and syringe pumps. *Syringe pumps* are small infusion pumps that use a syringe to gradually administer small amounts of medication to a patient. *Volumetric pumps* (also just known as *infusion pumps*) are electronic devices used to control the administration of intravenous fluids at a carefully regulated rate over long periods. Volumetric pumps are subdivided into two categories:

- **Pole-mounted volumetric pumps:** Used in most healthcare settings, these pumps are used to control the administration of IV fluids at a carefully regulated rate over long periods. Because these pumps are usually larger, they need to be hung on a pole to be used.

- **Ambulatory volumetric pumps:** These pocket-size pumps have a fluid container in the form of a small floppy bag or cassette (such as an insulin pump) that delivers the medication. These pumps allow your patient to remain mobile.

Another type of infusion pump is the patient-controlled analgesia (PCA) pump, which a patient can use to control (to some extent) the delivery of an amount of intravenous analgesic that's set in the pump by the nurse or doctor. The patient can administer a prescribed amount of medication by pressing a hand-held push button that tells the pump when to infuse. PCA pumps are available as pole-mounted or ambulatory (and PCA itself is even available in a syringe).

Characteristics of every infusion pump

Infusion pumps are programmed according to the manufacturer's instructions. Although each brand of pump is unique, they share similar characteristics:

- **Rate:** The volume of fluid infused over a period of time. Most pumps deliver in mL per hour; however, some use milligrams (mg) per hour.

- **Volume to be infused:** The amount of fluid, in mL, hanging in the IV solution container. It isn't always the same amount that you will infuse.

- **Volume infused:** The total amount of fluid, in mL, administered by the pump since it was last zeroed. This function isn't programmable; it's a feature of the pump.

- **Secondary rate:** The volume of fluid, generally set in mL per hour, infused over a period of time by the secondary line. Most pumps are designed so that the primary infusion will resume after the secondary infusion is complete.

More to Think About When Choosing IV Equipment

Generally speaking, *accessories* are items that contribute in some way to the effect, or result, of an activity or process. In IV therapy, accessory devices are designed to improve the functionality of your practice. They include things like inline filters, add-on devices, stabilization devices, and dressings.

Using an inline filter

Just as the filter in a swimming pool separates and then removes unwanted debris from the pool water, an *inline infusion filter* removes solid particles, microorganisms, and air from IV solutions and medications. All IV solutions and medications contain some degree of unwanted matter. The U.S. Pharmacopeia (USP) has developed a standard that regulates the amount of particulate matter allowed in any given solution. To date, a solution meets the standard if it contains less than 50 particles/mL of 10 microns or larger and 5 particles/mL of 25 microns or larger.

So does this mean you have to walk around with an electron microscope in your back pocket to measure the particle amount in every solution? Of course not! The facility you work for should have guidelines in place for using inline filters. Just make sure you follow them!

For your convenience, we've included a list of some of the more common medications that require a filter here:

- Amiodarone hydrochloride (Cordarone)
- Antithymocyte globulin (Thymoglobulin)
- Mannitol (Osmitrol)
- Total parenteral nutrition (TPN)
- Phenytoin sodium (Dilantin)
- Asparaginase (Elspar)
- Infliximab (Remicade)

When using an inline filter, keep in mind the following pointers:

- ✔ Place the filter at the most distal part of the tubing, closest to the patient.

- ✔ Prime the filter right along with the line to remove excess air. If you're adding a filter to an existing line, prime the filter separately before adding it to the existing line.

- ✔ Change the filter according to your facility's policy and the manufacturer's instructions. You may be required to change the filter as often as you replace the IV solution container.

You don't need to use a filter in every situation or for every patient. In fact, here are some instances when you should *not* use an inline filter:

- ✔ When using certain medications, like amphotericin B (Fungizone), that have a tendency to stick to the filter

- ✔ When infusing a very small volume of medication (because the filter ultimately retains some of the drug, which may alter its effect)

- ✔ When infusing through the arterial route (because the presence of a filter may alter central venous pressure monitoring)

Note: Inline filters for IV therapy can be used for antibiotic therapy, apheresis solutions, aqueous IV solutions, delivery of epidural anesthetic and analgesic solutions, lipid or TPN infusion, and neonate and pediatric IV therapy. Because filter materials differ, check with the manufacturer's instructions for use for drug incompatibilities or check with your facility's protocol for using inline filters.

Adding to your line with add-on devices

Add-on devices (devices that you can add to your infusion system) come in a myriad of sizes, shapes, and colors, and the healthcare market seems to offer a never-ending supply of them (see Figure 3-12 for just some of the options out there). The INS discourages the use of add-on devices as much as possible because they increase the risk of contamination in what is supposed to be a closed system. When used for a specific purpose and not convenience, however, an add-on device can increase the overall functionality of your entire infusion system.

The following add-on devices are some you may encounter in your facility:

- ✔ **Stopcocks:** These devices manually direct the flow of your IV solution. You can shut one port off while infusing or flushing through the other. Stopcocks come in three- or four-way varieties.

- ✔ **Extension sets:** These devices are used primarily to add length to an IV administration set.

- ✔ **J-loops and U-loops:** These small extension sets attach to the catheter hub, adding extra length and stability when securing the IV.

- ✔ **Multi-flow adapters, T-ports, and Y-connectors:** These devices allow two to three compatible infusions to flow at the same time into a single catheter lumen.

Use add-on devices sparingly and only when you can justify the need for them.

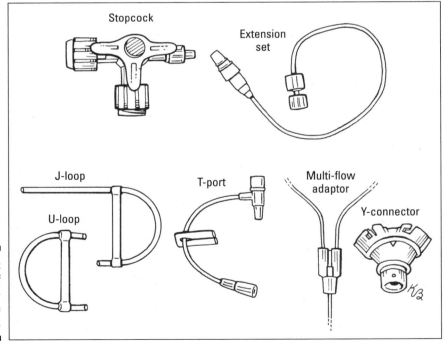

Figure 3-12: Some of the available add-on devices.

Illustration by Kathryn Born

Stabilizing your device

Two important areas that you need to address when inserting an IV are stabilizing the catheter itself and immobilizing your patient's joint (if you have to insert the catheter in an area of joint flexion). By stabilizing the catheter and immobilizing the joint, you help decrease the risk of catheter-related complications, which is extremely important in IV therapy.

Keeping your catheter safe and steady

Anytime you're dressing an IV insertion site, the INS recommends that you first stabilize the catheter and then cover and protect the skin. You can use several methods to stabilize a catheter:

- Sterile tape
- Surgical wound closure strips (Steri-Strips)
- A manufactured stabilization device like a StatLock, Grip-Lok, or Vital-Hold

Because studies have shown a significant reduction in catheter-related complications when using a manufactured stabilization device compared to other methods of stabilization, these types of devices are currently the preferred method of stabilization for any IV catheter.

Supporting your patient's joint

Immobilizing your patient's joint is critical when you're inserting an IV catheter into an area that would disrupt the secure placement of the catheter if movement occurred, such as in areas of joint flexion. The best way to hinder movement and thus immobilize the joint is to use an *arm board,* which is especially useful in stabilizing IV sites in small children, infants, or confused patients who may accidentally compromise the IV site. Arm boards should be padded for comfort and discarded after use. The tape securing the board shouldn't obstruct the view of the IV insertion site or restrict your patient's movement.

Whenever possible, avoid placing an IV near an area of joint flexion, such as the dorsal aspect of the hand, the cephalic vein of the wrist, or the antecubital fossa in the ventral aspect of the elbow joint. Placing an IV in these areas can cause the catheter to become dislodged, which can lead to infiltration.

Protecting the IV site

In keeping with the INS's *Infusion Nursing Standards of Practice,* you must always place an *occlusive dressing* over your patient's IV insertion site. An occlusive dressing is one that protects the IV site from air and bacteria. You can create occlusive dressings with gauze and tape, or you can use a premanufactured transparent dressing. Some facilities even use antimicrobial barrier products to help protect patients from infection.

Regardless of the type of dressing you use to protect the IV insertion site, always date, time, and initial every dressing.

To find out more about stabilization and dressing techniques for the peripheral line, refer to Chapter 12. To find out more about techniques for the central line, turn to Chapter 13.

Using a gauze dressing

Gauze sponges are made of natural cotton or synthetic cotton blends. Although gauze dressings are certainly more economic and absorbent than other types of dressings, they obscure the IV insertion site and prevent you from visualizing and monitoring it properly. Even so, sometimes gauze is your only option due to a patient's allergy to transparent dressings. When using a gauze dressing, keep in mind the following helpful tips:

- ✔ When observing an IV insertion site dressed with gauze, don't just lift the dressing up and then reattach it when you're done checking the insertion site. Remove it completely and then replace it after each observation.

- ✔ Tape across the entire surface of the gauze to make your dressing occlusive and not just around the edges. Doing so helps prevent moisture and microorganisms from penetrating the dressing.

- ✔ Change the dressing every 48 hours or when it becomes soiled, wet, or nonadherent to the skin.

- ✔ Use a protective skin barrier (such as Cavilon and Allkare) before applying tape to the skin to allow for better adherence of the tape and to prevent damaging the underlying tissue when you remove the tape. You apply both Cavilon and Allkare to the skin and then leave it there to dry; the barriers quickly dry to a nonsticky, protective, breathable waterproof coating.

Using a transparent dressing

Transparent dressings, like Tegaderm or Tegasorb, are more expensive than gauze, but when you apply them correctly, they last longer and may even provide better protection against contamination than other dressings. Transparent dressings are sterile and come in individually wrapped packages.

For over-the-needle catheters, change the transparent dressing when you change the catheter, usually every 72 hours, unless it becomes soiled, wet, or nonadherent before then. For midlines or central lines, change the sterile, transparent dressing at least every seven days and as needed. Also be sure to use a protective skin barrier product to help transparent dressings adhere more securely to the skin.

Going the extra mile with an antimicrobial barrier product

More and more facilities are using *antimicrobial barrier products,* as shown in Figure 3-13, at the insertion site of an IV catheter to reduce the risk of catheter-associated infections. Several antimicrobial barrier products are available, many of which feature a circular patch impregnated with anti-microbial agents, such as chlorhexidine gluconate or silver. (The Centers for Disease Control and Prevention recommends using a chlorhexidine-impregnated sponge disk dressing.)

Whether you use an antimicrobial barrier product is really up to the facility for which you work, but such a product is particularly helpful in reducing infections in certain high-risk populations.

Figure 3-13:
Anti-
microbial
barrier
products.

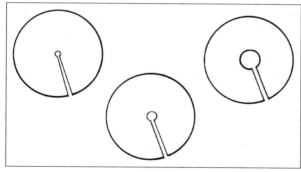

Illustration by Kathryn Born

Part II
What's Your Type? Components of IV Therapy

The 5th Wave   By Rich Tennant

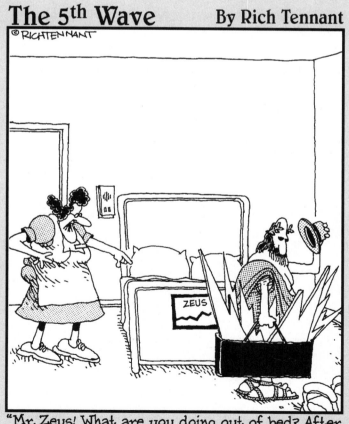

"Mr. Zeus! What are you doing out of bed? After your IV therapy, the doctor said you shouldn't even be shorting out lamps yet, let alone hurling thunderbolts!"

In this part . . .

*P*art II gives you a classroom-style introduction to the most common types of IV therapy. For those of you interested in infusing drugs, this part helps you discover how IV medications work to fight disease and restore health. It also covers the compatibility aspects of blood component transfusions and the different types of chemotherapy used to treat cancer. It provides insight into the delicate fluid and electrolyte balance needed to create physiologic equilibrium and the role IV therapy plays in restoring and maintaining that equilibrium. Finally, it explains the ins and outs of administering parenteral nutrition.

We cover the clinical, practical applications of these different types of IV therapy in Part IV.

Chapter 4

Medications Made to Order: Pharmacological IV Therapy

*W*hen an emergency medical team reaches a critically injured patient, one of the first things it does is assess the patient and attempt to get him stabilized. One of the steps of stabilization is to start an intravenous (IV) line and begin administering IV medications. These particular medications are vital to a patient's survival because they enable the team to quickly reverse low blood pressure in patients with shock, instantly dissolve clots in patients with heart attack or stroke, and correct life-threatening arrhythmias. But IV medications aren't used only in emergencies: They're a mainstay of treatment in everyday hospital settings, too.

This chapter is designed to guide you through the many aspects of pharmacological IV therapy. In it, you discover when and why medications are given intravenously, what clinical settings demand rapid IV infusion, and how you can identify and prevent adverse IV drug interactions. You're also introduced to *pharmacodynamics* and *pharmacokinetics* — the complex series of events and mechanisms triggered when medications enter the bloodstream — and you see how these complex events impact a medication's bioavailability and effectiveness. In short, you see how a medication works on the body and how the body works on a medication.

Understanding *how* to efficiently and accurately administer IV medications helps you save valuable time. Knowing *why* the medications are used and anticipating *which* medications work best in various clinical settings helps you save lives. This chapter arms you with the information you need to save both.

Understanding How Pharmacological IV Therapy Works

The use of pharmacological IV therapy has dramatically increased since the advent of modern IV drug therapy during World War I. Today, more than 80 percent of all hospitalized patients receive IV drug therapy for administration of fluids and medications. Intravenous medications are also widely used outside hospital settings in places like skilled nursing facilities (SNFs) and infusion centers and in some home healthcare situations.

To understand the growth and widespread use of this life-saving therapy, you need to recognize the reasons why IV medications are among the quickest, most effective treatments, and why, in some cases, IV administration is the only way a medication can be delivered to a patient. In the following sections, we explore how the body interacts with IV medications and how the drug is distributed throughout the body. We then explain how to know when using IV medication is the best treatment.

Pharmacokinetics: How the body works on a drug

When medications are introduced into the body, a fierce battle takes place between the protective mechanisms of the body and the survival mechanisms of the drug. The body's first line of defense is *pharmacokinetics* — a complex process that treats the medication as a foreign invader and tries to change it so it can be eliminated as quickly as possible. The four processes of pharmacokinetics are

- **Absorption:** This process transforms oral, intramuscular (IM), rectal, transdermal, or subcutaneous medications into agents that can enter the bloodstream. Intravenous medications bypass the absorption process and have rapid, near 100 percent bioavailability by directly entering the bloodstream.

- **Distribution:** Next, the medication disperses through body fluids and tissues, in which the body has a portion of free, active drugs and a portion of bound, inactive drugs.

- **Metabolism:** Metabolism is the irreversible conversion of a drug's parent compound into daughter metabolites. One of the goals of metabolism is to increase the drug's water or fat solubility so it can be more easily eliminated from the body. This process is also known as *biotransformation.*

> ✔ **Excretion:** Also known as *elimination* or *clearance,* this final process is the exit or removal of drugs from the body, primarily through the kidneys in urine or through the liver as bile in feces.

Pharmacodynamics: How a drug works on the body

The effects of medication appear rapidly after the IV injection is infused into the bloodstream. IV drugs relentlessly make their way to all parts of the body, including the major organs and tissues. When they reach the cellular level, the drugs go for the receptors on the cell's surface. When they reach their target receptors, drugs typically work in one of the following three ways:

✔ Binding to the receptor and blocking its action

✔ Mimicking and multiplying the receptor's action

✔ Creating a new receptor action

If a drug works in the first way, by binding to the receptor and blocking its action, the drug is called an *antagonist* because it switches off cell function. Examples of antagonists include heart Beta blockers, such as propranolol and atenolol.

If a drug works in the second or third way, by mimicking or creating a new action, the drug is called an *agonist* because it switches on cell function. Examples of agonists include morphine and albuterol.

Interfering with receptors, however, is only one way a drug works in the human body. Other drugs, called *activators,* target enzymes rather than receptors. Activators work by regulating chemical reactions in the cell to either increase or decrease cell activity. Examples of activator drugs include aspirin and some HIV medications.

Although most drugs act on cell receptors or enzymes, other drugs have different means of affecting cells. One example is a major class of antibiotics called *bactericidals;* drugs in this class kill bacteria by disrupting cell wall integrity and causing bacterial membranes to rupture.

Vitamins may also switch on or off cell function by interfering with cell signaling and communication. *Electrolytes* are another group of therapeutic agents that affect cell function in both direct and indirect ways. For details about electrolytes, check out Chapter 7.

Pharmacodynamics is a complex process that takes place at the cellular level, similar to the processes involved in cellular transport and osmosis, which we cover in Chapter 7. When medications enter the bloodstream and the cells, the drug's pharmacodynamics features cause the body to respond in many ways, including the following:

- ✔ Constricting and dilating blood vessels
- ✔ Constricting and dilating bronchial tubes
- ✔ Raising and lowering blood pressure, blood sugar, and heart rate
- ✔ Destroying bacteria cell walls
- ✔ Disrupting blood flow and destroying malignant cells

What's the point? Recognizing the reasons for IV medication administration

Identifying the reasons for giving medications by IV rather than by mouth or intramuscular (IM) injection is a key component in providing quality IV therapy. Being able to recognize when a patient needs to be switched from one medication form to an IV med is a critical part of tailoring the route of administration to match your patient's needs. Your goal is to always give the right medication to the right patient via the right route. If, for example, you give oral medications (by mouth or PO) to nauseated patients, whether or not it's the right medication may be meaningless because the patient may not be able to keep it onboard long enough for it to be effective.

The following sections cover the main reasons why you may need to use IV therapy to administer meds to your patient.

When your patient can't tolerate the oral route

No matter what diagnosis your patient has, he may not be able to take oral, rectal, or IM medications, or the medication he needs may not be indicated to be given via those routes. One of the remaining routes for most medications is IV. The rapid effects you get from delivering fluids directly into the bloodstream are necessary during emergencies or other situations in which IV medications are needed.

Recognizing and reporting that your patient needs to be switched from oral to IV medications leads to a quicker recovery and shorter hospital stay for your patient. Use the following symptoms as guidelines to help you determine when your patient can no longer tolerate oral medications:

✔ Vomiting or diarrhea after oral medication administration

✔ Nausea that requires multiple injections to control

✔ Fevers of undetermined origin

✔ Dry mouth, lack of tears, and minimal urination (in other words, dehydration)

You can identify dehydration in a patient who may have experienced diminished urine output (an early sign) by using the skin turgor test (a late sign) to gently pinch and release the skin on the top of the hand or on the forearm above the wrist. Normal skin turgor allows the skin to return to its original shape within three seconds. If the skin remains pinched or tented for three seconds or more, your patient has a lack of skin turgor, indicating dehydration and a need for IV fluid replacement (see Chapter 7 for more on fluid replacement).

When you need quicker access

Say you start your shift by going to assess a patient. When you enter the room, you find him unconscious and collapsed on the floor. You have no time to waste. You must react quickly and decisively. You quickly assess the patient, call a code blue, and initiate CPR. While other team members who responded to the code begin to administer oxygen, apply ECG leads, and take over CPR, the MD orders IV fluids and epinephrine. You grab the IV supplies and start an IV. When your patient is in the full throes of a cardiac arrest and his life hangs in the balance, you quickly identify the need for rapid access to IV medications.

Starting an IV on a critical patient provides the fastest route to deliver powerful medications directly into the patient's bloodstream. After hitting the bloodstream, IV medications go to work to alleviate symptoms and reverse the medical crisis.

When you administer an IV medication, you provide immediate *bioavailability* to the drug, meaning that 100 percent of the medication is in the bloodstream and ready for instant transport to organs and tissues.

Becoming proficient in administering IV therapy, even in the most daunting situations, will prove to be your most valuable asset in providing your patient with the quickest possible access to life-saving fluids and medications.

When you need better control

Giving medications intravenously provides more control of a drug's two basic pharmacological actions: intensity and duration. The *intensity* of a drug is how quickly the drug takes effect; the *duration* is how long the drug effect lasts. When a patient receives medications orally or intramuscularly, the drug's intensity isn't realized for about 30 to 45 minutes and the duration may last hours.

IV medications offer much more control because the drug's intensity is so rapid. Medications introduced directly into the bloodstream produce the rapid results that are often necessary during emergencies because the therapeutic levels of the medication are quickly reached. Better control is also achieved because IV medications produce more rapid effects through a process called pharmacodynamics, which we discuss in the earlier section "Pharmacodynamics: How a drug works on the body."

Another reason why IV administration provides more control is because IV meds don't have to go through the slow, time-consuming process of *absorption*. Absorption is part of a process that changes the structure of oral and other nonparenteral drugs to get them ready for distribution to the bloodstream. When you administer a medication intravenously, however, you save critical time by omitting all the absorption routes and injecting the medication directly into the bloodstream.

When you're dealing with IV meds, you must be aware of the signs and symptoms of overdose and frequently assess your patient for drug toxicity, particularly in elderly and pediatric patients. Elderly patients often have diminished liver and kidney functions, meaning medications can circulate in the bloodstream much longer than they do in an average healthy adult, without being eliminated through the kidneys or liver. Pediatric patients have smaller body surface areas and immature organs such as the kidney and require smaller doses and stricter monitoring for signs and symptoms of overdosing or drug toxicity.

To achieve maximum control with IV medications, you can use the *sliding scale method* of administration (if ordered by the doctor). The sliding scale method, also called *titration,* enables you to regulate your patient's vital signs by regulating the flow and drip rate of IV drugs. For example, a drop in your patient's blood sugar signals you to decrease insulin flow, and a rise in blood sugar signals you to increase insulin flow.

When titrating IV medications, monitor your patient's vital signs continuously until they reach the desired level of stability. Record and document your actions, and after titration is completed, monitor your patient frequently for signs of recurrent instability or adverse reactions (see the later section "Understanding Adverse Effects").

When you need to speed up drug delivery

Many patients are successfully treated every day with oral and IM medications, but frequently patients experience a crisis and need medications immediately. When you encounter a patient who requires medications *stat,* IV administration is the ideal way to go. After all, IV administration is one of the fastest, most efficient, and most effective methods of medication delivery.

To speed up medication delivery even more, physicians may order meds to be administered by *IV push* or *IV bolus,* which is when you deliver additional medication through an IV and administer it all at once over a period of a minute or two. IV push has the advantage of being able to give extra medicine, as needed, and because it's injected directly into the bloodstream, it can rapidly get the medicine into the body. IV push meds can be given per protocol, in situations such as cardiac arrest. (Chapter 11 offers a few more details on IV push administrations.)

The following list reflects a few of the many incidences that require rapid IV administration:

- Allergic reactions and anaphylactic shock
- Cardiac arrest
- Diabetic coma or insulin shock
- Hemorrhage
- Hypotension or malignant hypertension
- Respiratory distress
- Seizures
- Stroke
- Trauma

Blast from the past: A short history of IV therapy

Before the advent of infusion pumps, nurses inflated blood pressure cuffs around IV bags to speed up the infusion of medications and fluids.

Going back even farther in history: Before plastic IV bags, intravenous cannulas, and infusion pumps, IV fluids came in glass bottles, and IV fluids were delivered through stainless steel needles. IV push medications were administered very slowly to prevent dislodging the needle, puncturing the vein, and infiltrating the IV. When patients needed emergency treatment for life-threatening conditions such as anaphylactic shock or cardiac arrest, the physician slowly injected medication while the nurse stood on a chair and held the IV bottle to the ceiling to get maximum, safe IV push from gravity!

When the drug calls for the IV route

Knowing the correct route of administration is as important as giving the right medication to the right patient. Certain medications, such as insulin, can be given only by the parenteral route because stomach acids destroy them if taken by the oral route. Other medications, such as chemotherapy, can't be administered intramuscularly because they cause severe tissue damage. Anesthetic medications, such as propofol, and paralytic agents, such as succinylcholine, must be administered intravenously to maintain control of the drugs' intensity and duration.

The following medications and products must be given exclusively by IV administration:

- ✔ Blood transfusions (see Chapters 5 and 15)
- ✔ Blood-based products, such as plasma, blood factors, and artificial blood substitutes (see Chapters 5 and 15)
- ✔ Caustic medications, such as norepinephrine bitartrate (Levophed)
- ✔ Parenteral nutrition (see Chapters 8 and 18)

Becoming more familiar with the various agents administered in IV therapy helps you prevent medication errors by determining and using the safest route of administration.

Administering chemotherapy and caustic medications requires frequent monitoring of the IV site because these medications can cause extreme tissue damage if the IV becomes infiltrated. If the patient complains of pain or you note any redness or swelling at the infusion site, stop the medication immediately and report your findings to the physician. Because of the extreme complications caused by chemotherapy agents, infusion through a central vascular access device (CVAD) is recommended (see Chapters 6 and 16 for more on chemotherapy).

Understanding Adverse Effects

More than half of the most serious, life-threatening adverse drug events are related to IV administration, and the vast majority are caused by medication error. The most common medication errors include

- ✔ Missed or omitted dosing, particularly with insulin
- ✔ Too many or too frequent dosings, particularly with insulin
- ✔ Wrong interpretation of prescription

✔ Miscalculations in medication preparation

✔ Infusion-pump programming errors

✔ Wrong medication or route of administration

✔ Wrong patient

The risk for IV medication errors is so high that hospitals and infusion centers have adopted stringent guidelines requiring nurses to confer with other team members when calculating dosages and programming infusion pumps. To prevent distractions to nurses preparing medications, hospital medication rooms are off-limits to anyone other than authorized personnel.

Other efforts to decrease IV medication errors include the following:

✔ Hospitals have stepped up their morbidity and mortality committee meetings to review medication errors and develop prevention protocols.

✔ Nursing instructors are required to increase supervision of IVs administered by student nurses.

✔ IV manufacturers have begun creating distinctive packaging and labeling to help medical personnel distinguish between similar infusion products.

✔ Medical equipment manufacturers are working feverishly to produce smarter infusion pumps to identify, alarm, and shut down when human programming errors are suspected.

To prevent some of the most common IV medication errors, the Institute for Safe Medication Practices issued a high-alert medication list of drugs that pose the greatest risk for error and patient complications. The drugs on that list include the following:

✔ Vasodilators, such as epinephrine and norepinephrine

✔ Diabetic agents, such as insulin

✔ Anticoagulants, such as heparin

✔ Chemotherapy agents, such as carboplatin and cisplatin

✔ Narcotics, such as morphine

✔ X-ray contrast material

✔ Anesthetics, such as propofol and ketamine

✔ Cardiac drugs, such as propranolol, metoprolol, and lidocaine

Although medication errors account for the majority of adverse complications, many other complications can result from IV administration. Here are some of the most common complications, along with their definitions and causes:

- **Phlebitis:** Inflammation of the vein, resulting from an IV that isn't secured correctly or a caustic drug

- **Infiltration:** Fluid flowing into the tissues instead of the vein, most commonly caused by damage to the vein during IV insertion, catheter movement that leads to vein erosion, or a thrombus that restricts blood flow

- **Embolism:** A clot forming around the catheter in the vein that breaks off and winds up in the lungs

- **Air embolism:** A bolus of air that acts the same as a dislodged clot

- **Fluid overload:** The infusion of too much fluid over a short or long period of time, sometimes resulting in pulmonary edema or congestive heart failure

Even though infiltration, infection, and embolism can occur with IV therapy, medication error remains the most common cause of severe, adverse complications, which explains why more and more attention is directed toward error prevention. Technology may play a significant role in prevention by eliminating some of the common causes of errors, such as illegible handwritten prescriptions and math errors in calculating dosages. Following are some of the recent technology advances in the war on medication errors:

- Computerized physician order entry (CPOE)

- Electronic medication dispensers with bar code and radio frequency technology

- Online medication administration records

- Smart infusion pumps that recognize and report suspected errors

- Wireless technology enabling nurses to monitor IV pumps anywhere in the hospital

Technology, along with strict adherence to safety guidelines, can help reduce IV complications and make the healthcare environment a safer place for all patients.

Identifying Drug Incompatibilities

Knowing how to identify and prevent drug incompatibilities is a key component in providing safe, effective IV therapy to your patients.

Pharmaceutical references identify more than 600 different IV drugs and solutions, with more than 50,000 possible combinations. When you factor in complex drug prescriptions, called *admixtures,* and multiple types of IV lines, the potential for drug incompatibility is staggering.

More than 90 percent of all hospitalized patients receive IVs, and most of the IV fluids are administered by infusion pumps. Many of these pumps have internal drug listings and can calculate dosages and titrations automatically. The user only has to add parameters, and the pump does everything else.

However, medications aren't the only things that cause incompatibilities; IV fluids and diluents complicate the incompatibility picture because they frequently contain dextrose, sodium, vitamins, or electrolytes.

When you administer an IV medication, the simplest way to avoid drug interaction is to administer only one drug at a time. With today's IV pumps and complicated admixtures, however, avoiding infusing multiple drugs through multiple lines, particularly in critical care, is impossible.

Therefore, recognizing the visible *physical* signs and the subtle *chemical* signs of drug incompatibility is the first step in decreasing a patient's risk for adverse reaction caused by incompatibility. You can identify the following physical signs during drug preparation or administration:

✔ Change in color in the IV bag or tubing

✔ Development of haze or cloudiness caused by incompatible drugs

✔ Creation of gas or bubbles

✔ Difficulty in mixing

✔ Formation of solid particles, known as precipitates, which may cause embolus

If any of these signs appear during admixture preparation, don't administer the admixture and notify your pharmacy and supervisor immediately. If any of these signs appear during IV administration, discontinue the administration and notify your supervisor right away. Follow up to ensure that the patient receives orders for replacement meds, confirmed as compatible by the pharmacy, and follow standard guidelines to document the incident.

Chemical and biochemical signs are more difficult to identify and pose greater risk for your patient. Chemical and biochemical incompatibilities are frequently associated with the complex acid-base relationship in the patient's body and in the drug's composition.

To maintain acid-base or pH balance, the body is constantly moving electrolytes and chemicals within the cells (see Chapter 7 for more info). This constant movement is designed to keep the body in perfect biochemical balance, which is measured as pH 7.4. A measurement above 7.4 is alkaline or basic, and a measurement below 7.4 is acidic.

When disease or trauma disturbs the delicate pH balance of the body, causing the body chemistry to become too basic or too acidic, a number of potential drug incompatibilities can result, including the following:

- Decreasing or canceling drug effectiveness
- Diminishing drug half-life or duration
- Degrading drug composition
- Increasing drug potency

Drugs also have a delicate pH balance that must be maintained to prevent incompatibilities. Following the manufacturer's directions for dilution and storage is the best and safest practice for preserving a drug's pH balance. Use the following guidelines to ensure a medication's optimum effectiveness:

- Store in light or dark areas as directed by the manufacturer.
- Store in cool, warm, or refrigerated areas as directed by the manufacturer.
- Reconstitute with the correct type and amount of diluent.

Here are some additional tips for preventing incompatibilities:

- Use correct flushing solutions between multiple drug administrations.
- Check for compatibility with additives already in the IV bag or pump.
- Identify which meds are approved for intermittent piggyback infusion.
- Double-check compatibility of all piggyback meds.

Recognizing the drugs most commonly associated with incompatibilities is another line of defense in prevention. Some of the most frequent offenders are

- ✔ Diazepam (Valium)
- ✔ Furosemide (Lasix)
- ✔ Heparin
- ✔ Midazolam (Versed)
- ✔ Phenytoin (Dilantin)

Knowing which medications are compatible and can be given safely with other medications and which medications are incompatible and should never be given together is essential in pharmacological IV therapy. Being able to determine these differences is particularly important in critical care because so many different drugs are given through Y-site connectors on infusion sets. When patients are receiving multiple medications through multiple IV lumens, recognizing drug incompatibility is imperative.

To help healthcare workers identify drug incompatibilities and minimize the risk for adverse effects, pharmaceutical manufacturers provide easy-to-use IV medication compatibility charts. These handy reference guides compare frequently used medications and identify their high, medium, or low risk for compatibility or incompatibility. Busy healthcare workers use these charts for a quick, at-a-glance reference to help prevent incompatibility errors. Check out the sample chart in Table 4-1.

Use IV medication compatibility charts as learning tools for educational purposes only. Before administering any medication of questionable compatibility, check the current drug guide or call the pharmacist for the most current information on dosages and interactions. IV medication therapy is a constantly evolving process and new medications enter the healthcare arena every day. Compatibility charts are helpful reference guides, but they become quickly outdated in the competitive world of pharmaceuticals and should never be used as a stand-alone reference.

Table 4-1			Sample IV Medication Compatibility Chart					
	Albumin	**Atro-pine**	**Epinephrine (Adrenalin)**	**Diltiazem (Cardizem)**	**Phenytoin (Dilantin)**	**Dopa-mine**	**Fentanyl**	**Heparin**
Albumin	/			Y				
Atropine		/	Y		N	Y	Y	N
Epinephrine (Adrenalin)		Y	/	Y	N	Y	Y	Y
Diltiazem (Cardizem)	Y		Y	/	N	Y	Y	!
Phenytoin (Dilantin)		N	!	N	/	N	N	N
Dopamine		Y	Y	Y	N	/	Y	Y
Fentanyl		Y	Y	Y	N	Y	/	Y
Heparin		Y	Y	!	N	Y	Y	!
Insulin		Y	!	!	N	Y	Y	Y
Isoproterenol (Isuprel)		Y	Y	Y	N	Y	Y	Y
Furosemide (Lasix)		Y	Y	N	N	!	Y	Y
Lidocaine		Y	Y	Y	N	Y	Y	Y
Morphine		Y	Y	Y	N	Y	Y	Y
Potassium		Y	Y	!	N	Y	Y	Y
Procainamide (Pronestyl)		Y	Y	Y	N	Y	Y	Y
Verapamil		Y	Y	Y	N	Y	Y	Y

Y = physically compatible; N = not physically compatible; ! = caution, variable results; Blank — no information; / = same drug

Insulin	Isoproterenol (Isuprel)	Furosemide (Lasix)	Lidocaine	Morphine	Potassium	Procainamide (Pronestyl)	Verapamil
							N
Y	Y	Y	Y	Y	Y	Y	Y
!	Y	Y	Y	Y	Y	Y	Y
!	Y	N	Y	Y	!	Y	Y
N		N	N	N	N	N	N
!	Y	!	Y	Y	Y	Y	Y
Y	Y	Y	Y	Y	Y	Y	Y
Y	Y	Y	Y	Y	Y	Y	Y
/	N	Y	Y	!	Y	Y	Y
N	/	!	Y	Y	Y	Y	Y
Y	!	/	Y	Y	Y	Y	N
Y	Y	Y	/	Y	Y	Y	Y
!	Y	!	Y	/	Y	Y	Y
Y	Y	Y	Y	Y	/	Y	Y
Y	Y	Y	Y	Y	Y	/	Y
Y	Y	N	Y	Y	Y	Y	/

Original chart courtesy of IV Medication; `http://ivmedicationcompatibilitychart.com`*;*
October 26, 2011

Reconstituting IV Therapy Medications

IV medications frequently come from the manufacturer as dry medications, such as powders or crystals, because the dry medication is more stable and has a longer shelf life. Dry medications, however, must be reconstituted or dissolved into sterile liquids before they can be administered intravenously. Nurses and infusion specialists face the task of reconstituting medications, particularly when the hospital or facility has no pharmacy. We explore the ins and outs of reconstituting medications in the following sections.

IV medications aren't the only drugs that require reconstitution: Intramuscular, subcutaneous, and epidural drugs also come in powder form and must be reconstituted for use. To avoid mix-ups, labeling and separating the various types of reconstituted drugs is essential.

Understanding the basics

Figuring out how to reconstitute medications requires a few basic math skills to calculate dilution and dosage and a familiarity with the pharmaceutical's packaging of powder medications. The most common packaging is the single-dose or multi-dose rubber-capped vial. The single-dose package is a small, one-use-only vial, and the multi-dose vial enables the nurse to prepare several doses of medication at one time.

Reconstituting medications requires knowledge of the following key pharmaceutical terms:

- ✓ **Reconstitution:** Dissolving drug powder with liquid or diluent, as directed by a prescription, thus restoring it to an IV-compatible medication

- ✓ **Diluent:** Liquid added to a drug powder to dissolve it and prepare it for IV administration; usually 0.9 percent normal saline or bacteriostatic sterile water

- ✓ **Concentration:** Strength of a drug powder when it's dissolved in a known amount of fluid, reflecting the strength of each dose

- ✓ **Shelf life:** Length of time a medication can be safely stored and administered before it expires

Working with single-strength medications

Single-strength medications are the easiest to work with because they contain only one medication and they have the directions for dilution prominently displayed on the medication label. Single-strength medication labels typically provide the following information:

✔ Name of medication (brand or generic)

✔ Quantity of medication

✔ Concentration of the unit dose and the commonly prescribed dose

✔ Name of correct diluent and directions for reconstitution

✔ Storage temperatures and expiration date

✔ Name of pharmaceutical manufacturer

✔ Blank space for writing date of reconstitution

Working with multi-strength medications

Unlike the ease of working with single-strength medications, multi-strength medications require a little more math and decision making.

Multi-strength medications are meds that have multiple instructions for reconstituting different dosages, requiring the nurse to select the appropriate dosage and calculate the correct dilution to achieve that dosage. Although medication labels are helpful, they can't contain all the information necessary to select correct dosages. With complicated reconstitution instructions, you need to refer to the package insert, pharmacist, or physician to help ensure correct dilution and dosaging.

Storing leftovers

Reconstituted medications have a finite shelf life and must be stored according to manufacturer's recommendations to maintain optimum safety and effectiveness. Although most reconstituted medications require storage in a dry, dark area, some require refrigerated storage. Refer to the medication label or package insert for details on the shelf life and optimum refrigeration temperatures to ensure proper storage.

Practicing dosage calculations

Practice makes perfect, so use the ratio-proportion method to practice your problem-solving skills with the following practice problems (see Chapter 10 for more on the ratio-proportion method):

Sample single-strength medication problem

You're asked to administer 250 milligrams (mg) of amoxicillin from a 500-mg vial of amoxicillin powder, using the recommended diluent volume of 10 milliliters (mL). How many mL do you administer to achieve a dosage of 250 mg? Use the ratio-proportion method to solve this problem.

1. **Set up the following ratio-proportion:**

$$\frac{\text{Known equivalent of drug}}{\text{Known equivalent of diluent}} = \frac{\text{Known equivalent of prescription}}{\text{Desired equivalent}}$$

$$\frac{500 \text{ mg}}{10 \text{ mL}} = \frac{250 \text{ mg}}{x \text{ mL}}$$

2. **Cross-multiply.**

   $2,500 = 500x$

3. **Divide and solve.**

   $2,500 \div 500 = 5$ mL

   The mg cancel out, so you're left with mL.

You administer 5 mL to achieve a dosage of 250 mg.

Sample single-strength medication problem

You're asked to administer 80 mg of tobramycin from a 1.2-gram (g) vial of powder, using the recommended diluent volume of 30 mL. Convert the g to mg by multiplying the number of g by 1,000. Then use the same ratio-proportion method you use in the preceding example to calculate the dosage. (Gram conversion: 1 g = 1,000 mg; 1.2 g × 1,000 = 1,200 mg.)

1. **Set up the following ratio-proportion:**

$$\frac{1,200 \text{ mg}}{30 \text{ mL}} = \frac{80 \text{ mg}}{x \text{ mL}}$$

2. **Cross-multiply.**

   $2,400 = 1,200x$

3. **Divide and solve.**

   $2,400 \div 1,200 = 2$ mL

   The mg cancel out, so you're left with mL.

You administer 2 mL to achieve a dosage of 80 mg.

Sample multi-strength medication problem

You're asked to administer 20 mg IV of pantoprazole (Protonix) powder twice a day. Pantoprazole comes in a 40-mg vial and is a multi-strength med. According to the package insert, you reconstitute the med for both 2-minute and 15-minute infusions. For a 2-minute infusion, reconstitute 40 mg of pantoprazole with 10 mL of 0.9 percent saline (NS) to achieve a final concentration of 4 mg/mL. For a 15-minute infusion, dilute the medication by combining it with 100 mg of 0.9 percent NS to get a concentration of 0.4 mg/mL. How many mL do you administer for a 2-minute infusion and how many mL for a 15-minute infusion?

To calculate the mL needed for a 2-minute infusion, use the ratio-proportion method and follow these steps:

1. **Set up the following ratio-proportion:**

   $$\frac{4\ mg}{1\ mL} = \frac{20\ mg}{x\ mL}$$

2. **Cross-multiply.**

   $20 = 4x$

3. **Divide and solve.**

   $20 \div 4 = 5\ mL$

   The mg cancel out, so you're left with mL.

You administer 5 mL over 2 minutes.

To calculate the mL needed for a 15-minute infusion, use the same ratio-proportion method and follow these steps:

1. **Set up the following ratio-proportion:**

   $$\frac{0.4\ mg}{1\ mL} = \frac{20\ mg}{x\ mL}$$

2. **Cross-multiply.**

   $20 = 0.4x$

3. **Divide and solve.**

   $20 \div 0.4 = 50\ mL$

   The mg cancel out, so you're left with mL.

You administer 50 mL over 15 minutes.

Practicing for perfection

Most of the math involved in reconstituting medications is simple computational addition and division. However, some prescription situations demand a higher math skill level, including working with fractions and ratios. Referring to dosage calculation charts and online or offline dosage conversion tables proves invaluable in achieving the correct dilution and dosage.

Other helpful references are infusion textbooks. Most have practice problems like the examples in the nearby sidebar that walk you through various complicated reconstitution scenarios and provide the correct answers.

Practicing textbook sample problems will help improve your math skills and give you confidence in preparing correct dosages. (Check out Chapter 10 for details on calculating dosages and flow rates for IV therapy.)

 If you're uncertain about reconstituting highly complex drug admixtures, even after studying the drug label and accompanying information, never hesitate to consult with a knowledgeable colleague, pharmacist, or physician to ensure accurate dilution and dosing.

Familiarizing Yourself with Common Classes of Pharmacological Agents

Pharmacological agents are biologically active substances that produce a therapeutic response in the body. Knowing how to identify the various classes of pharmacologic agents helps you understand why certain classes of medications are routinely selected to treat certain clinical conditions. Some of the most common classes include

- **Antibiotics:** Medications such as penicillin and erythromycin that inhibit or destroy bacterial organisms.
- **Antifungals:** Medications such as amphotericin B that inhibit or destroy fungi.
- **Antivirals:** Medications such as acyclovir that inhibit the replication process of viral organisms.
- **Cardiovascular agents:** Medications such as digoxin that are used to affect heart rate, contraction, and rhythm.

✔ **Central nervous system (CNS) agents:** Medications such as diazepam (Valium) that impact brain activity by depressing it and meds such as caffeine that impact brain activity by stimulating it. CNS agents, such as phenytoin (Dilantin), are used to treat seizures, and antipsychotic meds, such as chlorpromazine (Thorazine), are used to treat mental illness.

✔ **Electrolyte and water-balancing agents:** Medications such as furosemide (Lasix) that are used to correct fluid imbalance, and electrolytes such as sodium, potassium, and chloride that are used to correct electrolyte imbalance.

✔ **Gastrointestinal (GI) agents:** Medications such as proton pump inhibitors (PPIs) that decrease gastric acid production and medications such as antiemetics that reduce nausea and vomiting.

✔ **Hematological agents:** Medications that act on blood and blood-forming organs. Hematological medication categories include anticoagulants such as heparin.

✔ **Hormones and synthetic substances:** Medications such as insulin that regulate the body's endocrine system and metabolism. An example of a synthetic hormone is levothyroxine (Synthroid), which is used to replace the natural thyroid hormone.

✔ **Respiratory agents:** Medications such as terbutaline and aminophylline that aid breathing by dilating bronchial tubes.

✔ **Vitamins and iron:** Vitamins are naturally occurring and synthetic nutritional substances essential for proper bone, muscle, and organ development in the body. Iron is an essential mineral that reverses anemia and supports oxygen transport to organs and tissues.

Chapter 5

Beefing Up on Blood Component Therapy Basics

In This Chapter

▶ Discovering the ins and outs of blood component therapy

▶ Understanding the stuff blood is made of

▶ Determining what blood is compatible with which patient

▶ Comparing the types of blood component therapies

*B*ritish obstetrician James Blundell performed the first successful human blood transfusion in 1818 to treat postpartum hemorrhage. Since that time, blood component therapy (the use of blood transfusions) has achieved a level of advancement far beyond what the pioneers of early transfusions could have ever imagined. More importantly, blood component therapy has come to know remarkable success as a means to save lives.

Unfortunately, some people who work in healthcare have come to take blood component therapy a bit too lightly — perhaps because the procedure isn't all that difficult to perform or because the process usually goes off without a hitch. Whatever the reasons for this mind-set, you need to look past them and approach blood component therapy with anything but complacency. After all, it's one of the most important tasks you'll ever have in healthcare.

In this chapter, we provide the basic principles of blood component therapy that you need to understand *before* you give a blood transfusion. We break down blood components into easy-to-understand parts. We tell you about the different types of blood transfusions and the role that blood compatibility plays in the transfusion process. We discuss ABO, Rh, and HLA blood groupings and explain why they're important for you to know. Finally, we explain the various types of blood components used during a transfusion, giving you a clear picture of which ones to use when. To find out how to administer blood component therapy, turn to Chapter 15.

Defining Blood Component Therapy

Blood component therapy (commonly referred to as a *blood transfusion*) is a method of introducing whole blood or blood products directly into your patient's bloodstream. You can administer blood component therapy through one of two access devices:

- **Peripheral vascular access device (VAD):** A catheter (small, flexible tube) placed into a peripheral vein of the hand, arm, or foot (or scalp for pediatric patients) to administer medication, fluids, or blood products.

- **Central vascular access device (CVAD):** A catheter placed into a large vein in the neck, chest, groin, or upper arm (or scalp or leg veins for pediatric patients). The tip of the central catheter should end in the central venous system, preferably the superior vena cava (SVC) or inferior vena cava (IVC).

We talk more about each of these devices in Chapter 3. In the following sections, we explain when you may need to administer blood component therapy and what risks you need to be aware of.

Knowing when blood component therapy is necessary

The circulatory system is the blood's primary mover and shaker. Not only does it carry blood filled with oxygen and nutrients to all the body's cells, but it also transports carbon dioxide, the waste product of metabolism, out of the cells so the body can excrete it.

When patients become ill or get injured, the circulatory system often suffers. When the circulatory system suffers, patients lose the following:

- Blood volume
- The oxygen-carrying capacity of the blood
- The capability for the blood to coagulate

Whatever the reason for a circulatory system compromise, patients who lose blood volume may be in serious danger unless they receive a blood transfusion.

Understanding the risks involved

Because blood now goes through a careful screening process before a patient receives it, the process of receiving a blood transfusion is safer than ever before. Nevertheless, complications from blood transfusions are still possible, and as a healthcare professional, you must be aware of them. Here are some of the most common complications related to blood component therapy:

✔ Immunologic complications, such as hemolysis, immune-mediated platelet destruction, febrile nonhemolytic reactions, allergic reactions, anaphylactic reactions, transfusion-related acute lung injury, and delayed hemolytic reactions

✔ Non-immunologic complications, such as transmission of infectious disease, bacterial contamination, circulatory overload, hypothermia, and metabolic complications

Every healthcare provider must discuss the benefits and risks associated with a blood transfusion with the patient prior to the administration of the transfusion. Patients must then sign a consent form, verifying that they're fully aware of the purpose, benefits, and risks involved with the procedure.

Every time you administer a transfusion, make sure the provider has discussed the risks and benefits with the patient and answered any questions *before* the patient signs the consent.

Breaking Down Blood Composition

Before you administer blood products to any patient, you need to understand the basic composition of blood so you know what you're giving and why. Blood is an extraordinary body fluid composed of cellular elements (that is, red blood cells, white blood cells, and platelets) suspended in blood plasma. About 45 percent of the blood's volume consists of these cellular elements, and each element has a specific purpose:

✔ **Red blood cells:** The most abundant cells in the blood are the *erythrocytes,* or red blood cells. Erythrocytes contain *hemoglobin,* an iron-rich protein that facilitates the movement of oxygen through the bloodstream.

✔ **White blood cells:** *Leukocytes,* or white blood cells, are cells of the immune system that fight infection. Leukocytes are divided into two subgroups and are present in the blood and the lymphatic system:

• *Granulocytes* have granules in their cytoplasm and include eosinophils, basophils, and neutrophils.

• *Agranulocytes,* which are granule-free, include monocytes and lymphocytes.

✔ **Platelets:** *Thrombocytes,* better known as platelets, are responsible for the blood's ability to coagulate. If blood were unable to coagulate, you could bleed to death from a relatively minor injury.

The remaining 55 percent of your blood's volume is made up of *plasma*, the liquid part of the blood. Plasma is mostly water, but it's also rich with plasma proteins like albumin, globulin, and fibrinogen and other elements, such as:

- Glucose
- Electrolytes
- Vitamins and minerals
- Lipids
- Carbohydrates
- Gases (carbon dioxide and oxygen)

Figure 5-1 shows the different components of the blood.

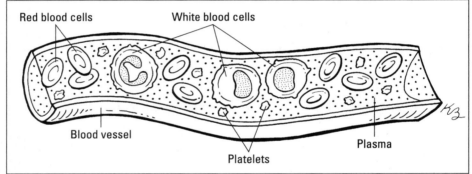

Figure 5-1: Blood composition.

Illustration by Kathryn Born

Finding a Match: Compatibility Is Key

Compatibility is important with any kind of relationship, but it's particularly important when donor blood meets recipient blood. Before a patient can receive a blood transfusion, both the donor's blood and the recipient's blood must undergo a screening process to make sure they're compatible. If a patient receives blood from a donor that isn't compatible with the patient's blood, serious, adverse reactions may result in fatal consequences for the patient.

Donor plus recipient: A match made in heaven

Before your patient receives a blood transfusion, the following screening tests must take place to determine whether or not donor and recipient blood are compatible:

✔ **ABO and Rh blood typing:** This test tells the blood bank which ABO blood group your patient belongs to and whether he's Rh-positive or Rh-negative (see the next section for details on these blood types).

✔ **Cross-matching:** This test is performed after blood typing to find donor blood that's compatible with recipient blood.

✔ **Antibody screening:** This test screens for the presence of unexpected antibodies that may be clinically important (refer to the next section for details on antibodies).

✔ **Screening for transmissible diseases:** This test screens the donor's blood for such diseases as Hepatitis B, Hepatitis C, and HIV/AIDS.

When you assume care of a new patient, you may need to get an order for a *type and screen.* This lab test identifies the patient's ABO and Rh blood grouping *without* cross-matching donor blood, a step that's necessary only if the patient requires a transfusion. If you type and screen the patient's blood when he's admitted to the hospital, then his blood type will already be known in case he eventually needs blood products.

Identifying antigens and antibodies in the blood

Blood cells have substances called *antigens* (or *agglutinogens*) that rest on their surfaces. Your body recognizes many substances as antigens, including bacteria, viruses, and allergens. Antigens are capable of stimulating the production of *antibodies* (also known as *immunoglobulins*). Antibodies are special proteins created by the immune system to help identify and then neutralize antigens. Antibodies are named after the antigens responsible for their formation and with which they react.

Some antigens are more commonly found in the blood than others. We explore the three antigen systems that are most important to blood component therapy in the following sections.

The ABO system

The most significant group of antigens is associated with red blood cells. This system, known as the *ABO system,* was the first set of antigens to be discovered more than a century ago.

The four blood types in the ABO system are named for their corresponding antigens:

✔ A

✔ B

✔ AB

✔ O

The ABO system also contains two antibodies — anti-A and anti-B — that occur naturally without any stimulation from an antigen. A person can have one, both, or neither of these antibodies present in his plasma.

When performing a transfusion, the recipient must not have antibodies to antigens in the blood product being transfused (in other words, antigens in the donor blood must be compatible with antigens in the recipient's blood). If antibodies are present and the patient receives mismatched blood, those antibodies in the patient's blood will instigate a transfusion reaction. We talk more about transfusion reactions in Chapter 15.

Table 5-1 shows the four ABO blood groups and their compatibilities. *Note:* When used in conjunction with blood types, the plus (+) and minus (–) signs refer to the presence or absence of *antigen D*, the most important antigen in the Rh system, which we discuss in detail in the next section.

Table 5-1	ABO Blood Compatibilities		
Blood Group	**Antibody in Plasma**	**Can Give Blood To**	**Can Receive Blood From**
A	Anti-B	A, AB	A, O
B	Anti-A	B, AB	B, O
AB	Neither	AB	A, B, AB, O
O	Both	A, B, AB, O	O

People with type O– blood are considered *universal donors.* Because O– lacks A and B antigens, you can give it (in limited amounts) to patients from any blood group in emergency situations with little risk of complications. People who are AB+ are considered *universal recipients.* Because neither A nor B antibodies are present in the plasma of people with AB+ blood, a patient with this blood type may receive blood from any other blood group.

The Rh system

The second most important antigen system is the *Rhesus* or *Rh* system. Named after the Rhesus monkey in which the substance was first discovered, the Rh system consists of two groups:

✔ Rh-positive

✔ Rh-negative

As we mention in the previous section, the terms *Rh-positive* (+) and *Rh-negative* (−) refer to the presence or absence of *antigen D,* the most important antigen in the Rh system. Although a small percentage of the population has Rh-negative blood, most people are Rh-positive. A person who has Rh-positive blood may receive blood from both Rh-positive and Rh-negative donors, but a person who is Rh-negative can receive blood only from an Rh-negative donor.

Whether a patient is Rh-positive or Rh-negative is particularly important during pregnancy. If a pregnant mom is Rh-negative but the father is Rh-positive, the fetus can inherit the Rh factor from the father. If the fetus is Rh-positive and the mother is Rh-negative, the mom can develop antibodies as if she were allergic to her own baby. These antibodies can cross the placenta and attack the unborn child's red blood cells, possibly leading to serious illness, injury, or death of the fetus. To prevent this attack from happening, Rh-negative moms may require an injection of *Rh immunoglobulin,* a blood product that can prevent *sensitization* (antibody production) in an Rh-negative mother.

The HLA system

Human leukocyte antigens (HLA antigens, for short) exist on the surface of lymphocytes, granulocytes, monocytes, and platelets. Although they're best known for their role in the rejection of transplanted organs, HLA antigens also contribute to some basic transfusion complications, such as febrile nonhemolytic transfusion reaction (NHFTR), transfusion-related acute lung injury (TRALI), and immunological refractoriness to random platelet transfusions (we discuss blood transfusion complications in Chapter 15).

When antigens and antibodies go to war: The hemolytic hazards of a mismatch

When a patient receives blood that doesn't match his own blood, the antibodies and antigens in the two blood supplies pick up their swords and go to war. The only problem is neither of them wins. The most serious consequence related to a mismatch is the *hemolytic reaction,* a reaction that occurs when antibodies from mismatched donor blood stick to the surfaces of a recipient's red blood cells. This causes *hemolysis,* or the destruction of the red blood cells. Hemolysis damages the kidneys, leading to kidney failure. Chapter 15 talks about hemolytic reactions in greater detail.

Types of Blood Component Therapies

Transfused blood comes in two types, depending on where it originates:

- ✔ *Autologous* blood is derived from the recipient.
- ✔ *Homologous* blood is taken from a donor.

The best kind of blood transfusion is autologous because it reduces the risks normally associated with donor blood. In an emergency, though, autologous blood may not be readily available, in which case donor blood is your patient's only option.

Regardless of whether you infuse autologous or homologous blood, you can use either whole blood or individual blood components, depending on the particular situation.

The whole in every part: Whole blood versus individual blood components

Whole blood contains the whole enchilada: red blood cells, white blood cells, platelets, plasma, and all the vital nutrients that go along with that plasma. You may give a patient whole blood when she has lost a massive amount of blood (more than 25 percent of her blood volume) in a relatively short period of time. This loss could be a result of severe hemorrhage, trauma, or surgery.

Most patients don't receive whole blood and instead receive individual blood components derived from whole blood. These components include

- ✔ Packed red blood cells (PRBCs)
- ✔ Modified PRBCs
- ✔ Leukocyte-filtered RBCs
- ✔ Platelets
- ✔ Fresh frozen plasma (FFP)
- ✔ Cryoprecipitate
- ✔ Albumin and plasma protein fraction (PPF)
- ✔ Granulocytes

Table 5-2 shows you a quick comparison of blood and blood products, and the rest of this section explains each blood product in greater detail:

Table 5-2 **Guide to Blood and Blood Products**

Blood Component	Indications	Compatibility	Considerations
Whole blood	To replace massive blood loss due to hemorrhage, trauma, or surgery	Must be ABO identical and Rh compatible (see the section "Finding a Match: Compatibility Is Key")	Use blood administration tubing. Use only with normal saline. Must use blood within 4 hours after it leaves blood bank. Monitor patient closely for complications and fluid volume overload. Use a blood warmer if giving large amounts.
Packed red blood cells (PRBCs)	To restore or maintain the oxygen-carrying capacity of the blood. To replace severe blood loss due to surgery. To correct symptomatic anemia in patients	Must be ABO compatible	Use blood administration tubing. Must use PRBCs within 4 hours after they leave blood bank. Use only with normal saline.
Leukocyte-filtered RBCs	Same indications as PRBCs, plus the following: To prevent febrile nonhemolytic transfusion reactions. To treat the patient who is immunocompromised	Same as PRBCs	Use blood administration tubing. Use a special filter if necessary. Must use RBCs within 4 hours after they leave blood bank. Use only with normal saline.

(continued)

Table 5-2 (continued)

Blood Component	Indications	Compatibility	Considerations
Platelets	To treat bleeding due to low platelet count or abnormally functioning platelets	Must be ABO identical	Must use a special filter.
		Rh-negative recipient must have Rh-negative donor	Must use platelets within 4 hours after they leave blood bank.
	To improve presurgical platelet count		Pre-medicate patient with *anti-pyretics* (fever-reducer) and antihistamines if ordered by healthcare provider.
			If repeated transfusions are required, use single-donor platelets.
Fresh frozen plasma (FFP)	To reverse anticoagulant effects of warfarin (Coumadin)	Must be ABO compatible	Use as soon as possible after thawing.
		Rh compatibility not required	Use blood tubing and administer rapidly.
	To provide clotting factors for patients with clotting disorders or liver disease		
	To treat some forms of hereditary angioedema		

Blood Component	Indications	Compatibility	Considerations
Granulocytes	To treat patients who are infection resistant or unresponsive to antibiotics To treat patients with neutropenia	Must be ABO compatible Must be Rh compatible	Administer over 2–4 hours with blood tubing and standard blood filter. Monitor closely as adverse effects are common. Pre-medicate patient with anti-pyretics and antihistamines if ordered by healthcare provider.
Albumin	To replace blood volume lost due to shock caused by burns, trauma, or surgery To restore volume in patients undergoing high-volume paracentesis (the most common use)	ABO and Rh compatibility not required	Use specialty administration set as provided by the manufacturer. Use with caution in patients with heart failure and lung disease because of the possibility of fluid volume overload.
Cryoprecipitate	To treat factor VIII deficiency and fibrinogen disorders To treat factor XIII deficiency	Must be ABO compatible Rh compatibility not required	Administer with blood tubing and administration set. Administer within 6 hours of thawing. Confirm diagnosis of specific clotting factor deficiency before infusion.

Blood and blood products *must only* be administered with normal saline (0.9 percent sodium chloride). See Chapter 15 for details.

Sending them packing: Packed red blood cells

Packed red blood cells (PRBCs) contain red blood cells from which most of the plasma has been removed. You may use PRBCs to

- ✔ Replace severe blood loss
- ✔ Improve the oxygen-carrying capacity of blood in patients who have symptomatic anemia unresponsive to medication

Cleaning up their act: Modified packed red blood cells

Modified packed red blood cells are prewashed in normal saline to remove platelets, cellular debris, most of the plasma, and some of the leukocytes. You use modified PRBCs in

- ✔ Patients who have had recurrent or severe allergic reactions to previous blood transfusions
- ✔ Neonates
- ✔ Mothers who need transfusions *in-utero* (while the fetus is still in the womb)

Skipping the leukocytes: Leukocyte-reduced packed cells

Some patients react negatively to blood transfusions that contain leukocytes; as a result, the blood bank must remove them or filter them out of some of the blood they collect. The blood bank prepares *leukocyte-reduced packed cells* through a process involving centrifugation or filtration or by washing the cells with a special solution.

Leukocyte-filtered red blood cells are used primarily when your patient has had a *nonhemolytic transfusion reaction* (a transfusion reaction that isn't associated with hemolysis) that involves a fever, a common type of transfusion reaction. When the blood doesn't contain any leukocytes, the patient has a better chance of tolerating a blood transfusion without any adverse effects.

Pass the platelets, please

Platelets, which are made in the bone marrow, allow your blood to coagulate. If your patient's platelet count is low, excessive bleeding can occur because the blood has difficulty clotting. On the other hand, if the platelet count is too high, the blood can become too thick and plug the blood vessels.

You may need to do a transfusion of platelets in the following cases:

✔ When your patient has excessive bleeding associated with a decreased platelet count or abnormally functioning platelets

✔ To increase the platelet count before surgery

Keeping it fresh: Fresh frozen plasma

Fresh frozen plasma (FFP) is plasma that has been removed from whole blood and then frozen. After FFP is frozen, the blood bank can store it for up to one year. FFP is rich with clotting factors, so you can use it when platelet concentrations aren't readily available.

You may need to use FFP in patients who

✔ Have coagulation disorders secondary to severe liver disease

✔ Have *disseminated intravascular coagulation* (a bleeding disorder, commonly referred to as DIC)

✔ Have *dilutional coagulopathy* (a condition that occurs when fluids are replaced in large amounts)

✔ Have been hypo-coagulated because of warfarin (Coumadin) therapy and the effects need to be reversed

✔ Are experiencing a hereditary form of angioedema

Cryoprecipitate

Cryoprecipitate, also referred to as *cryoprecipitated antihemophilic factor,* is a frozen blood product made from FFP. Like FFP, cryoprecipitate can be frozen and stored for up to one year.

You may use cryoprecipitate when a patient has one of the following conditions:

- ✔ Hemophilia
- ✔ Von Willebrand disease
- ✔ Fibrinogen deficiency
- ✔ Factor XIII deficiency
- ✔ DIC

Albumin and plasma protein fraction

Albumin and *plasma protein fraction* (PPF) are blood products derived from human plasma. In fact, they're two of the most abundant elements in the plasma.

Albumin, as we discuss in detail in Chapter 7, comes in two strengths — 5 percent, which is isotonic, and 25 percent, which is hypertonic. Both are indicated for hypovolemic shock.

PPF is an isotonic solution that's made up of albumin and two other types of plasma proteins. You use it in the emergency treatment of shock or other conditions in which a circulatory fluid volume deficit exists.

Adding granules with granulocytes

Granulocytes are white blood cells with granules in their cytoplasm. The granulocytes, along with the lymphocytes, platelets, and red blood cells, are contained in a suspension of anticoagulant and plasma. Donor granulocytes must be ABO and Rh compatible with the recipient. Granulocytes are rarely given, but you may administer granulocytes when your patient has

- ✔ A fever that's unresponsive to antibiotics
- ✔ A life-threatening infection, like *septicemia,* that's resistant to antibiotics
- ✔ *Neutropenia* (an abnormally low number of neutrophils)
- ✔ *Myeloid hypoplasia* (decreased granulocyte production)

Chapter 6

Chemotherapy 101

*F*acing chemotherapy for the first time is a frightening prospect for cancer patients and their families. Most patients have heard of the devastating side effects of chemotherapy and fear the treatment as much as the cancer itself. This chapter helps you understand the basics of chemotherapy and the goals of treatment so that you can help direct your patients through the scary and sometimes isolated journey of cancer treatment.

Here, you enter the microscopic cellular world to see how normal cells rest, grow, and multiply in regular cycles so you can compare that process to how cancer cells never rest and never stop multiplying. You also get a rundown of the different types of chemotherapy, most of which you administer intravenously, and find out how it attacks cancer cells when they're most vulnerable. Finally, you get a quick overview of the main classifications of chemotherapy drugs so that you know what to expect in terms of treatment and side effects when you're administering intravenous (IV) therapy to cancer patients.

Getting with the Program: The Principles of Chemotherapy

Scientists accidentally discovered chemotherapy in the 1940s during World War II when they were working with the chemical weapon mustard gas. Physicians began using derivatives of mustard gas in medicine and found that therapeutic doses shrank malignant tumors and slowed the growth of cancer.

Over the years, chemotherapy evolved into a multi-million-dollar pharmaceutical industry. Today, more than half of all cancer patients receive chemotherapy of some type, and it has become an indispensable weapon in the fight against cancer.

Although chemotherapy is associated with many risks, it has greatly improved over the past seven decades and is still considered a frontline defense against cancer. Used alone and in combination with other treatments, chemotherapy is credited with saving thousands of lives every year.

Defining chemotherapy

Chemotherapy is the systemic treatment of cancer with drugs, called *cytotoxins,* that kill rapidly dividing cells. Unfortunately, cytotoxic drugs can't tell the difference between rapidly dividing malignant cells and rapidly dividing normal cells like gastrointestinal cells and hair follicles. The killing of these normal cells along with the cancerous cells leads to common side effects, including nausea, vomiting, and hair loss. We discuss these and other debilitating side effects of chemotherapy later in the section "Considering the risks."

The most common route of administration for chemotherapy is intravenous, but you can also give it orally or by direct infusion into tumors, organs, or extremities. In most cases, chemotherapy consists of a combination of drugs administered in cycles over a period of weeks or months. Doctors use it in conjunction with surgery, radiation, and other cancer treatments.

Taking a closer look at cell cycles

Chemotherapy is designed to kill cancer cells at the most vulnerable phase of their cell cycle — when they're in the rapidly multiplying phase of cell division. Before you can understand how chemotherapy kills cancer at specific times during the cell's growth, you need to understand the activities and changes that take place during the cell cycle.

The five phases of the cell cycle

All cells have cycles during which they rest, grow, and reproduce to replace cells that are lost to injury or old age. The cell cycle is a series of five phases, beginning with the resting phase and ending with the *mitosis* or division phase, during which the cell actually divides and produces two identical

cells. Each cell then repeats the same process, known as *replication,* to reproduce new cells and replace old ones.

Proteins called *cyclins* are required to help cells move through the complete
cell cycle; they work by signaling the cells to either reproduce or stop reproducing. At different points in the cell cycle, critical control points called
checkpoints are set up, where cyclins transmit stop and go signals to regulate
the cycle. Three major checkpoints are found in the cell cycle (particularly in
the G1, G2, and M phases; see the list that follows for details) and are set up
to keep normal cells from mutating as cancer cells do.

Here's a quick look at the five phases of the cell cycle (shown in Figure 6-1):

- ✔ **G_0 phase:** The *G_0 phase* is the resting phase of the cycle; the cell has
  not yet started to divide. This phase is the longest in the cell cycle, and
  depending on the type of cell, it can last from a few hours to a few years.

- ✔ **G_1 phase:** During the *G_1 phase,* cyclins send a signal to the cell to reproduce, and the cell starts making proteins and growing. This phase is also
  known as the *growth phase* and lasts about 18 to 30 hours.

- ✔ **S phase:** During the *S phase,* cyclins activate chromosomes that contain
  the genetic code DNA used to create two new cells with identical DNA.
  This active phase lasts about 18 to 20 hours and is also known as the
  synthesis phase.

- ✔ **G_2 phase:** During the *G_2 phase,* cyclins signal the cell to check DNA and
  get ready to split into two new cells. This phase lasts between two and
  ten hours.

- ✔ **M phase:** The *M phase* or *mitosis* takes place when the cell actually
  divides into two new identical cells. This phase is also known as the *division phase* and lasts between 30 and 60 minutes.

If the cells are normal, the two new cells return to the resting phase after the
M phase or continue reproducing, depending on the signal they receive from
the cyclins.

In contrast, cancer cells continue to multiply because they never receive a
signal to stop. Cancer cells have a mutation in the gene that stimulates cell
cycles, leading to erratic, uncontrolled cell division that never allows the cell
to grow to maturity or stop multiplying. As a result, malignant cells continue
to divide and pile on top of each other, destroying healthy cells and forming
a tumor of malignant immature cancer cells — until an outside agent, such as
chemotherapy, disrupts cell division and halts tumor growth.

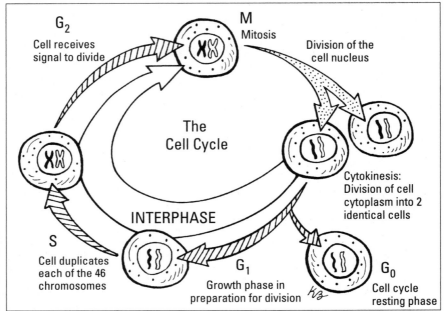

Figure 6-1:
Cell cycle division and replication.

Illustration by Kathryn Born

Chemotherapy: The drug that disrupts the cell cycle

Chemotherapy drugs are designed to take advantage of cell cycle phases by attacking cancer cells at specific, vulnerable phases of the cycle. Scientists divide these designer drugs into two categories based on their optimum killing power during cell cycle phases:

- ✔ **Cell-cycle-specific:** *Cell-cycle-specific drugs* target cancer cells during certain phases of the cell cycle, such as the S or M phase.

- ✔ **Cell-cycle-non-specific:** *Cell-cycle-non-specific drugs* target cancer cells at all phases of the cell cycle.

Targeting rapidly dividing cells with cell-cycle-specific drugs is desirable because these cells have the highest uptake of chemotherapy drugs, leading to maximum destruction of cancer cells. On the other hand, cell-cycle-nonspecific drugs offer greater flexibility because they can be effective at any phase of the cancer cell cycle.

Combining these two categories of chemotherapy drugs (through *combination chemotherapy*) is the best of both worlds, enabling *oncologists* (physicians who specialize in cancer treatment) to customize drug regimens that act both at specific phases and at all phases of the cell cycle. Combination chemotherapy attacks cancer by using different mechanisms of action during different cell phases: One drug may disrupt DNA at the S phase, while another interferes with protein synthesis at the G_1 phase. The overall goal of combination chemotherapy is not only to kill cancer cells but also to prevent them from mutating and becoming resistant to future treatment.

Although most cancer cells grow rapidly and uncontrollably, others grow slowly. For example, melanoma is a rapidly growing, aggressive skin cancer that must be treated immediately, whereas basal cell carcinoma is a skin cancer that grows slowly and may not even be detected for years. This difference in cancer cell growth explains why scientists design different types of chemotherapy agents to target different phases of the cell cycle. Each drug has its own unique method of action and is effective at a specific time during the cell cycle.

Slowing down cancer: How chemotherapy works in the body

Chemotherapy drugs kill cancer cells by stopping cell division and replication. Typically, chemotherapy works by changing or damaging cancer genes (RNA and DNA). RNA and DNA tell cancer cells how to duplicate. When chemotherapy damages these genes, the cells can't replicate, which slows cancer growth and shrinks tumor size.

Oncologists select chemotherapy drugs and customize drug regimens for each patient based on the following factors:

- Condition of the patient
- Presence of *metastasis,* or spread of cancer to other organs
- Rate at which cell division takes place
- Time of the drug's greatest effectiveness
- Type of cancer cell
- Stage of cancer

To take advantage of a drug's specific action, doctors design chemotherapy schedules to administer drugs in cycles, targeting periods of rapid cell division and cancer cell growth. A typical chemotherapy cycle can be one or more days, administered over a period of one to six weeks. Average treatment regimens consist of multiple cycles of administration given over a period of several weeks or months.

Because chemotherapy destroys healthy cells along with malignant cells, treatment schedules are usually spaced at intervals, allowing the patient to rest. Proper rest between treatments gives normal cells a chance to recover and lessens the severity of side effects.

Considering the risks

The risks of chemotherapy sometimes greatly overshadow the benefits. It is, after all, a systemic poison that can't differentiate between the good cells and the bad cells. Chemotherapy kills healthy cells with as much destructive force as it kills malignant cells, leading to moderate to severe side effects. Some of these side effects, from most common to least common, include

- Nausea, vomiting, diarrhea, and anorexia (weight loss)
- Fatigue and debilitation
- Hair loss
- Fevers
- Mouth sores
- Easy bruising
- Bone marrow depression
- Immune system suppression
- Delayed reactions and fuzzy thinking (also known as *chemo-brain*)

Body cells that normally experience rapid cell division are at the greatest risk and suffer the most destruction from chemotherapy. A few of the cells at greatest risk and the resulting clinical symptoms include

- **Gastrointestinal cells:** Damage to gastrointestinal cells causes the most common symptoms of nausea, vomiting, and diarrhea. Less common symptoms include mouth sores and loss of taste.
- **Scalp and hair follicles:** Damage to the scalp and hair follicles causes loss of scalp hair, eyebrows, eyelashes, and body hair.
- **Bone marrow:** Damage to bone marrow leads to bone marrow depression, which causes anemia, increased susceptibility to infection, and bleeding.

Chemotherapy protocols attempt to minimize the destructive effect on healthy cells while maximizing the destructive effect on malignant cells. Late-generation medications have really helped relieve severe symptoms, but much work is still needed to decrease the debilitating side effects of chemotherapy.

In addition to the side effects we list earlier in this section, chemotherapy also causes late-developing side effects that don't become apparent for months or even years after treatment. These late-developing side effects include

- **Damage to lung tissue:** Can lead to asthma, lung cancer, and other respiratory illnesses
- **Damage to cardiac tissue:** Can lead to cardiomyopathy, arrhythmias, and heart block
- **Damage to kidney tissue:** Can lead to nephrotoxicity and acute renal failure
- **Damage to reproductive tissue:** Can lead to infertility and birth defects
- **Damage to nerves:** Can lead to peripheral neuropathy
- **Damage to all tissues:** Can lead to risk for a second primary cancer

Scientists have long looked for a magic chemotherapy bullet that kills cancer cells without harming healthy cells. The search continues today, and many areas of current investigation are inspiring hope. A few of the most promising cancer-fighting agents include the following:

- **Kinase inhibitors:** Agents that interrupt the ability of cancer cells to stay together and form tumors
- **Apoptosis agents:** Agents that cause cancer cells to commit suicide and kill themselves
- **Targeted therapy agents:** Agents that are designed to target and disrupt specific molecules within a cancer cell

Although these new agents show promise of improved treatment outcomes and fewer side effects, standard chemotherapy drugs remain a central component in the treatment of cancer. Despite all of its risks and debilitating side effects, chemotherapy saves lives. You need to understand chemotherapy's vital role in the fight against cancer so you can help your patients weigh the risks and benefits of this life-extending therapy.

Determining the Goals of Treatment

Chemotherapy's primary treatment goal is to eliminate cancer, but doctors also use it to halt tumor growth, shrink tumor size, and eradicate cancer cells that *metastasize* (spread) to other parts of the body after primary treatment. Each type of chemotherapy has a particular goal.

To help you provide patients with a realistic concept of what to expect and what not to expect from their chemotherapy, you need to have a working knowledge of the basic types of chemotherapy. Here are the most common types:

- **Neoadjuvant chemotherapy:** Neoadjuvant chemotherapy is administered before surgery or radiation to help shrink the cancerous tumor to make surgery or radiation more effective and less extensive. (Check out the section "Controlling the spread" for more details on neoadjuvant chemotherapy.)

- **Adjuvant chemotherapy:** The goal of adjuvant chemotherapy is to destroy microscopic cells that may be present after the primary tumor is removed by surgery. It helps prevent a possible cancer recurrence. (See the section "Controlling the spread" for more details on this type of chemotherapy.)

- **Induction chemotherapy:** Induction chemotherapy is given in high doses in the initial treatment especially of advanced cancers in order to make subsequent treatment (surgery or radiotherapy) more effective. It's also administered to induce remission. This type of chemo is most commonly used in the treatment of acute leukemias. (See the section "Using chemo to cure" for details on remission.)

- **Consolidation chemotherapy:** Doctors order consolidation chemotherapy, also called _intensification therapy,_ when remission is achieved. The goal of this therapy is to sustain a remission, and it's commonly used in the treatment of acute leukemias.

- **Maintenance chemotherapy:** Maintenance chemotherapy is given in lower doses to assist in prolonging a remission. Maintenance chemotherapy is used only for certain types of cancer, most commonly acute leukemias.

- **First-line chemotherapy:** First-line chemotherapy has the best probability of effectively treating a certain cancer. First-line therapy, also known as _standard therapy,_ is considered the best treatment based on its effectiveness during clinical trials.

- **Second-line chemotherapy:** Doctors order second-line chemotherapy if a disease hasn't responded to treatment or has recurred after first-line chemotherapy. Second-line chemotherapy, sometimes referred to as _salvage therapy,_ has been tested in research studies and clinical trials and has been found to be effective in treating unresponsive or recurring cancers.

- **Palliative chemotherapy:** Palliative chemotherapy is given to relieve symptoms and provide pain management without expectations of significantly reducing the cancer.

Using chemo to cure

Chemotherapy is usually given in combination with surgery and radiation, but it's also effective in curing several different cancers on its own. Cancers such as leukemia and mesothelioma are frequently treated with stand-alone chemotherapy because they're so widespread that they can't be removed with surgery or blasted with radiation. In these cases, chemotherapy is given as a single-drug treatment or in combination with two or more chemo drugs.

Oncologists make their decision to use stand-alone chemotherapy based on the type and stage of cancer, plus the following factors:

- ✔ Metastasis (the spread of cancer to other organs)
- ✔ Chemotherapy drug effectiveness
- ✔ Dissemination (or spread) of cancer cells
- ✔ Inability to identify the primary source of cancer

As we mention earlier, the goal of chemotherapy is to cure the patient or to achieve a state of complete remission. _Complete remission_ is the disappearance of evidence of cancer after treatment with chemotherapy. Remember that remission doesn't always mean the patient is cured; it simply means the cancer is no longer detected on X-rays or lab tests. Remission becomes a cure when the cancer doesn't recur after a five-year period.

For millions of people, chemotherapy as a stand-alone treatment cures their cancer and extends their lives. For millions of others, chemotherapy combined with surgery or radiation enables them to enjoy full, productive lives.

Controlling the spread

When used in combination with surgery or radiation, chemotherapy is called _adjuvant_ or _additional therapy._ The goals of adjuvant therapy are to prevent recurrence, prevent resistance to future treatment, and eradicate the spread of cancer cells remaining in the body after primary treatment.

Adjuvant chemotherapy is the treatment of choice for metastasis — when disseminated cancer cells remain in the bloodstream or lymphatic system and spread to other parts of the body. Unfortunately, these disseminating cancer cells aren't easy to detect after resection or radiation of the primary tumor, and they're difficult to identify on routine tests, such as computerized tomography (CT) scans and magnetic resonance imaging (MRI). However, they can be identified on microscopic exams of the margins of the primary tumor or in the lymph nodes removed during surgery.

Without adjuvant chemotherapy, disseminated cancer cells continue to grow and can metastasize to other parts of the body. From the first site of metastasis to the last, the most common sites are

- Local structures adjacent to the primary tumor
- Lymph nodes, particularly those near the primary tumor
- Lungs
- Liver
- Brain
- Bones

To provide maximum effectiveness against metastasis, adjuvant chemotherapy typically begins three to five weeks after the surgical removal or radiation of the primary tumor. Length of treatment varies based on the type of cancer cell. Oncologists commonly use adjuvant chemotherapy for the following cancers:

- Breast cancer (especially when the patient has cancer cells in the lymph nodes removed during primary surgery, large tumors that indicate a high probability of metastasis, the presence of aggressive, high-grade tumor pathology, or tumors with negative hormone receptors)
- Colon cancer
- Lung cancer
- Lymphoma
- Ovarian cancer
- Pancreatic cancer
- Testicular cancer

Doctors sometimes use another form of adjuvant treatment, called *neoadjuvant chemotherapy,* before the primary treatment to shrink tumors and decrease the tumor load. By shrinking the tumor before surgery or radiation, neoadjuvant chemotherapy reduces the number and strength of remaining cancer cells and gives the primary treatment a better chance to eradicate the cancer.

Although adjuvant chemotherapy isn't guaranteed to prevent cancer from spreading or recurring, studies indicate that patients benefit significantly from it. In breast cancer patients, for example, adjuvant chemotherapy in women under 50 reduced their risk of recurrence by 35 percent, and it reduced the risk in women over 50 by 20 percent.

Still, accurately tracking the success of adjuvant chemotherapy is difficult, especially because treatment is sometimes administered in the absence of detectable amounts of cancer cells. The decision to undergo adjuvant chemotherapy, with its inherent risks and debilitating side effects, is a personal one that doctors have to discuss with their patients. But when you compare the downsides of adjuvant chemotherapy to the possibility of a longer life, most patients decide that the benefits outweigh the risks.

Providing comfort: The palliative side of chemotherapy

The main goal of _palliative chemotherapy_ is to relieve pain caused by the ever-increasing sizes of late-stage malignant tumors. However, some doctors also use it to extend life, even when there's no hope for cure or survival.

The use of palliative chemotherapy when a cure isn't possible is a controversial subject among physicians. To deal with the moral and ethical dilemmas associated with palliative therapy, many oncologists use a series of considerations to determine whether a patient should or shouldn't receive palliative chemotherapy. These considerations include

- ✔ **Response rate:** _Response rate_ is the rate at which the tumor improves with treatment by either shrinking or not growing.

- ✔ **Median duration of response:** _Median duration of response_ is the amount of time that doctors can expect cancer to respond to therapy before it starts growing again.

- ✔ **Side effects:** The number and severity of unwanted side effects that doctors can expect from treatment are an important factor when deciding whether to use palliative chemo.

- ✔ **Length of treatment:** The duration of treatment and the number of treatment cycles, based on the tumor's response to treatment, is another consideration in deciding to give palliative therapy. Standard practice is to wait for one to two full cycles of treatment (a typical cycle lasts three to four weeks) before evaluating the tumor's response to treatment. If the tumor is responding, treatment may continue until the cancer stops growing or until side effects become severe enough to interfere with further treatment.

In tumors that have a good response rate, palliative chemotherapy provides the following benefits:

- Halted tumor growth
- Tumor shrinkage
- Pain relief and alleviation of other debilitating symptoms
- Improved quality of life and life extension

Although the use of palliative chemotherapy remains controversial, most physicians agree that it shouldn't be recommended for the following people:

- Patients who have received multiple treatments and are still declining
- Patients who have multiple sites of metastasis
- Patients who aren't responding to a trial use of chemotherapy
- Patients with poor performance status (PS) scores, who are bedridden or confined to a chair more than half the time

The central issues surrounding palliative therapy are quality of life and life extension. These issues, especially when a cure is no longer possible, are deeply personal ones that the patient, family, and physician must ultimately decide.

It's Classified: Classifying Chemotherapy Drugs

Understanding the classification of chemotherapy drugs helps you become aware of which drug class doctors prescribe for specific cancers and what side effects you can expect to see from a particular drug. The most commonly used chemotherapy drug classifications include the following (all of which can be administered through IV therapy):

- **Alkylating agents:** *Alkylating agents* are cell-cycle-non-specific drugs that work most effectively during the resting phase of the cancer cell cycle. These agents prevent cancer from reproducing by directly damaging the cell's genetic DNA material. Some alkylating agents are derivatives of mustard gas, while others are made from metal salts. Still others are plant-based; for example, vinca alkaloids are made from the periwinkle plant, and taxanes are made from the Pacific yew tree.

- **Antimetabolites:** *Antimetabolites,* agents with cell structures that are very similar to those of normal cells, trick cancer cells into allowing them to enter the cancer cell's structure. When accepted inside the cancer cell, antimetabolites disrupt reproduction and prevent the cancer cells from dividing. Examples of antimetabolites include methotrexate (Trexall) and 5-fluorouracil (5-FU).

- **Anti-tumor antibiotics:** *Anti-tumor antibiotics* are agents that act during multiple phases of the cancer cell cycle to block enzyme production and cause cell structure changes. They're made from natural substances produced by microorganisms. Examples include doxorubicin (Adriamycin) and mitomycin (Mutamycin).

- **Topoisomerase inhibitors:** *Topoisomerase inhibitors* are drugs that interfere with the action of enzymes by manipulating the cancer cell's DNA to prevent reproduction. Examples include irinotecan (Camptosar) and topotecan (Hycamtin).

- **Mitotic inhibitors:** *Mitotic inhibitors* slow cancer growth by preventing cell division or mitosis. These drugs disrupt the microtubules of cancer cells, preventing them from pulling the cell apart when it attempts to divide and reproduce. Mitotic inhibitors, also known as *antimicrotubule agents,* are derived from natural substances, such as plant alkaloids. Examples are eribulin (Halhaven) and paclitaxel (Abraxane).

- **Corticosteroids:** Corticosteroids are hormone-like agents that kill or slow the growth of cancer cells and shrink tumor size. Although doctors don't completely understand the exact mechanism of action, corticosteroids appear to disrupt cancer cells' DNA and RNA, preventing the cells from reproducing. Examples of these agents include prednisolone (Delta-Cortef) and dexamethasone (Decadron).

- **Miscellaneous agents:** Scientists are currently studying and developing several agents for use in the treatment of cancer. Some of the most promising agents are

  - **Enzymes and enzyme inhibitors:** Enzymes and enzyme inhibitors, such as ribonucleotide reductase inhibitors, disrupt the genetic capability of cancer cells to reproduce.

  - **Retinoids and vitamin A:** These derivatives show promise for suppressing growth in malignant and premalignant cells. They're also being studied for potential cancer prevention because they help destroy *oncogenes,* or genetic mutations known to promote cancer.

  - **Targeted therapies:** Targeted therapies are drugs or other substances that block the growth of cancer by interfering with specific molecules in the cancer cell. By focusing on specific cancer cell molecules, targeted therapy results in less damage to normal cells.

✔ **Immunotherapy agents:** *Immunotherapy* is a treatment that boosts and enlists the body's own immune system in the fight against cancer. Immunotherapy involves extracting disease-fighting T-cells from a cancer patient's immune system, multiplying them in the laboratory, and infusing them in large quantities back into the patient. Patients who are immunocompromised and have ineffective T-cells are also candidates for immunotherapy. They just get infused with donor T-cells from a mini-stem-cell transplant.

Another form of immunotherapy, called *vaccine immunotherapy,* involves developing a vaccine from the patient's malignant tumor. After the doctor removes the tumor, scientists prepare the vaccine by using tumor cells, and the patient receives an injection of the tumor vaccine to prevent recurrence or relapse.

Chapter 7

Maintaining Equilibrium with Fluids and Electrolytes

· ·

In This Chapter

▶ Understanding fluid and electrolyte basics

▶ Seeing how fluids move in and out of compartments in the body

▶ Evaluating how much fluid your patient really needs

▶ Getting to know IV solutions and their specific characteristics

▶ Recognizing and fixing imbalances in fluids and electrolytes

▶ Understanding acid-base balance and correcting imbalances

· ·

*I*magine, for a moment, the amazing internal functions of your body. Your cells, harmoniously bathing in a sea of extracellular fluids, work like a well-oiled machine to maintain that delicate balance known as *equilibrium*. Your body maintains equilibrium by keeping a vigilant watch over fluid and electrolyte balance, enlisting the help of various organ systems and endocrine glands when this balance is threatened.

Maintaining equilibrium is a constant balancing act — it never occurs at one given point in time. When pathological processes affect the body's physiology, body systems go into overdrive, commanding millions of reactions to try to restore balance — a complex process, indeed, but one that's fundamental to the practice of infusion therapy.

In this chapter, we break down the walls that stand between you and the principles of fluid and electrolyte balance. We simplify the processes, showing you how body systems work together to maintain equilibrium. We discuss different IV solutions and the role tonicity plays in correcting fluid and electrolyte imbalances. Finally, we talk about acid-base balance and the part it plays in maintaining equilibrium.

Getting Your Fill: Introducing Fluids and Electrolytes

If you're a typical, average-sized adult male, approximately 60 percent of your body weight is composed of body fluids, a little less if you're female. Although water (a *solvent,* or substance that can dissolve other substances) is their primary component, body fluids also contain *electrolytes* (the active chemicals in the fluids) and other dissolved particles (known as *solutes*).

A number of factors influence the amount of body fluids that you have. These factors include things you can control, such as how much body fat you have, and things you can't control, such as your age and gender. In general, men have more body fluids than women, younger people have more than elderly folks, and thin people have more than people with a few extra pounds.

Body fluids work in conjunction with electrolytes to maintain equilibrium. In fact, you often hear them referred to concurrently because they're *interdependent:* When one of them is altered for any reason, the other one is likely to be altered, too, and vice versa.

Appreciating your body fluids' full-time job

Body fluids are lucky because they have a full-time job and often get to work overtime. They're also excellent multi-taskers that function in five distinct ways:

- To stabilize body temperature
- To deliver nutrients and gases to and from cells
- To remove cellular waste products and products of metabolism
- To maintain a balance with electrolytes
- To maintain adequate blood pressure

Under normal circumstances, your body strives continuously to make your daily intake match your daily output. An alteration in either of these processes leads to fluid and electrolyte disturbances that disrupt equilibrium.

To help maintain balance, your body acquires fluids and electrolytes through eating and drinking and loses fluids and electrolytes through the following organs:

- **Kidneys:** The kidneys are the driving force behind equilibrium. The average adult loses about 1 to 2 liters of fluid a day through normal urination. However, if your patient is bed-bound and suffering from illness or injury, his urinary output may be much less — 500 to 700 milliliters (mL) per day.

- **Skin:** A person can lose between 350 to 450 mL of fluid per day from water that passes through the skin. Fever, increased sweating, and major burns can increase this loss.

- **Lungs:** While the body is in its resting state, a person can lose 300 to 400 mL of fluid per day to water vapor from the lungs. However, the amount can be much less for patients who are on a ventilator and much greater in patients with breathing aberrations such as tachypnea.

- **Gastrointestinal (GI) tract:** Because the intestines reabsorb most of the fluids a person takes in, only 100 to 200 mL of fluid are lost through the GI tract. This loss increases, however, if your patient has diarrhea or other abnormalities, such as an excessively draining fistula.

The loss of water through the skin and lungs is known as *insensible water loss.* It's insensible because you don't always know you're losing it.

To keep the volume and concentration of body fluids within their normal range, the body enlists the help of regulatory organs such as the brain, kidneys, heart, lungs, and adrenal and parathyroid glands. Together, these organs work with regulatory transport mechanisms to achieve equilibrium (we explain these mechanisms in the later section "On the Move: Following Fluids between Compartments"). Two hormones — aldosterone and antidiuretic hormone (ADH) — also play an important role, as does your thirst mechanism.

Even with all these organs and hormones working together, fluid balance isn't constant, however, and is affected by the following factors:

- Fluid volume gains and losses (Figure 7-1 gives you a summary of daily fluid gains and losses in a normal, healthy adult)

- The distribution of body fluids within the cells

- The concentration of particles (solutes) in the fluids

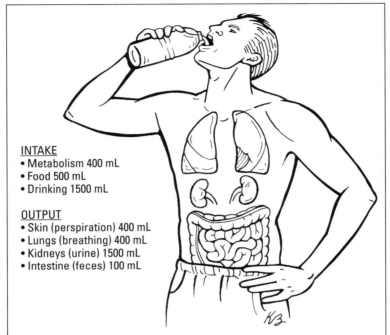

INTAKE
• Metabolism 400 mL
• Food 500 mL
• Drinking 1500 mL

OUTPUT
• Skin (perspiration) 400 mL
• Lungs (breathing) 400 mL
• Kidneys (urine) 1500 mL
• Intestine (feces) 100 mL

Figure 7-1:
Typical adult daily fluid gains and losses.

Illustration by Kathryn Born

Getting a charge out of electrolytes

Alas, the body doesn't live by fluids alone. As we mention earlier, active chemicals in your body fluids are known as *electrolytes*. Because electrolytes bear an electrical charge, they're also referred to as *ions*. These ions carry either a positive charge (making them *cations*) or a negative charge (making them *anions*).

Body functions depend on electrolytes. If electrolyte balance is compromised, body functions often pay the price. IV therapy involves six important electrolytes: sodium, potassium, calcium, and magnesium, which are cations, and chloride and phosphorus, which are anions.

Electrolyte concentrations vary, depending on where in the body they're located: inside the cells (in the *intracellular fluid,* or ICF) or outside the cells (in the *extracellular fluid,* or ECF). Electrolyte disturbances can wreak havoc on the body very quickly, so you need to have a basic understanding of each electrolyte's properties.

Here are a few important tidbits to remember about the four principal cation electrolytes:

- ✔ **Sodium:** Sodium is the major extracellular cation. It influences water distribution in the body and helps maintain fluid volume. It's also a key player in cellular activity. Retention of sodium can result in fluid volume overload.

- ✔ **Potassium:** Potassium is the most abundant intracellular cation. It maintains equilibrium inside the cell and is influenced by changes in acid-base balance.

- ✔ **Calcium:** In general, 99 percent of the calcium in the body is found in the teeth and bones; the rest is found mostly in the ECF. Calcium is important for the promotion of neuromuscular activity, normal cardiac electrophysiology, bone development, and normal blood coagulation.

- ✔ **Magnesium:** About 50 to 60 percent of the magnesium in the body is found in the bones; the rest is in the ICF, where it's the second most abundant electrolyte. Magnesium is responsible for activating enzymes involved in metabolism and activating the sodium-potassium pump (see the later section "Going against the grain with active transport" for info on this pump).

Here's what the two most important anion electrolytes do to help maintain equilibrium:

- ✔ **Phosphorus:** Phosphorus is the major intracellular anion; it's found mostly in teeth and bones but also in cells. Phosphorus occurs as phosphate, it helps maintain acid-base balance, and it's important for cellular energy metabolism and bone formation.

- ✔ **Chloride:** Chloride is the most abundant extracellular anion. It's influenced by acid-base changes, is important in balancing cations in the ICF and ECF, and is a component of the hydrochloric acid in the stomach that helps the body digest food. Along with sodium, chloride also helps maintain blood osmotic pressure (see the later section "Understanding the big 'O': Osmosis" for details on this type of pressure).

On the Move: Following Fluids between Compartments

A person's body fluids are distributed between two main fluid compartments, as shown in Figure 7-2. When you infuse an IV solution, it moves into one of these two compartments, depending on the type of solution you're using. Here's a quick look at the difference between the two fluid compartments:

✔ **Intracellular space:** This space contains the fluid inside your cells. Approximately two-thirds of your body fluids (40 percent of your body weight) are swimming around inside your intracellular fluid compartment.

✔ **Extracellular space:** This space is made up of the fluid outside of your cells. The remaining one-third of your body fluids (or 20 percent of your body weight) is here. The extracellular fluid compartment is further divided into two main areas:

- **Intravascular space:** The intravascular space contains the *plasma,* which is the fluid inside your blood vessels. Approximately half of your blood volume is made up of plasma, and the other half consists of red blood cells, white blood cells, and platelets.

- **Interstitial space:** The interstitial space contains fluid surrounding the tissues and cells, including your lymph fluid. The average-sized adult has about 8 liters of interstitial fluid.

The breakdown of body fluids in the body is known as the *60-40-20 rule:* 60 percent of a person's body weight is water; 40 percent is intracellular fluids and 20 percent is extracellular fluids.

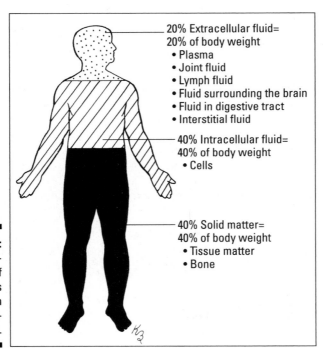

Figure 7-2:
The distri-
bution of
body fluids
between
compart-
ments.

20% Extracellular fluid=
20% of body weight
• Plasma
• Joint fluid
• Lymph fluid
• Fluid surrounding the brain
• Fluid in digestive tract
• Interstitial fluid

40% Intracellular fluid=
40% of body weight
• Cells

40% Solid matter=
40% of body weight
• Tissue matter
• Bone

Illustration by Kathryn Born

But body fluids don't just sit there looking pretty. To maintain balance, they have to shift to and from the various fluid compartments. How do they do this? With a little help from their regulatory friends.

Regulatory transport mechanisms help body fluids and electrolytes get to where they need to go. These mechanisms are either active or passive, depending on whether they require energy to get the job done. By constantly exchanging particles and fluids within the compartments, the body maintains an equal concentration and an acid-base balance (we discuss acid-base balance later in the section "Acid-Base Balance Made Easy").

Catching a free ride with passive transport

In *passive transport,* fluids and solutes move freely between compartments to balance the concentration on either side of a cell membrane. Three important passive transport mechanisms move fluids and solutes through the membrane: diffusion, filtration, and osmosis.

Taking on diffusion: The movement of solutes from a high to low concentration

Most solutes move from an area of higher concentration to an area of lower concentration. For example, if you place a drop of food coloring in a glass of water, it disperses evenly in a short period of time to color all the contents of the glass. This process is known as diffusion. *Diffusion* is a passive transport mechanism (meaning that it doesn't require any energy) that occurs along a concentration gradient. When the diffused particles are evenly distributed, the concentration gradient no longer exists, resulting in an equal concentration on either side of the membrane. Figure 7-3 shows what diffusion looks like.

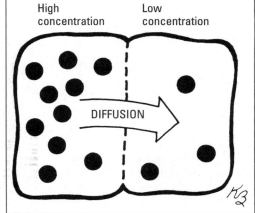

Figure 7-3:
Diffusion of solutes through a cell membrane.

Illustration by Kathryn Born

Having fun with filtration: The movement of solutes from high to low pressure

Suppose you pour vegetable soup into a strainer. The liquid broth, which contains water and other small, nutrient-rich particles, passes through the strainer, and the vegetables, which are too large to pass, stay behind. This is a common example of filtration. *Filtration* is the movement of solutes (like the small particles in soup broth) and water through a membrane (like a strainer) from an area of higher pressure to an area of lower pressure.

The body's primary filtration system, known as *capillary filtration* (see Figure 7-4), occurs when fluids and solutes are filtered through the capillary walls (an area of higher pressure) and into the interstitial fluid (an area of lower pressure).

Left on its own, however, capillary filtration would eventually cause all your plasma to move out of your capillaries. You can imagine the harmful effects this would have — severe hypovolemia, shock, and eventually death. Fortunately, when capillary filtration threatens equilibrium by doing what comes naturally, *capillary reabsorption* steps in to keep capillary filtration under control. Put simply, the capillaries reabsorb fluid when the intracellular *albumin,* a plasma protein that can't filter through the membrane because it's too large, draws fluid back into the cells by osmosis. (See the later section "Cozying up with colloids" for more on albumin and the next section for more on osmosis.)

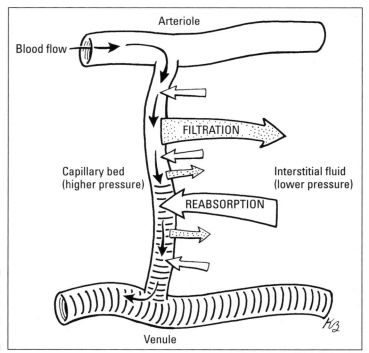

Figure 7-4:
Capillary filtration at its finest.

Illustration by Kathryn Born

Understanding the big "O": Osmosis

Have you ever wondered how a plant's roots draw water from the soil? They do so through a passive transport mechanism known as osmosis. *Osmosis* refers to the movement of water through a membrane from a region of low solute concentration to a region of high solute concentration until both solutions are relatively equal. Fluids in the body move between fluid compartments by osmosis. Figure 7-5 helps you visualize this concept more clearly.

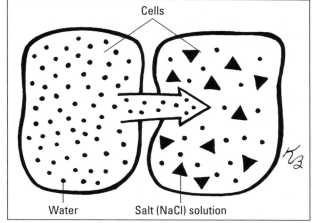

Figure 7-5: Osmosis in action.

Water   Salt (NaCl) solution

Illustration by Kathryn Born

The degree to which osmosis occurs depends on the concentration of the solution, also referred to as its *osmolarity*. Osmolarity, which you express as milliosmoles per liter (mOsm/L), influences the way water moves between fluid compartments. Osmolarity is important when you're considering the best IV solution for your patient because the concentration of a solution determines how the solution will ultimately be distributed to the compartments.

Two opposing forces provide for normal movement of fluids and diffusible solutes across the capillary membrane:

- ✔ **Hydrostatic pressure:** The pressure exerted by fluid against the walls of the blood vessel
- ✔ **Osmotic pressure:** The pressure created by the pulling force of the protein albumin

Hydrostatic pressure, which is usually stronger than osmotic pressure due to its higher concentration, pushes fluid out of the capillaries and into the interstitial space, and osmotic pressure tries to hold onto fluids by pulling them back in. Both play tug-of-war on a dynamic continuum at the arterial and venous ends of the blood vessel to maintain equilibrium (Figure 7-6 shows what this tug-of-war looks like).

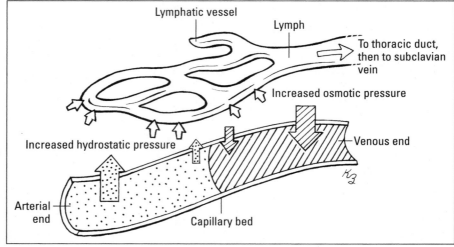

Illustration by Kathryn Born

Figure 7-6:
The
tug-of-war
between the
pressures.

An *osmole* is a standard unit of osmotic pressure based on the molecular weight of a solute, in grams (g), divided by the number of ions or particles into which it dissociates in solutions.

Going against the grain with active transport

Sometimes a cell needs to have a higher concentration of one ion on one side of the membrane than it does on the other, as is the case with sodium and potassium. Uneven concentrations are possible thanks to *active transport,* the movement of a substance across a membrane from a region of lower concentration to a region of higher concentration against a concentration gradient, using energy.

Figure 7-7 shows the *sodium-potassium pump,* which is located within the cell membrane. This pump actively moves the sodium and potassium ions across the cell membrane back to where they're supposed to be.

Picture sodium and potassium standing on opposite sides of a fence. The right side of the fence is the extracellular fluid, and the left side is the intracellular fluid. When sodium tries to wander back across the fence line and into the cell, the sodium-potassium pump steps in and pushes it back so the extracellular fluid can maintain its high sodium concentration. The same goes for potassium in the intracellular fluid.

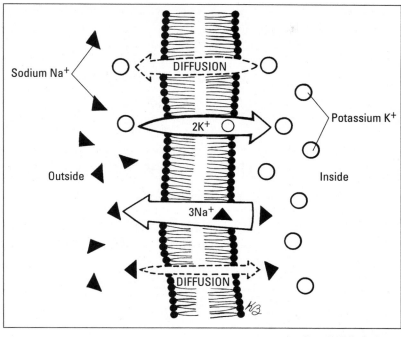

Figure 7-7:
The sodium-potassium pump in a cell membrane.

Illustration by Kathryn Born

Assessing Your Patient's Fluid Requirements

To understand how IV solutions work to preserve equilibrium in your patient, you need to be aware of the rationale behind the healthcare provider's choice of solutions and the characteristics of the solution that you have to infuse. Based on the patient's diagnosis and a thorough physical assessment, the provider orders IV fluids for maintenance or for replacement of existing or ongoing fluid losses.

Taking a peek at the labs

Before administering IV therapy, you need to assess your patient's baseline laboratory values. That way, you have a foundation on which to determine whether the treatment you administer is effective or needs to be adjusted in any way. Here are some laboratory values that are significant to fluid maintenance or replacement therapy.

Lab Test	What the Test Evaluates
Blood urea nitrogen (BUN)	Kidney function during fluid therapy
Creatinine	Kidney function during fluid therapy
Urine specific gravity	Water balance and concentration of particles in the urine, which reflects the concentration of body fluids and hydration status
Urine osmolality	Changes in fluid volume and concentration
Serum electrolytes	Deviations from normal values
Complete blood count (CBC)	Hemoglobin status before and during fluid therapy, which can reflect hydration status
Arterial blood gases	Acid-base balance
Coagulation studies	Baseline status before administering blood products
Blood glucose	*Osmotic diuresis* (increased urination that results when substances like glucose enter the kidney tubules)
Lactate dehydrogenase	Carbohydrate metabolism

Maintenance fluids: Accounting for everyday losses

The average, healthy adult needs between 2,400 and 3,200 mL of fluid each day to maintain equilibrium. When your patient is *NPO* (*nil per os,* or nothing by mouth) or her oral intake is restricted for another reason, she can't meet her daily requirement for fluids and electrolytes. She also continues to incur losses from normal bodily functions, such as urination and sweating. This is where maintenance IV therapy comes into play.

Maintenance fluids help your patient replace water and electrolytes lost to normal, everyday processes. The amount of IV solution needed to replace normal losses depends on an evaluation of intake and output and your patient's age, height, weight, percentage of body fat, existing kidney and heart function, and current electrolyte status.

Replacing existing and ongoing losses from illness or injury

An acute injury or illness often causes your patient to suffer sudden deficits of fluid, electrolytes, and/or blood products. *Replacement therapy* replaces existing fluid losses due to stressors such as hemorrhage, vomiting, diarrhea, and starvation. The amount of fluid restoration needed is based on intake and output and a thorough analysis of your patient's complete blood count and metabolic panel.

On the other hand, when your patient has ongoing losses from abnormalities such as fistulas, nasogastric tubes, burns, or excessively draining wounds, you must review her fluid status and then replace any lost fluid on an *ongoing* basis. You accomplish ongoing replacement therapy through evaluation of intake and output followed by replacement with the appropriate solution.

Fluid imbalances can occur in the blink of an eye, so be sure to establish your patient's baseline fluid status before beginning any type of maintenance or replacement therapy.

Restoring Volume with Crystalloids and Colloids

Whether your patient needs maintenance or replacement therapy, the type of IV solution the healthcare provider orders depends on the type of body fluids and electrolytes lost from illness, injury, or normal everyday occurrences. IV solutions come in two main types — crystalloids and colloids — each of which has an important role in restoring or expanding volume.

IV solutions (both crystalloids and colloids) fall into three categories according to their tonicity. *Tonicity* basically refers to the concentration (or osmolarity) of a solution. Blood plasma has an osmolarity of approximately 300 milliosmoles per liter (mOsm/L), and IV solutions are often categorized according to whether their osmolarity is less than, greater than, or equal to that of blood:

- **Isotonic:** This type of electrolyte solution has an osmolarity of 250 to 375 mOsm/L, about equal to that of blood.

- **Hypotonic:** This type of electrolyte solution has an osmolarity that's less than 250 mOsm/L.

- **Hypertonic:** This type of electrolyte solution has an osmolarity that's greater than 375 mOsm/L.

Figure 7-8 gives you a basic rundown of the different IV solutions and how they work in the body after they're infused.

In terms of fluid resuscitation, neither crystalloids nor colloids are inherently better than the other. In a landmark clinical trial known as the Saline versus Albumin Fluid Evaluation (SAFE) Study, researchers evaluated 6,997 patients who needed fluid replacement due to a critical illness. Half of the group received albumin (a colloid), and the other half received normal saline (an isotonic crystalloid). Results concluded that after 28 days, the mortality rate was 21 percent regardless of which solution patients received. In another example, after reviewing 63 eligible clinical trials, the Cochrane Database System Review reported that there's no evidence that a colloid solution is any better than a crystalloid solution at reducing the risk of death.

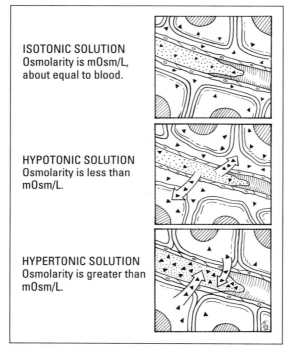

Figure 7-8:
Under-
standing
how IV
solutions
work in the
cells.

ISOTONIC SOLUTION
Osmolarity is mOsm/L,
about equal to blood.

HYPOTONIC SOLUTION
Osmolarity is less than
mOsm/L.

HYPERTONIC SOLUTION
Osmolarity is greater than
mOsm/L.

Illustration by Kathryn Born

Getting acquainted with crystalloids

Crystalloids are electrolyte solutions that can pass freely between the intra-vascular compartment and the interstitial space; these solutions work in either area to expand volume.

Isotonic crystalloids

The crystalloid solution of choice is often the *isotonic solution* because it has the same electrolyte concentration as the extracellular fluid, which means the solution doesn't alter the electrolyte balance in the plasma. When you infuse an isotonic solution, it doesn't move into the intracellular fluid com-partment by osmosis but rather stays where it's infused — in the blood ves-sels (within the intravascular compartment).

The job of the isotonic fluid is to expand volume. Because the isotonic fluid doesn't enter the cells, the red blood cells don't increase or decrease in volume.

Isotonic solutions are administered to treat fluid volume deficit resulting from hemorrhage, severe vomiting, or diarrhea and heavy drainage from GI suction, fistulas, or wounds. You can also use them to supply free water or to treat an abnormally high serum osmolarity.

Table 7-1 gives some examples of isotonic IV solutions and their uses.

Table 7-1	Isotonic Solutions	
Solution	*Osmolarity and Behavior*	*Purpose*
Normal saline (0.9% sodium chloride)	Normal saline has a total osmolarity of 308 mOsm/L, but because it contains only sodium and chloride, it doesn't totally mimic the extracellular fluid (ECF). Because water goes where sodium goes, when administered, it remains in the ECF.	This solution is used to treat ECF volume deficit, which occurs as a result of severe vomiting or diarrhea, hemorrhage, burns, excessive drainage from GI fistulas and wounds, and dehydration. It's also sometimes used as adjunct treatment for high concentrations of various electrolytes to help the kidneys flush out the excess.
D5W (5% dextrose in water)	D5W starts off as an isotonic solution with an osmolarity of 278 mOsm/L, but it disperses into a hypotonic solution after you administer it (when glucose from the solution enters the cells), with one-third moving to the ECF and two-thirds moving to the intracellular fluid (ICF).	D5W's primary role in IV therapy is to supply water and decrease a high serum osmolarity resulting from dehydration.
Lactated Ringer's solution (LR)	This solution, which has an osmolarity of 274 mOsm/L, is most similar to plasma. LR contains sodium, chloride, potassium, and calcium ions, along with lactate, which metabolizes into bicarbonate.	This solution is used primarily to treat *hypovolemia* (fluid volume deficit, or FVD) and to provide electrolytes. It's also commonly used to resuscitate burn victims.

Hypotonic crystalloids

IV solutions that are *hypotonic* have an osmolarity that's less than plasma. When you administer a hypotonic solution, fluid moves by osmosis out of the blood vessels and into the cells, causing the cells to increase in size.

Half-normal saline (0.45 percent normal saline) has an osmolarity of 154 mOsm/L. It's the most commonly used hypotonic solution for IV therapy, and it's used to replace cellular fluid loss in patients who are dehydrated and require water replacement. Other hypotonic solutions, such as 0.33 percent sodium chloride, 0.2 percent sodium chloride, and 2.5 percent dextrose in water, typically get additives before they're infused to increase their osmolarity; these solutions are generally used for pediatric patients.

Never give hypotonic solutions to patients who are at risk for increased intracranial pressure (ICP) because of the potential for a fluid shift to the brain tissue, which can cause or exacerbate cerebral edema.

Infuse hypotonic solutions slowly. Administering them too rapidly can lead to cell damage and *cellular edema* (an abnormal accumulation of serous fluid in the cells).

Hypertonic crystalloids

When the total osmolarity in a solution exceeds that of the extracellular fluid, the solution is called *hypertonic*. Hypertonic solutions draw water from the intracellular fluid compartment (inside the cells) into the extracellular fluid compartment, causing the cells to decrease in volume. Table 7-2 gives some examples of hypertonic fluids and their uses.

Hypertonic solutions can be irritating to veins, so administer them slowly.

Table 7-2	Hypertonic Solutions	
Solution	*Osmolarity*	*Purpose*
3% NaCl (hypertonic saline)	1,026 mOsm/L	This solution is used primarily in emergency situations to treat hyponatremia, especially when the condition causes seizures; 3% NaCl is extremely hypertonic and must be administered slowly and with great caution because rapid infusion may lead to fluid volume overload.
D5NS (5% dextrose in 0.9% sodium chloride)	550 mOsm/L	D5NS can be given peripherally to expand volume in varying situations.
D10W (10% dextrose in water)	556 mOsm/L	D10W is a more concentrated formula that you can give peripherally to treat hypoglycemia (low blood sugar).

Cozying up with colloids

Unlike crystalloids, *colloid solutions* are volume expanders that contain large molecules — in fact, the molecules are so large that they're unable to pass through the capillary membrane. Through osmotic pressure, they pull fluids into the intravascular space, expanding intravascular volume (see the earlier section "Understanding the big 'O': Osmosis" for details on osmotic pressure).

Because the molecules in colloids are so large, less fluid volume is required during administration than with crystalloids. Colloids also last longer because their large molecules remain warm and cozy inside the intravascular fluid compartment much longer than their crystalloid counterparts.

Colloid solutions come in two types — those derived from natural sources within the body and those derived through synthetic means. Here are the two most common types of colloid solutions used in IV therapy:

- ✔ **Plasma protein (albumin):** Albumin, a naturally occurring protein in the body, is the most commonly used colloid solution. It's used to treat hypovolemic shock, and it's prepared directly from human plasma. Before it can be used in IV therapy, it undergoes rigorous heat processing to reduce its potential for transmitting disease.

  Using albumin presents some disadvantages, including its high cost and limited availability. Because albumin is a blood product, its manufacture is dependent on a human donor.

- ✔ **Synthetic solutions:** *Synthetic colloid solutions,* such as hetastarch, dextran, and gelatins, are commonly used to increase plasma volume in the early management of shock — or impending shock — due to burns, hemorrhage, surgery, sepsis, or trauma. Besides being readily available, long-lasting, and inexpensive, synthetic colloid solutions are generally acceptable to people of all religious groups, unlike products that are derived from human blood.

Table 7-3 compares common types of colloid solutions.

Table 7-3	Colloid Solutions			
Solution	*Tonicity*	*Maximum Volume Expansion*	*Duration of Expansion*	*Major Side Effects*
Albumin 5%	Isotonic	70–100%	12–24 hours	Allergic reactions
Albumin 25%	Hypertonic	300–500%	12–24 hours	Allergic reactions

(continued)

Table 7-3 *(continued)*

Solution	Tonicity	Maximum Volume Expansion	Duration of Expansion	Major Side Effects
Hetastarch	Isotonic	100–200%	8–36 hours	Renal dysfunction
Dextran 40	Isotonic	To maximum volume, usually within several minutes after the end of infusion	Varies but decreases more rapidly than dextran 70	Anaphylaxis
Dextran 70	Isotonic	Increases plasma volume in excess of amount infused within an hour	Can last up to 24 hours	Anaphylaxis
Gelatins	Isotonic	70–80%	Less than 6 hours	Anaphylaxis

Correcting Fluid and Electrolyte Imbalances

In this section, we discuss various types of fluid and electrolyte imbalances and explain how to correct them. Table 7-4 gives you the normal serum levels and the names of the imbalances.

Table 7-4 Normal Levels and Imbalances in Fluids and Electrolytes

Imbalance In	Normal Serum Levels	Deficit	Excess
Fluid volume	N/A	Hypovolemia	Hypervolemia
Sodium (Na^+)	135–145 mEq/L	Hyponatremia	Hypernatremia
Chloride (Cl^-)	96–106 mEq/L	Hypochloremia	Hyperchloremia
Potassium (K^+)	3.5–5.0 mEq/L	Hypokalemia	Hyperkalemia
Calcium (Ca^{2-})	8.9–10.1 mg/dL	Hypocalcemia	Hypercalcemia
Phosphate (PO_4^{2-})	2.5–4.5 mg/dL	Hypophosphatemia	Hyperphosphatemia
Magnesium (Mg^{2+})	1.5–2.5 mg/dL	Hypomagnesemia	Hypermagnesemia

Disorders related to imbalances in fluid volume, electrolytes, and pH seldom exist in a vacuum. Pathological states frequently involve most, if not all three, of these elements. Restoring equilibrium, or at least getting patients back to their usual, steady state, is the goal of fluid and electrolyte therapy. (See the later section "Acid-Base Balance Made Easy" for details on pH imbalances.)

Correcting disturbances doesn't occur in a short period of time. On the contrary, constant monitoring and adjusting may take hours, if not days, to ensure that the patient is no longer in danger. During electrolyte replacement therapy, for example, you may have to monitor your patient's metabolic panel frequently, at least every six hours, to avoid complications that may arise from an under- or overcorrection of electrolytes.

Note: In the following sections, we list signs and symptoms of the various fluid and electrolyte disorders in order of severity, from mild to moderate to severe.

Hypovolemia: Getting low on fluids

Hypovolemia, commonly referred to as *fluid volume deficit* (FVD), occurs when the body loses excessive (but relatively equal) amounts of fluids and electrolytes from the extracellular compartment. Don't confuse the term with *dehydration,* which refers only to the loss of water accompanied by increased levels of serum sodium.

The causes of hypovolemia include vomiting, diarrhea, excessive GI suctioning or an exceedingly draining fistula, severe burns, trauma resulting in hemorrhage, and decreased fluid intake, especially in patients who are at risk.

When hypovolemia is severe, it's often easier to recognize. In fact, the clinical picture of hypovolemia depends on how severe the deficit is and how rapid its onset is. Here are some signs and symptoms that should alert you to a possible diagnosis of hypovolemia, from mild to severe:

- Thirst
- Acute weight loss
- Decreased *skin turgor* (the skin's ability to return to its normal shape when stretched)
- Tenting of the skin
- Clammy skin
- *Oliguria* (decreased urine output)
- Dark, concentrated urine
- Weak, rapid pulse

- ✔ Flattened jugular veins (when lying down)
- ✔ Altered mental status
- ✔ Decreased central venous pressure
- ✔ Low-normal blood pressure

One of the most important goals for treating hypovolemia is correcting the underlying cause of the disturbance. Encourage oral fluids, but when they're insufficient and the deficit is severe, initiate IV therapy based on a thorough patient assessment and a doctor's order.

The most appropriate IV solution for treating hypovolemia is an isotonic solution such as lactated Ringer's solution or normal saline. After the patient's fluid volume is restored, however, you can change the solution to one that provides free water (such as half-normal saline or D5W), which helps the kidneys excrete metabolic waste. (See the earlier section "Getting acquainted with crystalloids" for details on these solutions.)

During replacement therapy, you need to monitor your patient closely, particularly for fluid volume overload. This monitoring includes careful assessment and accurate recording of intake and output, vital signs, hemodynamic pressures (if applicable), breath sounds, and daily body weight.

Hypervolemia: Having excess fluid

Hypervolemia, also referred to as *fluid volume excess* (FVE), occurs when extracellular fluid volume increases. Hypervolemia is usually the result of an increase in sodium that causes the body to retain fluids. The many causes of hypervolemia range from simple fluid overload to the more serious congestive heart failure, kidney failure, and cirrhosis of the liver. Whatever the cause, early identification is key to restoring balance and improving patient outcomes.

Similar to hypovolemia, symptoms of hypervolemia depend on the degree of the overload and the rapidity of its onset. Here are the symptoms of hypervolemia, from mild to severe:

- ✔ Edema, especially in dependent areas
- ✔ Weight gain
- ✔ *Ascites* (abnormal accumulation of fluid in the abdomen)
- ✔ Increase in urine specific gravity
- ✔ *Polyuria* (increased urination)
- ✔ Decrease in hematocrit and BUN (blood urea nitrogen)
- ✔ Decrease in serum sodium and osmolarity

Pulmonary edema, a condition in which fluid builds up in the lungs, is one of the consequences of hypervolemia. In pulmonary edema resulting from hypervolemia, you may see additional symptoms such as *dyspnea* (shortness of breath) and wheezing; hypertension; crackles or "rales" on lung exam; distention of neck veins; a rapid, bounding pulse; and pulmonary congestion, as seen with a chest X-ray.

To manage hypervolemia, you have to manage its underlying cause. If the cause is unknown, you may treat it symptomatically by using dietary restriction of sodium and fluids and/or administration of diuretics. Having the patient elevate his extremities and wear supportive stockings may also help mobilize fluids and reduce edema in dependent areas.

When the kidneys are impaired and the patient's body can't rid itself of fluids with the help of dietary and/or pharmacological interventions, you can use hemodialysis or peritoneal dialysis to remove waste, excess sodium, and water and to control potassium levels and acid-base balance.

Treatment for hypervolemia includes careful monitoring of your patient's vital signs, intake and output, pulmonary status, daily body weights, and response to diuretic therapy.

Simplifying sodium imbalances

Sodium has two important jobs: to control water distribution throughout the body and to maintain fluid volume in the extracellular compartment. Imbalances of sodium occur when intake and output don't match or when kidney and/or hormonal control mechanisms fail.

Hyponatremia: Low sodium

Hyponatremia is defined by serum sodium levels below 135 mEq/L. This decrease may be related to a predisposing condition, or it may result from excess vomiting, diarrhea, fistulas, sweating, or diuretic use, especially when combined with a low-salt diet.

When the intravascular fluid has a low concentration of sodium, water is pulled from the intravascular space and into the cells. What does this look like, clinically? When the sodium levels decrease gradually, you're likely to see mild to moderate symptoms of hyponatremia, including nausea, headache, fatigue, loss of appetite, tachycardia, and vomiting. In people whose deficit is acute and more severe (particularly when sodium levels drop below 115 mEq/L), you may see the following more serious neurological changes that are related to increased intracranial pressure:

- ✔ Confusion
- ✔ Lethargy
- ✔ Muscle twitches
- ✔ Stroke-like symptoms, such as *hemiparesis* — slight paralysis or weakness affecting one side of the body
- ✔ Seizures

When hyponatremia is caused by a fluid volume disturbance, you should also look for signs and symptoms related to hypovolemia or hypervolemia (see the earlier sections "Hypovolemia: Getting low on fluids" and "Hypervolemia: Having excess fluid").

The method for correcting a sodium deficit is pretty obvious: Replace the sodium. A patient who can still eat and drink can replace sodium orally by consuming foods and fluids with high salt contents, such as beef broth or tomato juice. When diet alone doesn't correct the deficit, you can give oral supplements, which are the preferred method of sodium replacement for most patients.

But what about the patient who is NPO (nothing by mouth) or who can't take oral supplements for some other reason? That's where IV therapy comes in.

If the primary problem is water retention, restricting fluids is far easier — and safer — than administering sodium. Depending on the degree of the overload, you may also be able to use a loop diuretic, such as furosemide (Lasix), to decrease volume and, therefore, increase serum sodium levels.

When your patient's sodium deficit is severe, you may administer hypertonic saline slowly in small amounts. Carefully monitor your patient in an intensive care setting for signs of hypervolemia; see the earlier section "Hypervolemia: Having excess fluid" for details.

When you replace sodium in a patient who has normal fluid volume or who is overloaded with fluid, you predispose him to an even greater degree of fluid volume overload. That's why you must carefully monitor your patient for signs and symptoms of hypervolemia whenever you replace sodium.

Hypernatremia: Excess sodium

Hypernatremia is defined as serum sodium levels above 145 mEq/L. This increase can be the result of excessive sodium intake or abnormal losses of fluid.

Under normal circumstances, when sodium levels increase, the thirst mechanism kicks in, leading you to drink more water to normalize the sodium concentration in your body. But what about infants, the elderly, the cognitively impaired, or the unconscious patients who can't respond adequately (or at all) to the thirst mechanism? These patients are at even greater risk for fluid and electrolyte disturbances.

The symptoms you see in a patient with hypernatremia occur because fluid is being drawn out of the cells and into the intravascular space in an attempt to decrease the intravascular sodium concentration. This process causes cellular dehydration.

Be on the lookout for early signs of hypernatremia, such as thirst, reduced urine, nausea, vomiting, and unusual restlessness, weakness, or fatigue. As the condition worsens, signs and symptoms become more obvious and may include the following:

- *Polydipsia* (excessive thirst)
- Dry, sticky mucous membranes
- An elevated temperature and flushed skin
- Agitation, mental status changes, seizures, and coma

The primary goal of correcting hypernatremia is decreasing elevated serum sodium levels:

- If excess sodium intake is to blame, then initially restrict dietary sodium.
- When serum sodium levels are elevated because of fluid loss, the goal of treatment is replacing fluid volume, which also corrects the sodium imbalance. Typically, it's done with isotonic or slightly hypotonic saline to make sure the correction of sodium is done slowly.

 D5W disperses as a hypotonic solution in the plasma (see the earlier section "Getting acquainted with crystalloids" for details). Take care when administering hypotonic solutions because infusing them too rapidly may lead to an overcorrection, resulting in cerebral edema, seizures, and death. Doctors sometimes order diuretics together with IV therapy to prevent this situation.

Catching on to chloride

As the major anion in the extracellular fluid, chloride helps maintain serum *osmolarity* (the concentration of a solution in terms of osmoles of solutes per liter of solution), acid-base balance, and the balance of intracellular and extracellular cations. Serum chloride levels depend on bicarbonate (HCO_3) concentration and various acid-base disturbances. The kidneys and gastrointestinal system help to keep chloride, which is normally found in gastric and pancreatic secretions, in check. Normal values of chloride range between 96 and 106 mEq/L. A shift in either direction leads to an imbalance.

Chloride and sodium imbalances often occur *in tandem,* meaning that when there's a deficiency in one, there's a deficiency in the other, and conversely, when there's an excess of one, there's an excess of the other. See the earlier section "Simplifying sodium imbalances" for info on hyper- and hyponatremia.

Hypochloremia: Low chloride

Hypochloremia occurs when a patient has a serum chloride level of less than 96 mEq/L. This condition is normally caused by vomiting, fistulas, diuretics, or prolonged nasogastric suctioning. But you may also see hypochloremia in a patient who drinks massive amounts of water or whose dietary intake is compromised.

Symptoms of hypochloremia are often related to other electrolyte disturbances or acid-base changes and can include excess fluid loss or dehydration (diarrhea or vomiting), muscle weakness, sweating, or high fever. If the deficit is severe, you also need to watch out for the following symptoms:

- ✔ Increased muscular excitability
- ✔ *Tetany* (muscle spasms, tremors)
- ✔ *Bradypnea* (decreased respiratory rate)
- ✔ Metabolic alkalosis

Hyperchloremia: Excess chloride

Hyperchloremia occurs when your patient's serum chloride levels rise above 106 mEq/L. Common causes include hypernatremia and *metabolic acidosis* (when the body produces too much acid or when the kidneys aren't removing enough acid from the body).

Symptoms of hyperchloremia are often related to its underlying cause — too much chloride — and symptoms of hypernatremia may be the most prevalent (see the earlier section for details). In severe cases, you may also see the following:

- ✔ *Tachypnea* (increased respiratory rate)
- ✔ Respiratory alkalosis
- ✔ Respiratory failure

Correcting hypochloremia and hyperchloremia

You correct hyperchloremia and hypochloremia by correcting the primary electrolyte and/or acid-base disturbance that caused them. For example, when you have a patient with hypovolemia due to vomiting, the first thing you need to do is replace volume, which will subsequently correct the hypovolemia *and* the chloride imbalance.

Playing it safe with potassium imbalances

Potassium imbalances are relatively common in healthcare, and even a slight deviation from normal can negatively impact cellular activity. Potassium, the major intracellular cation, is important to a person's heart and muscles. In fact, imbalances frequently manifest themselves in a patient's abnormal EKG.

Normal serum values of potassium range from 3.5 to 5.0 mEq/L. Potassium levels below or above normal lead to potassium imbalances for which treatment is necessary.

Hypokalemia: Low potassium

Hypokalemia refers to a serum potassium level that dips below 3.5 mEq/L. Common offenders that contribute to this imbalance include vomiting, diarrhea, use of loop diuretics such as furosemide (Lasix), heart failure, excess serum calcium or magnesium levels, metabolic alkalosis, and certain hormonal disorders.

Here are some of the most common signs and symptoms that you may see in a patient with hypokalemia:

- ✔ Constipation
- ✔ Fatigue
- ✔ Lethargy
- ✔ Muscle cramps
- ✔ *Parathesis* (numbness and tingling)
- ✔ Diminished reflexes
- ✔ *Paralytic ileus* (paralysis of part of the intestines)
- ✔ EKG changes, such as flattened T-waves and prominent U-waves
- ✔ Cardiac arrhythmias
- ✔ Hypoventilation

Hypokalemia is best served when prevented. That said, when it does occur, the doctor may order your patient to eat a potassium-rich diet and/or take oral potassium supplements on a daily basis. When your patient can't tolerate oral potassium, you have to use IV therapy to correct the deficit.

Intravenous potassium should be premixed, and you have to administer it slowly at a rate no higher than 20 mEq per hour and a concentration no greater than 40 mEq/L. If your patient has a central line and a severe deficit, you may need to increase the concentration to 60 to 100 mEq/L. Because of the potential for complications, cardiac monitoring is recommended when you have to administer potassium in higher concentrations.

When you're evaluating for hypokalemia, always evaluate for hypomagnesemia first. If the patient's magnesium is low, you need to correct it in order to correct the hypokalemia. (See the later section "Managing magnesium imbalances" for details.)

Never give potassium via IV push (it can cause cardiac arrest), and make sure the potassium is diluted, mixed thoroughly, and properly labeled before you administer it. In addition, never exceed 20 mEq/L of potassium in 1 hour in an unmonitored patient.

Hyperkalemia: Excess potassium

Hyperkalemia occurs when a patient's serum potassium level exceeds 5.0 mEq/L. Hyperkalemia is almost always associated with kidney disease and is the result of the kidney's inability to excrete enough (or any) potassium. Aside from decreased excretion, hyperkalemia can also occur from an increased intake of potassium or a shifting of potassium from the cells to the blood.

Here are the signs and symptoms of hyperkalemia:

- ✔ Muscular weakness
- ✔ Muscular flaccidity (when the condition progresses to severe)
- ✔ EKG changes, such as peaked T-waves
- ✔ Cardiac arrhythmias, including heart block and ventricular fibrillation

In cases of mild hyperkalemia, dietary restriction of potassium and of medications that contain potassium may be all your patient needs to correct the imbalance. For more severe cases, you may also administer sodium polystyrene sulfonate (Kayexalate) orally or by enema, especially in patients with kidney impairment.

When potassium levels are excessive, you may need to administer IV insulin together with glucose to move potassium from the extracellular fluid back into the cells and to prevent hypoglycemia. If serum potassium levels are greater than 6.5 mEq/L, you may need to administer intravenous sodium bicarbonate, which also causes potassium to shift back into the cells. Just keep in mind that the effects of these therapies are only temporary because they don't actually remove potassium from the body.

In extreme emergencies, you may need to give the patient calcium gluconate or calcium chloride, which act quickly to reduce serum potassium levels and can help stabilize cardiac arrhythmias associated with hyperkalemia. However, the effects last for only 30 to 60 minutes.

Before you treat an abnormal potassium level, you may want to recheck the patient's blood to make sure the results are accurate. After you verify the results, patients who are being treated with IV therapy to correct a potassium deficiency must be placed on continuous cardiac monitoring because potassium helps regulate the cardiac muscle.

Making calcium less complicated

Remember when your mother told you to drink all your milk? She may have been on to something. Calcium, the fifth most abundant substance in the body, is vital to the formation of teeth and bones, not to mention its calming, sedative effect on your nerves. Normal serum calcium levels run between 8.9 and 10.1 mg/dL.

The parathyroid hormone, or PTH (released by the parathyroid gland), and calcitonin (released by the thyroid gland) regulate calcium levels in the body. When serum calcium levels drop below normal, the parathyroid gland secretes PTH, causing calcium to move from your bones to your blood. When serum calcium levels get too high, the parathyroid gland secretes calcitonin to help bring them down.

Calcium and phosphate have an inverse relationship, meaning that when one is up, the other is down, and vice versa. Read more about this relationship in the section "Picking apart phosphate imbalances."

Hypocalcemia: Low calcium

Hypocalcemia occurs when the serum calcium level drops below 8.9 mg/dL. The most common causes of hypocalcemia are not eating enough calcium-rich foods and not getting enough vitamin D, which is necessary for intestinal absorption of calcium. Other causes may be related to hypoparathyroidism, hyperphosphatemia, alkalosis, pancreatitis, hypomagnesemia, burns, and the use of certain medications, including overuse of loop diuretics.

Active vitamin D is synthesized in your skin from exposure to UV light, or you can obtain it by dietary supplementation. Vitamin D is metabolized by your liver into biologically active 25-hydroxyvitamin D, which is needed for dietary calcium absorption and regulation of bone calcium.

Symptoms of hypocalcemia may start off mild, whereby general fatigue and muscle cramps are common. As the condition progresses, the following symptoms may occur:

- Parathesis (numbness and tingling) involving the fingers and toes and/or the area around the mouth
- Abdominal cramps
- Increasing muscle cramps in the extremities
- Hyperactive tendon reflexes
- Positive Trousseau's sign (muscular contraction, including flexion of the wrist and metacarpophalangeal joints, hyperextension of the fingers, and flexion of the thumb on the palm) and Chvostek's sign (twitching of the ipsilateral facial muscles, suggestive of neuromuscular excitability)
- Tetany (muscle spasms and tremors)
- Bronchospasm (constriction of the airways of the lungs)
- Seizures
- Cardiac arrhythmias, prolonged QT interval
- Congestive heart failure (CHF) and shock

Treatment of hypocalcemia begins with identifying and then eliminating the cause. You can treat mild cases with oral calcium supplements in patients who can tolerate them. When the deficit is severe, IV therapy may include calcium gluconate (the drug of choice for peripheral infusions) or calcium chloride.

Too rapid injection of calcium may decrease blood pressure or cause cardiac syncope. Intravenous calcium should be restricted to acute symptomatic patients who require prompt therapy.

Calcium chloride and calcium gluconate may irritate the tissues. Monitor the IV site carefully for signs of *extravasation*, which occurs when IV solutions leak from the blood vessel into the tissues.

Hypercalcemia: Excess calcium

If your patient has been immobilized for a long period of time, takes far too many antacids, has cancer or hyperparathyroidism, or overuses thiazide diuretics, chances are he may also have *hypercalcemia,* or a serum calcium level above 10.1 mg/dL.

Hypercalcemia may cause your patient to exhibit the following signs and symptoms:

- Fatigue
- Gastrointestinal disturbances, such as nausea, vomiting, and anorexia
- Weakness and decreased tendon reflexes
- Confusion
- Polyuria (increased urination)
- Cardiac complications, such as decreased heart rate and arrhythmias
- Shortened QT interval
- Atrioventricular (AV) block

First-line treatment of hypercalcemia includes hydration therapy. If your patient can't tolerate oral fluids, then IV therapy with normal saline at 200 to 300 mL per hour is appropriate. Normal saline helps dilute overly high calcium concentrations in the blood and facilitates the flushing of calcium via urinary excretion.

In more severe cases, you may need to accompany hydration therapy with other forms of IV therapy, such as calcitonin, to help prevent the bones' reabsorption of calcium. If the patient is hypervolemic, an IV push of furosemide (Lasix) may accompany hydration therapy to accelerate the excretion of calcium from the kidneys.

Picking apart phosphate imbalances

Phosphate is important for normal energy metabolism, and it plays a role in maintaining nerve and muscle function. It's also one of the primary buffers in acid-base balance (see the later section "Acid-Base Balance Made Easy" for details). Normal phosphate levels range from 2.5 to 4.5 mg/dL.

As we mention in the previous section "Making calcium less complicated," phosphate and calcium have an inverse relationship, meaning that when one is up, the other is down, and vice versa. Additionally, both are regulated by the parathyroid glands, and both require sufficient levels of vitamin D to be absorbed by the intestines.

Hypophosphatemia: Low phosphate

Hypophosphatemia occurs when serum phosphate levels drop below 2.5 mg/dL. Common causes include vomiting, vitamin D deficiencies, hypercalcemia, diabetic ketoacidosis, chronic alcoholism, and alcohol withdrawal.

Signs and symptoms of hypophosphatemia are similar to the symptoms I list for hypercalcemia and include fatigue, GI disturbances, weakness, decreased tendon reflexes, confusion, polyuria, cardiac disturbances, and EKG changes (see the earlier section "Hypercalcemia: Excess calcium" for details).

The best treatment of hypophosphatemia is prevention. Advise your patient to avoid using antacids that may contain phosphorus-binding compounds and other medications that may decrease phosphate levels in the blood. Having a patient eat a diet sufficient in phosphorus and take oral supplements is also helpful in prevention. IV phosphorus solutions, such as sodium phosphate or potassium phosphate, are available, but they're reserved for the most severe deficits.

When administering IV solutions that contain phosphorus, be sure to give the medication slowly over a period of four to six hours to prevent phosphate intoxication. And don't forget to monitor the IV site for signs of tissue necrosis and sloughing.

Hyperphosphatemia: High phosphate

Hyperphosphatemia occurs when the serum phosphorus level is greater than 4.5 mg/dL. In most cases, it's related to kidney disease, both acute and chronic. Other causes include hypocalcemia, *rhabdomyolysis* (the breakdown of skeletal muscle), and *hemolysis* (the destruction of red blood cells).

Hyperphosphatemia is generally asymptomatic; however, it can occur in conjunction with hypocalcemia, the symptoms of which are numbness and tingling in the extremities, muscle cramps and spasms, depression, memory loss, and convulsions (see the earlier section "Hypocalcemia: Low calcium" for more details).

Like any electrolyte imbalance, treatment for hyperphosphatemia aims to identify and then eliminate the cause. You can use IV normal saline in mild to moderate cases to increase urinary excretion. But you may need to treat severe cases of hyperphosphatemia with intravenous calcium acetate, which binds with phosphorus to help lower the increased serum phosphate level.

Managing magnesium imbalances

Among other functions, magnesium helps activate enzymes involved in metabolism and is important in the activation of the sodium-potassium pump (see the section "Going against the grain with active transport" for details). The normal range for serum magnesium runs from 1.5 to 2.5 mg/dL.

Hypomagnesemia: Low magnesium

Hypomagnesemia occurs when the serum magnesium level is less than 1.5 mg/dL. Patients at high risk for hypomagnesemia include those who are malnourished, are alcoholics, have severe diarrhea, or take too many diuretics.

Signs and symptoms of hypomagnesemia depend on the degree of the deficit and may include any of the following:

- Parathesis (numbness and tingling)
- Weakness
- Increased tendon reflexes
- Tetany (muscle spasms and tremors)
- Positive Trousseau's and Chvostek's signs (see the earlier section "Hypocalcemia: Low calcium" for details on these signs)
- Mild to severe mood changes
- Cardiac arrhythmias
- Seizures
- EKG changes, such as prolonged PR and QT intervals, widened QRS complex, depressed ST segment, and inverted T-waves

After eliminating the cause of hypomagnesemia, the goal of treatment is to correct the deficit. In mild cases, you can correct the deficit through dietary or supplemental means. But you may need to administer IV therapy for more severe cases. The drug of choice for correcting hypomagnesemia is magnesium sulfate, diluted to a concentration of 20 percent or less for IV administration. The actual dose depends on the degree of the deficit.

Monitor your patient for signs of magnesium toxicity during replacement therapy. Initially, watch for a decrease in the knee-jerk reflex, which disappears before respiratory depression (the most serious side effect of magnesium toxicity) sets in.

Hypermagnesemia: Excess magnesium

Hypermagnesemia, which is less prevalent than hypomagnesemia, occurs when serum magnesium levels exceed 2.5 mg/dL. The major cause of hypermagnesemia is kidney failure, but overuse of antacids and/or laxatives, endocrine disorders, and lithium toxicity may also contribute to this imbalance.

Usually, mild cases of hypermagnesemia are asymptomatic. As serum magnesium levels increase, so do the symptoms, which may include the following:

- ✔ Nausea
- ✔ Muscular problems, such as weakness, paralysis, and decreased tendon reflexes
- ✔ Facial parathesis
- ✔ Respiratory depression, which may lead to respiratory arrest
- ✔ Bradycardia and cardiac arrest

Treatment for mild hypermagnesemia includes eliminating foods high in magnesium (such as tuna, artichokes, and nuts) and any medications that may be contributing to an increased magnesium level. In moderate cases, you may use IV therapy with half-normal saline to flush the system. In the most severe cases, you may administer IV calcium gluconate until the patient no longer exhibits symptoms.

Acid-Base Balance Made Easy

The human body is an acid-making machine and, as such, it continuously produces acids in the form of hydrogen ions. You measure hydrogen ion concentration by *pH,* or potential hydrogen. Figure 7-9 shows the pH scale.

The normal range of pH in a person's blood is 7.35 to 7.45. A lower pH means the blood is too *acidic,* and a higher pH means the blood is too *alkaline* (also called *basic*). Staying in either direction for too long without treatment can be dangerous and even life threatening.

Under normal circumstances, when pH shifts from its usual range, the body enlists the help of compensatory mechanisms in the lungs and kidneys to help restore balance. If the body can't correct pH through normal, compensatory mechanisms, medical professionals implement therapeutic interventions that often include IV therapy.

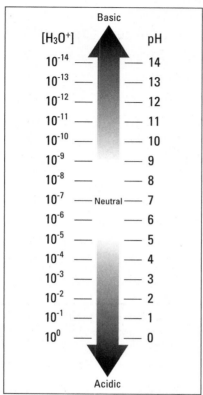

Basic

$[H_3O^+]$ pH

10^{-14}	14
10^{-13}	13
10^{-12}	12
10^{-11}	11
10^{-10}	10
10^{-9}	9
10^{-8}	8
10^{-7} — Neutral —	7
10^{-6}	6
10^{-5}	5
10^{-4}	4
10^{-3}	3
10^{-2}	2
10^{-1}	1
10^{0}	0

Acidic

Figure 7-9:
The pH
scale.

Illustration by Wiley, Composition Services Graphics

Sorting out types of acid-base imbalances

Acid-base alterations are characterized as either respiratory or metabolic and either acidotic or alkalotic. A *respiratory* acid-base imbalance occurs when there's an alteration in the CO_2 (carbon dioxide) levels of the blood. Any acid-base disturbance that is *not* caused by an alteration in CO_2 is essentially *metabolic*. Metabolic acid-base disturbances occur when there's an increase of acid (lowering pH) or a loss of bicarbonate (HCO_3^-) or when there's an increase of bicarbonate and a loss of acid.

To identify specific acid-base imbalances, healthcare providers can draw and then analyze arterial blood gases (ABGs) and/or a basic metabolic panel. Here are the normal values for arterial blood gases (for patients' breathing room air) that you should use as a reference point when identifying acid-base imbalances:

✔ **Acidity (pH):** 7.35–7.45

✔ **Partial pressure of oxygen (PaO$_2$):** 80–100 mmHg

✔ **Partial pressure of carbon dioxide (PaCO$_2$):** 35–45 mmHg

✔ **Bicarbonate (HCO$_3^-$):** 22–26 mEq/L

✔ **Base excess:** –2 to +2

Partial pressure refers to the part of the total gas pressure exerted by an individual gas, like oxygen or carbon dioxide, against the arterial walls. *Base excess* measures the metabolic component in acid-base disturbances. It calculates the amount of acid or alkali required to return the pH back to normal.

Table 7-5 gives you a quick reference guide to interpreting acid-base disturbances based on pH and arterial blood gases.

Note: *Compensation* occurs when the body tries to make up for an imbalance by using some form of innate compensatory mechanism (like breathing faster to rid the body of excess CO$_2$), which sometimes reflects in the ABGs.

Table 7-5	Interpreting Acid-Base Disturbances		
Acid-Base Disturbance	*Change in pH*	*Change in PaCO$_2$*	*Change in HCO$_3^-$*
Respiratory acidosis	Down (below 7.35)	Up (above 45 mmHg)	Normal (22–26 mEq/L) or up (above 26 mEq/L)
Respiratory alkalosis	Up (above 7.45)	Down (below 35 mmHg)	Down (below 22 mEq/L) unless compensated
Metabolic acidosis	Down (below 7.35)	Down (below 35 mmHg) unless compensated	Down (below 22 mEq/L) unless compensated
Metabolic alkalosis	Up (above 7.45)	Up (above 45 mmHg)	Up (above 26 mEq/L)

Here's how the four main types of acid-base disturbances compare:

✔ **Respiratory acidosis:** When the PaCO$_2$ (partial pressure of carbon dioxide as measured by ABGs) rises above 45 mmHg, the end result is respiratory acidosis. Respiratory acidosis is usually caused by *hypoventilation* (decreased respiratory rate and/or shallow breathing), which, in turn, causes the CO$_2$ levels to rise, leading to a drop in pH.

✔ **Respiratory alkalosis:** Respiratory alkalosis occurs when the $PaCO_2$ falls below 35 mmHg. It's generally caused by *hyperventilation* (increased ventilatory rate), which, in turn, causes the pH to rise above normal because the patient has blown off too much CO_2.

✔ **Metabolic acidosis:** A bicarbonate concentration lower than 22 mEq/L leads to metabolic acidosis. Metabolic acidosis is generally a direct result of the buildup of metabolic acids, and it has many causes, including severe dehydration, starvation, acute kidney failure, and diabetic ketoacidosis.

✔ **Metabolic alkalosis:** In contrast to metabolic acidosis, metabolic alkalosis is defined as a bicarbonate concentration in the blood that increases to more than 26 mEq/L. As a result, the pH also rises to above 7.45. Diuretic therapy is one of the most common causes of metabolic alkalosis, but it can also occur because of corticosteroid use, excessive vomiting or nasogastric suctioning, and ingestion of certain alkaline drugs.

Your patient may also have a mixed acid-base imbalance, whereby she exhibits two acid-base disturbances at the same time. A mixed imbalance may contain a combination of these disturbances and usually occurs when compensatory mechanisms fail to correct the initial disturbance. Mixed disturbances may be difficult to recognize when you're looking only at blood gases, so the healthcare provider may want to evaluate your patient and her lab work systematically.

Correcting acid-base imbalances

Just like body fluids and blood, every solution that you infuse has a pH. The hydrogen ion concentration in a solution determines whether that solution is acidic or basic. If a solution has a low pH, it's acidic. If it has a high pH, it's alkaline.

Treatment for metabolic acid-base disturbances is likely to include IV therapy. Two known agents used in IV therapy to correct metabolic acid-base disturbances are

✔ **Alkalinizing agents:** Alkalinizing agents used in IV therapy help buffer excess acid and return the pH to normal. The most common of all alkalinizing agents is sodium bicarbonate, which medical professionals use to treat various forms of metabolic acidosis. You frequently use bolus doses in cardiopulmonary resuscitation while using more dilute solutions in nonemergencies. Side effects from sodium bicarbonate are rare if you use them with caution.

✔ **Acidifying agents:** These days, doctors rarely use acidifying agents, such as ammonium chloride and hydrochloric acid, in clinical practice to treat metabolic alkalosis. If the cause of the alkalosis is hypovolemia, then treatment aims to replace fluid volume with IV normal saline. If metabolic alkalosis is severe or in the presence of normal volume or volume overload, you may need to use other types of agents, including acetazolamide (Diamox) and spironolactone (Aldactone), to increase urinary excretion of HCO_3.

Acetazolamide and spironolactone are used in metabolic alkalosis as diuretics. Treating your patient with these agents may accelerate urinary losses of potassium and phosphorus. So you need to make sure you monitor your patient's electrolytes frequently when administering these drugs.

Chapter 8

Serving Up Parenteral Nutrition

● ●

In This Chapter

▶ Outlining some parenteral nutrition basics

▶ Mixing up a parenteral recipe to meet your patient's nutrient needs

● ●

An astounding number of patients are malnourished before they're even admitted to the hospital. Other patients have abdominal surgery and aren't able to eat food by mouth. In these cases, you may need to administer parenteral nutrition (PN) solutions to help increase nutrients such as glucose, amino acids, lipids, vitamins, and minerals. This chapter explains the importance of assessing your patient's nutritional status and providing nutritional support if needed.

This chapter won't make you a registered dietician, but it will give you plenty of tools to help you understand and safely administer life-saving meals of intravenous (IV) nutrition through parenteral nutrition. For how-to information on PN administration, turn to Chapter 18.

From Soup to Nuts: Reviewing Parenteral Nutrition Basics

Although many advances have been made in nutritional therapies, malnutrition still exists in hospitalized patients. Surveys indicate that 30 to 50 percent of all hospitalized patients are at some degree of risk for malnutrition, and 12 percent are at risk for severe malnutrition. Not to mention that as many as 60 percent of patients over the age of 65 have some evidence of malnutrition when they're admitted to the hospital. (Older patients, in general, are at risk of malnutrition because their dietary intake is often insufficient to meet the increased nutritional requirements associated with illness or surgery.)

Older patients aren't the only ones at risk. Patients who are overweight and even those who have ideal body weight also suffer from milder forms of malnutrition, but unfortunately, they're often overlooked for nutritional assessment and treatment.

The prevalence of malnutrition in hospitalized patients prompted the Joint Commission (previously known as the Joint Commission on Accreditation of Healthcare Organizations) to require nutritional assessment on all patients within 24 hours of hospital admission. Since this requirement became mandatory in 1995, the overall nutritional status of hospitalized patients has improved, but malnutrition remains a serious health issue, occurring everywhere in the world and impacting patients from neonates to geriatrics.

Enter parenteral nutrition. When patients are malnourished, doctors usually prescribe some form of parenteral nutrition (PN), which, simply put, is nutrition through an IV.

Knowing when to use parenteral nutrition

When a patient can't eat food the normal way, clinicians frequently try using *enteral nutrition* (EN) through a feeding tube that they place directly into the patient's stomach or small bowel. When the patient can't tolerate or metabolize EN feedings, however, doctors turn to *parenteral nutrition* (PN), which they administer by a peripheral or central IV route.

Because PN poses the same risks and complications as any other IV therapy (see Chapter 18 for details), doctors prescribe PN only after they've thoroughly evaluated the patient's clinical condition, type of disease, nutritional status and laboratory values, and failure of alternative nutritional support therapies.

PN is particularly appropriate for the following conditions:

- ✔ Bowel obstruction or a malfunctioning, nonfunctioning, or inaccessible gastrointestinal (GI) tract
- ✔ GI problems that aren't expected to resolve within seven days
- ✔ Severe malnourishment
- ✔ Crohn's or Whipple's disease exacerbations
- ✔ Exudative, ulcerative, or inflammatory bowel disease
- ✔ Mesenteric ischemia or paralytic ileus
- ✔ Sepsis or major trauma

What happens when starvation goes untreated?

Starvation triggers a series of biochemical and physiological events known as the *starvation response*. The starvation response occurs when the intake of calories, vitamins, and nutrients is less than the daily energy requirement of the body for a prolonged period of time. When the starvation response kicks in, a metabolic process called *catabolysis* begins to break down fat and muscle to replace dietary calories and protein.

Catabolysis uses calories from fat and protein breakdown to keep vital systems and organs properly functioning. Fat breakdown, called *lypolysis,* and protein breakdown, called *proteolysis,* continue until some type of intervention, such as parenteral nutrition (PN), interrupts the destructive cycle.

In hospitalized patients, early symptoms of starvation include the following:

✔ Anorexia and dehydration

✔ Anxiety, irritability, and fatigue

✔ Decreased response to treatment

✔ Delayed wound healing

✔ Infection and prolonged hospital stays

✔ Weight loss

Left untreated, catabolysis continues until fat and muscle stores are depleted, leading to organ failure, system shutdown, and death. Hence, two of the primary goals of PN are to prevent and treat starvation before it enters the destructive catabolysis stage.

Doctors also use PN in postoperative patients to help accelerate healing in nonhealing wounds, as well as in burn patients to restore protein and maintain electrolyte balance.

Although the risks associated with PN are much greater than those associated with nasogastric (NG) and enteral feedings, the risks of withholding PN are far more serious. Without nutritional assessment and early intervention with PN, patients with a compromised GI system can experience serious complications, including the following:

✔ Impaired recovery and delayed wound healing

✔ Impaired immune, respiratory, and circulatory systems

✔ Increased time in the hospital

✔ Starvation and catabolysis (see the nearby sidebar for details)

✔ Increased morbidity and mortality

Identifying the many nutrients of PN

The macronutrients and micronutrients required by the body to maintain health and metabolic equilibrium are the building blocks of PN. *Macronutrients* include protein (amino acids), carbohydrates (glucose), and lipids (fats). *Micronutrients* include vitamins, minerals, and trace elements, as well as electrolytes and medications. When you mix these ingredients with sterile water or normal saline, the nutritious IV solution accomplishes the three main goals of PN:

- ✔ Prevention of *malnutrition* (a condition that occurs when your body doesn't get enough nutrients)

- ✔ Replenishment of body tissue and restoration of organ function

- ✔ Prevention and correction of *nutritional deficiency* (a condition that occurs when a person's nutrient intake consistently falls below the recommended requirements)

Fortunately for your patients' sake, the basic components of PN can be mixed, matched, and customized to fit each patient's clinical condition and nutritional requirements. Typically, the pharmacy, along with a nutritional support team made up of a registered dietician (RD) and a pharmacist, evaluates the patient's chart and prepares PN solutions based on the patient's nutritional status. The following sections provide more details about the basic components of PN.

Starting with the body's primary building block: Protein

Protein is part of every cell in the body. No other single nutrient plays as significant a role in maintaining health and well-being as protein. After all, the body uses protein to grow and repair all its major structures (bones, muscles, and skin), promote immune function, create enzymes and hormones, and produce energy. Not to mention, protein is essential to maintaining metabolic equilibrium and sustaining life.

Because protein malnutrition is the most common form of malnutrition in hospitalized patients, protein (usually in the form of amino acids) is a central ingredient in many PN solutions. The protein in PN fulfills these major roles:

- ✔ Replaces protein stores depleted by malnutrition

- ✔ Prevents the breakdown of skeletal muscle

- ✔ Increases metabolic nitrogen in order to maintain *nitrogen balance* (the difference between the amount of nitrogen ingested from dietary protein and the amount of nitrogen excreted through the kidneys) in the body

Healthy people need approximately 0.8 grams (g) of protein per kilogram (kg) of body weight per day (g/kg/day), or 8 percent of their total energy requirements, to maintain nitrogen balance. But when patients' bodies are stressed because of illness or surgery, those protein requirements must increase to meet the needs for wound healing, immune function, and nitrogen replacement. Critically ill patients typically need additional protein requirements up to 1.5 to 2.0 g/kg/day. As a result, doctors often prescribe PN solutions that contain enough protein to account for 15 to 20 percent of the patient's total energy requirements immediately following a physical trauma such as surgery.

Higher intake and lower output of nitrogen places patients in a positive nitrogen balance or *anabolic state,* in which the body builds up and stores protein. In contrast, negative nitrogen balance places patients in a *catabolic state,* in which the body breaks down protein and depletes protein stores, leading to protein malnutrition.

Left untreated, protein malnutrition causes a depletion of the body's stores of visceral proteins, which, in turn, leads to muscle breakdown, wasting, and weakening. Find more details on protein depletion in the sidebar "What happens when starvation goes untreated?"

Note: Along with increased protein and nitrogen requirements, critically ill patients also need an increased calorie intake. To increase calories without interfering with nitrogen balance, you need to maintain the optimal calorie-to-nitrogen ratio — 150 carbohydrate calories to 1 g of nitrogen — in PN infusions.

Because PN is individually dosed according to the nutritional needs of each patient and because protein is a major ingredient in PN, special consideration must be made for patients with renal disease or hepatic failure and those on protein-sparing diets.

Energizing the body: Simple and complex carbs

The body digests and converts carbohydrates (often called *carbs*) to *glucose* to provide its primary source of energy. Carbohydrates come in two types:

- ✔ **Simple carbs:** Also called *simple sugars,* these carbs consist of no more than one or two sugars. The body rapidly digests, absorbs, and converts them into energy. Although many simple carbs are sweet treats, such as candy, cola, and syrups, simple carbs also include healthier foods, such as fruit and milk. Unlike candy and cola, simple carbs like fruit and milk contain important nutrients like vitamins, fiber, and calcium, which your body needs to stay healthy.

- ✔ **Complex carbs:** Also known as *starches,* complex carbs are made of three or more linked sugars and take longer than simple carbs to digest, absorb, and convert into energy. You find them in grains, nuts, seeds, and vegetables.

Although complex carbs provide better glucose control and are preferred over simple carbs in regular diets, PN can't use complex carbs because they require breakdown and conversion into simple sugars, which the body does using an enzyme called *amylase.* You find amylase in saliva and pancreatic secretions. Along with the digestive tract, amylase helps break down complex carbs into simple sugars to be absorbed into the bloodstream for energy.

As a result, simple carbs (glucose) are the primary source of calories and nonprotein energy in PN. Glucose is a vital component of PN because it supplies calories, spares protein, is the primary source of energy used by all cell types and organs, and can bypass the digestive tract and go directly into the bloodstream. Glucose is especially essential in PN because it's the only source of energy for the following:

- Brain
- Kidney
- Red blood cells

To satisfy the minimum energy requirements needed by the brain and central nervous system, PN must provide 150 to 200 g of glucose, infused at a rate of no more than 5 to 7 milligrams per kg per min (mg/kg/min). Optimum glucose oxidation and effectiveness are achieved with 5 to 7 g/kg/day. Exceeding these amounts may result in conversion of excess glucose into fat, stressing the body by requiring more energy and oxygen to metabolize fat.

Note: In patients with diabetes, hyperglycemia, or critical illness, the maximum glucose usually doesn't exceed 4 g/kg/day.

Providing calorie-dense nutrients: Lipids

Lipids, also called *intravenous fat emulsions* (IVFEs), are created when fats and oils are suspended within each other. They're second to glucose in providing the highest source of nonprotein calories, typically providing 20 to 30 percent of PN-supplied nonprotein calories, although they may supply as many as 50 percent of nonprotein calories when dictated by the patient's condition. IVFEs offer an isotonic, calorie-dense energy source that can be delivered alone or with glucose and amino acids. When delivered alone, IVFEs provide energy without glucose, decreasing the need for insulin in patients on PN.

In PN, lipids have the following key roles:

- To provide life-supporting *fatty acids,* which contain nutrients that maintain the health of the *cellular membrane,* a structure that regulates everything that enters and leaves the cell

✔ To provide nonprotein calories that convert into energy, regulate inflammation-producing hormones in the system, and promote cardiac and circulatory system health

✔ To prevent *fatty acid deficiency,* which, if left untreated, can cause abnormal liver function values, arthritic changes and cardiac disease, delayed wound healing and impaired immune function, and decreased blood platelets

The body synthesizes many fatty acids, but certain fatty acids, known as *essential fatty acids,* must be either ingested or supplied as IVFEs via nutritional support therapy — that is, PN. The two essential fatty acids that patients whose nutritional statuses have been compromised by disease or surgery need to get through PN are

✔ Linoleic acid or omega-6

✔ Alpha-linoleic acid or omega-3

Most IVFEs contain enough omega-6 to cover 1 to 2 percent of a patient's daily energy requirements and enough omega-3 to cover 0.5 percent of the patient's daily energy requirements. In ICU or critically ill patients, it's recommended to provide 9 to 12 g/day of omega-6 and 1 to 3 g/day of omega-3.

Most IVFEs are administered slowly through piggyback infusions. Piggyback infusion enables lipids to enter the distal section of IV tubing, minimizing interaction with amino acids and dextrose in the primary PN mixture. Piggyback infusions are also hung higher, preventing backup of fat emulsions into the primary IV line. See Chapter 3 for details on piggyback infusions.

Patients tend to tolerate IVFEs better when they're infused slowly, not exceeding 1.7 mg/kg/min. Fast lipid infusions are associated with pulmonary problems and impaired immune function. In addition to these adverse reactions from rapid infusion of lipids, other reactions to IVFEs include the following:

✔ Allergic reactions

✔ Altered inflammatory responses

✔ Increased triglyceride levels

✔ PN-associated liver disease (PNALD)

Egg-product emulsifiers cause most allergic reactions related to IVFEs, but not all IVFEs are egg-product produced. To avoid allergic reactions, be sure to ask your patient whether they're allergic to eggs before administering IVFEs.

Hospital pharmacies prepare many of the IVFEs you use in PN, but several different formulations are available commercially. A few of the most common commercially prepared IVFEs include

- Soybean-based emulsions (called *long-chain triglycerides* or LCTs)
- Soybean, fish, and olive oil (omega-9) oil emulsions
- Soybean and safflower oil emulsions
- Soybean and medium-chain triglyceride oils, such as coconut oil
- Triglyceride mixtures made of fatty acids with varying chain lengths

Pointing out the two types of PN

PN comes in two types, depending on how many nutrients it provides and how you administer it:

- **Total parenteral nutrition (TPN):** TPN is IV nutrition for patients who can't tolerate or metabolize nutrients from any other source. TPN provides all of a patient's fluid, macronutrient, and micronutrient requirements. You usually administer TPN to patients with a longstanding history or a severe degree of nutritional deficit. It's intended for use in patients who require nutritional support for more than seven to ten days.

  Because TPN is the sole source of nutrient requirements for the patient, it contains much higher concentrations of nutrients than peripheral parenteral nutrition (see the next bullet point) and must be administered through a large central venous line. For this reason, TPN poses greater risk for serious complications than nutrition administration through a peripheral line. We cover the complications associated with central lines in Chapter 13.

- **Peripheral parenteral nutrition (PPN):** Also called *partial parenteral nutrition,* PPN delivers only a portion of a patient's daily required nutrients and is administered through a peripheral IV. PPN is intended for short-term use as a nutritional supplement to other forms of nutrition, such as oral, enteral, or nasogastric feedings.

  PPN contains macronutrients and micronutrients that are similar to the ones in TPN, but the concentrations are much lower because it's not the sole source of the patient's nutrition. When patients require higher concentrations of nutrients over longer periods of time, you should switch from PPN to TPN through a central line.

Creating a Balanced PN Recipe for Success

PN solutions typically can be customized for individual patients in hospital pharmacies, but in many cases, you can meet the patient's nutritional needs with a premade formulation that contains standard concentrations of macronutrients and micronutrients.

Whether you're infusing a premade solution or a customized version, ensuring that the macronutrients and micronutrients meet the energy, protein, and fatty-acid needs of the patient, without exceeding the recommended maximum daily intake, is the key to creating a successful, balanced recipe for PN.

Incorporating the main ingredients

Macronutrients, such as protein, carbohydrates, and lipids, form the basis for all PPN and TPN formulations. Micronutrients, such as vitamins, minerals, and electrolytes, round out the nutrients needed to meet daily energy requirements.

Adding in some protein, carbs, and lipids

Protein requirements for patients who are receiving PN therapy usually start out at 0.83 g/kg/day. Requirements may increase because of stress, injury, or other factors, but the daily intake shouldn't exceed 2.5 g/kg/day.

As we mention earlier in this chapter, carbohydrates provide the major energy source in PN. Hence, glucose or dextrose usually provides 50 to 70 percent of daily nonprotein calories, or approximately 1,000 to 1,600 calories per day. Because a typical liter of 5 percent dextrose in water contains only 170 calories, glucose concentrations of 10 to 70 percent are typical in parenteral formulations. However, glucose should reach a final diluted concentration of no more than 10 percent for peripheral infusions and no more than 35 percent for central venous infusions.

Lipid emulsions supply essential fatty acids and a significant portion of daily requirements of nonprotein energy. (Check out the earlier section "Providing calorie-dense nutrients: Lipids" for more on lipid requirements.)

Garnishing with a pinch of vitamins and minerals

Vitamins and minerals are important micronutrients in PN solutions because they help maintain normal metabolism, cellular function, and musculoskeletal health. Just how many vitamins and minerals are added to any PN mixture depends on the patient's degree of illness and energy requirements.

The vitamins most commonly used in PN include

- **Vitamin A:** Works as an antioxidant to help maintain vision as well as skin, bone, and epithelial cell health
- **Vitamin B-1 (thiamine):** Plays a key role in the metabolic process of creating energy through carbohydrate digestion
- **Vitamin B-2 (riboflavin):** Plays a key role in the body's metabolism of fats, carbohydrates, and protein and in the maintenance of red blood cell health
- **Vitamin B-3 (niacinamide):** Improves the circulatory system and decreases cholesterol
- **Vitamin B-5 (pantothenic acid):** Helps retrieve energy from nutrition and improves immune function
- **Vitamin B-6 (pyridoxine):** Plays an essential role in the synthesis of amino acids (the building blocks of protein)
- **Vitamin B-9 (folic acid):** Plays a necessary role in the synthesis of DNA and RNA, which play a part in the reproduction of all body cells
- **Vitamin B-12 (cobalamin):** Aids in the formation and regeneration of red blood cells
- **Biotin (a B vitamin):** Works with other B vitamins to synthesize and utilize protein
- **Vitamin C (ascorbic acid):** Improves protein synthesis, antioxidant activity, plaque repression, and immune system function
- **Vitamin D:** Works with sunlight exposure to promote calcium absorption and maintain bone health
- **Vitamin E:** Provides antioxidant activities that destroy free radicals and improve cardiovascular health
- **Vitamin K:** Plays an essential role in producing blood clot formation

In addition to vitamins, PN commonly includes the following major minerals:

- **Calcium:** Promotes and maintains bone and muscle health
- **Magnesium:** Plays an essential role in the synthesis of protein, fat, and nucleic acid
- **Potassium:** Plays a key role in the overall health of body cells and tissues
- **Sodium:** Regulates the transmission of fluid into and out of the body's cells and determines the total amount of water in the body

Other minerals, such as chromium, selenium, and iodine, are known as *minor minerals* or *trace elements* and are used sparingly in nutritional support.

Note: Minerals that carry an electric charge are known as electrolytes. Minerals such as calcium, potassium, and sodium are also electrolytes and help balance and maintain the body's blood chemistry. See the next section for details.

Seasoning with a spark of electrolytes

Electrolytes are micronutrient components of PN that are essential to maintaining biochemical equilibrium within the body. They're usually added to PN after labs are drawn to get a baseline for each patient. The most common electrolytes used in PN include the following:

- ✔ Calcium
- ✔ Chloride
- ✔ Potassium
- ✔ Sodium

Daily monitoring of electrolytes is essential for patients on PN because their micronutrient levels (including those of electrolytes) fluctuate depending on changing cellular needs caused by disease and stress. By monitoring electrolytes with daily lab results, electrolyte dosing can be adjusted to match the patient's changing needs for replacement.

Moistening the mix with fluids

Fluids, usually in the form of sterile water or physiologic saline with dextrose, are essential components in any PN solution because they provide the liquid medium for IV delivery of nutrients and hydration. After all, average adults require approximately 2,450 milliliters (mL) of liquid per day to maintain proper hydration and fluid and electrolyte balance (see Chapter 7 for details).

When you're administering standard or commercially prepared PN solutions, subtract the volume of PN solution from the daily fluid requirement of 2,450 mL. The difference is the amount of fluid or sterile water that needs to be added to the PN solution. Refer to product instructions and prescribing information for infusion recommendations. For more details, check out Chapter 18.

Keep in mind that patients with fever, fistulas, vomiting and diarrhea, and nasogastric suction have increased fluid requirements and must be closely monitored for fluid loss and dehydration. In contrast, patients with renal failure, congestive heart failure, ascites, and pulmonary disease have reduced fluid requirements and must be monitored for fluid overload. In either clinical situation, make sure you report any signs of dehydration or fluid overload to the attending physician.

Mixing in a little medication

Patients who require PN also usually require medications. As a result, most successful nutritional support plans include medications that address the underlying illness causing the patient's malnutrition.

The primary difficulty you face when administering medications with PN is the potential for drug interactions. Some medications are compatible with nutritional products, but others cause serious drug interactions. Multiple-lumen vascular access devices (VADs) alleviate some of the problem by allowing medication administration through one port and PN administration through another, but the potential for drug interactions remains high.

When administering medications with PN, you must know which medications are compatible and which medications aren't. To further minimize risk for interactions, refer to medication tables that identify known drug incompatibilities with 2-in-1 and 3-in-1 nutrition *admixtures* (mixtures of ingredients), the manufacturer's instructions for use, and your institution's guidelines for PN/medication administration. Be sure to consult the pharmacist if you still have questions.

Preparing the finished product

The finished PN is usually prepared by trained personnel, using laminar-flow equipment and strict adherence to aseptic technique. All admixtures are prepared according to guidelines for preparation, storage, quality assurance, and other safe-practice recommendations found in the National Advisory Group on Standards and Practices Guidelines for Parenteral Nutrition.

To ensure patient safety and to optimize patient outcomes, refer to these guidelines or your institution's standardized protocols whenever you administer PN products.

Part III

Getting Down to IV Therapy Business

The 5th Wave   By Rich Tennant

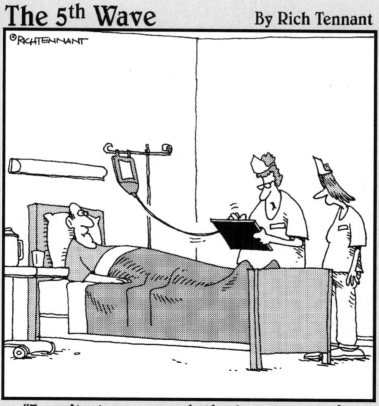

"I can't stress enough the importance of documenting everything."

In this part . . .

Part III covers some of the most essential components of IV therapy. It starts by discussing the importance of accurately documenting your actions throughout the infusion process. Then it breaks down IV dosing and flow rates into simple, easy-to-understand calculations and introduces you to infusion pump technology and other methods of delivering IV therapy. Next, it walks you through the steps of starting, monitoring, and discontinuing a peripheral IV line. Finally, this part describes the aseptic techniques associated with central vascular access devices and explains the critical role that IV nurses play in preventing bloodstream infections.

Chapter 9

Documenting Diligently: The Backbone of Infusion Therapy

....

....

An old saying among nurses goes something like this: "If it wasn't documented, it wasn't done." Not only does accurate documentation keep you out of the courtroom, but it also contributes to continuity of care and gives insurance companies the information they need to reimburse for payment. Not all documentation is created equal, however, especially in the eyes of the law. Because sloppy documentation draws attention to the possibility of error, it's important that your documentation rises above the rest. In other words, you need to be fully aware of the information you include in the medical record and make sure you completely document essential facts that are pertinent to patient care.

But let's face it: Documentation is tedious. You didn't get into healthcare to spend the entire day documenting. Nor did you enter a caring profession to care little for your patients, which sometimes happens because you're too busy documenting. In truth, documentation in healthcare is like paying taxes — there's no getting around it. What makes it tolerable is knowing that diligent documentation is the backbone of your practice. It speaks loudly to the prudent actions you take to lead your patients to successful outcomes.

In this chapter, we give you a recipe for success in documentation. We tell you why accurate documentation matters and how you can make your documentation as comprehensive as possible. Finally, we give you some basic guidelines on how to document all aspects of intravenous (IV) therapy, including the insertion, your ongoing monitoring, and the discontinuation of the vascular access device (VAD), the central vascular access device (CVAD), and the IV infusion itself.

Seeing Why Accurate Documentation Matters

Accurate documentation provides a clear, concise, permanent record of what you did, what happened when you did it, and what the outcome was after you did what you did. The following sections explore the four primary reasons that complete and accurate documentation is so important in healthcare.

Improving communication for continuity of care

Documentation acts as a means of communication among all members of the healthcare team, from the healthcare provider in charge to the nursing assistant who takes the patient's vital signs. Not only does accurate documentation help you and other team members provide continuity of care, but it also validates that everyone on the team followed the standard of care specific to his discipline, which is an important part of the patient's overall treatment and legal record.

Consider Mr. Jones, a 79-year-old man who was admitted to the ICU with acute respiratory failure secondary to chronic obstructive pulmonary disease (COPD). He has been intubated, was placed on a ventilator, and is receiving several IV medications, including a *vasopressor,* an agent that causes a rise in blood pressure. During the first few days of his hospitalization, he's being seen not only by nurses but also by the attending physician, the pulmonologist, the respiratory therapist, the physical therapist, and the dietician.

As each team member evaluates Mr. Jones, their documentation, like tiny pieces of a puzzle, reveals the entire clinical picture of the patient. But what if one of the attending nurses omits documentation that a medication was given and another nurse comes along and gives the same medication twice? Imagine the possible consequences this error could have for Mr. Jones. And what if the healthcare provider doesn't document parameters for blood pressure regulation? This could make the titration of Mr. Jones's IV blood pressure medication even more challenging, especially to an inexperienced nurse. Because patient care goes on 24 hours a day, documentation may be the only way in which many of the healthcare team members communicate. This fact alone makes accuracy in documentation even more important.

Acting as your insurance policy: The importance of legal records

Today, protecting yourself — and your license — with proof of competent practice is more important than ever. Precise documentation serves as your insurance policy, protecting you from charges of negligence, the most common form of malpractice. Healthcare professionals on the wrong end of a lawsuit face the loss of their jobs, their licenses, and their personal assets; they may even face possible jail time.

In *Pellerin v. Humedicenters,* failure to document nursing procedures led to an award of more than $90,000 in damages. The plaintiff in the case alleged that the emergency room nurse gave an injection of hydroxyzine (Vistaril) and meperidine (Demerol) via a substandard manner, which resulted in *cutaneous gluteal neuropathy,* a condition caused by nerve damage. Although how the patient attained the injury was never proven, the nurse's failure to document the site and mode of injection was found to reflect care below the usual standard of care, resulting in a breach. Had the nurse documented the site, injection mode, and the patient's response to the injection, she may have kept herself — and the case — out of the courtroom.

Following protocol: Outlining steps to reach successful patient outcomes

The steps you take when performing a specific task should comply with agency protocol and be clearly outlined in your documentation. Your documentation is proof-positive that you followed agency protocol, which is generally based on the legal standard of care designed to protect your patient against medical errors.

For example, the Infusion Nurses Society (INS) states that, in general, if a nurse administers a blood transfusion, the blood must be verified at the patient's bedside in the presence of another qualified clinician. This means checking and rechecking the blood by

- Asking the patient's full name and date of birth and verifying the armband and the medical record number, especially if the patient is unable to respond

- Checking the order, blood type, Rh group, expiration date, and blood unit number

- Observing the blood for any abnormalities (such as clumping or gas bubbles) and returning it to blood bank if you notice any issues

Following protocol and documenting each step of the transfusion process ensures that the nurse won't be found negligent if the patient suffers injury and the case is eventually litigated.

Providing info necessary for insurance reimbursement

Many insurance companies, including Medicare, reimburse for costs based on patient outcomes. As a result, patient care that results in outcomes that negatively impact the patient often leads to little or no reimbursement. Proper documentation provides insurance companies with justification as to why specific medical services are necessary and protects the patient from having to assume financial responsibility if a claim is denied.

Consider Tim, a day-shift nurse who admits a morbidly obese female to his floor. On the initial assessment, he neglects to do a skin check. He asks the patient whether she has any wounds, and the patient says no. In truth, the patient has a Stage II decubitus ulcer that she can't yet feel because of her obesity and poor health. When the admitting nurse gets to the part of the health assessment that asks about wounds, he checks the box that says the skin appears normal. The next nurse comes in and she, too, fails to do a skin check or document that the skin is abnormal. This continues for a week or so, until finally on your shift, the patient begins to complain that her backside is sore. You turn her on her side and notice that, indeed, she now has a Stage III decubitus. You look through the chart and find that nothing has been previously documented. You notify the physician and he orders wound care. Who do you think is going to pay for the wound care supplies and any other important care or equipment that may be needed for the wound? The hospital! Because the nurse didn't document the wound on the initial assessment or during subsequent assessments, Medicare and other insurance companies aren't likely to reimburse the hospital, because existing documentation doesn't support that the patient had the wound upon entering the hospital.

Making Your Documentation Rise above the Rest

The Infusion Nurses Society (INS) has set a standard of care for documentation before, during, and after infusion therapy. Your mission, if you choose to accept it, is to incorporate the following principles into your documentation as you chart throughout the day.

Just the facts: Keeping it accurate and focused

In order for your infusion therapy documentation to be accurate, it must be factual. This means your documentation should contain objective data based on reality, not personal opinion, though subjective data that's supplied by the patient is also important to include in your charting. Just keep in mind that writing down what the patient actually says rather than rephrasing it in your own words is generally a better approach.

What should you include in your documentation to make it more accurate? As a general rule, be sure to incorporate the following:

- ✔ Factual information about your patient's condition, diagnosis, and primary complaint
- ✔ The actions you took before, during, and after treatment
- ✔ Your patient's response to the treatment provided
- ✔ Your continued plan of care

When documenting, try to keep your focus. Refrain from including opinion or negative comments about your patient. If you discontinue a peripheral IV, base your documentation on what actually happened during the procedure, not on how rude your patient was when you removed the tape from her arm. If you tried to start an IV on a patient who was refusing it, stick to the facts and not that she called you every name in the book when you tried to approach her. Legally, however, you can quote what the patient stated if you feel it's necessary to protect yourself or to further explain your actions.

At no time should you use your documentation as a coverup or to demonstrate that you provided care that you didn't actually give. If you make a mistake, check with your organizations' risk management team and policies and procedures manual to find out how to handle the incident. Generally, mistakes in patient care are documented in a separate occurrence report, not added to the patient's chart.

Making it complete

Before you push yourself away from the computer or put down your pen and call it a day, ask yourself whether your documentation is complete and has the ability to stand alone. Anyone reading it should be able to get a clear picture of what you observed, what treatment you provided, and how the patient responded to the treatment.

If you infuse a medication that results in patient injury and neglect to document the precise steps you took before, during, and after the infusion — identifying your patient; verifying allergies; obtaining baseline vitals; identifying the drug, dose, rate, time, and method of administration; and noting the patient's response to treatment — you could face serious legal consequences.

Ensuring it's legible and correcting writing mistakes

Despite the advent of computer technology, a wealth of handwritten information remains part of a patient's medical record. In fact, poorly written medical documents are becoming increasingly popular as the basis for litigation. Your handwriting should be legible no matter what you're documenting — from the way you label your IV site down to the signature following your clinical notes.

Check with organizational policies and procedures to determine how to handle errors in patient charting. If you make an incorrect entry in the medical record, never erase it or use correction fluid to cover it up. Most organizations want you to draw a single line through the incorrect entry, initial it, and then continue with the correction immediately after the word or phrase that you crossed out. Avoid crossing out a word and writing *error* or *mistake* above it; this is a red flag for savvy litigators, even if no actual mistake was made in patient care.

Building on timeliness

Lawyers in malpractice cases often use the documented time of treatment to determine whether the healthcare professional acted judiciously and in a timely manner based on the standard of care. Keeping legal issues in mind, you should make entries to the patient record in real time, as you go along, not at the end of the day, hours after you've completed a task. Include the date and time with every entry and accurately record the sequence of events. Sometimes, however, a late entry is necessary. In such cases, be sure to follow your agency's policies and procedures on how to document late entries in the medical record, bearing in mind that excessive late entries may draw negative attention to your documentation if patient care is ever questioned.

Make sure your documentation accurately reflects when you gave a medication. Most hospitals and other healthcare organizations give you a window of time in which to give your medications. Never document that you gave a medication at a time in which you did not to hide the fact that you were late (or early) in administering it.

Making sure it's accessible and easily retrievable

More and more healthcare organizations are switching to electronic health records. Not only is an electronic record more secure than paper charts, but it reduces medical errors, eliminates excess paperwork, is far more legible, and allows patient data to be readily accessible and easily retrievable.

When a patient suffering from cardiopulmonary arrest is brought to the ICU from another unit, what would happen if the nurse accompanying her was unable to find the chart and knew little about the patient because she just started her shift and didn't get an adequate report? Fortunately, this type of scenario seldom takes place when organizations use electronic charting, because patient data is just a click away and easily retrievable to all who require access to it.

If your organization has not yet made the switch, your documentation should still comply with these principles. That said, always make sure that you keep patient data in the patient's chart, where anyone involved in patient care can have access to it.

Putting It into Practice: Documenting IV Therapy

Now that you know why accurate documentation matters in healthcare and how principles of good documentation can help protect you and the agency you work for, you need to know how to apply all this info to what you do in your everyday clinical practice.

The following sections walk you through proper documentation of specific tasks involved in administering IV therapy, including insertion of a VAD, administration of the IV infusion, continued monitoring of the IV site, and removal of a peripheral or central line.

Before you begin

Before you provide infusion therapy, you need to complete a thorough patient assessment to ensure that the device you're using and the treatment you're about to give is appropriate. When documenting your patient assessment, always include pertinent information that describes the following:

- Your patient's primary problem for which you're providing infusion therapy
- Any allergies the patient may have
- The patient's diagnosis
- What you found in your initial and ongoing assessment
- Your patient's baseline vital signs

In addition, be mindful of your organization's policy for documenting IV therapy. To save time and clearly identify trends in patient status, many organizations ask that you chart *by exception,* meaning you chart only events that stray from the norm. Another common form of documentation uses an IV therapy flow sheet like the one shown in Figure 9-1. An IV therapy flow sheet allows you to maintain accurate, ongoing documentation of your IV infusion. Whichever method you use, the goal is to be as thorough as possible so that your documentation accurately reflects what was done.

Anytime you hang IV fluids, electrolytes, or medications, follow your institution's policy and procedures. Standard procedures usually include writing your initials, the date and time of the infusion, and any medications that you add to the infusion on every solution container.

Patient: Mrs. Jones
Dx: L Total Knee Replacement
Venipuncture Limitations: Rt mastectomy; Left arm only
Permanent Access: PICC line inserted 05/01/12 0900

Intravenous care action codes: C = cap; T = tubing; F = filter; D=dressing change

Date/ Time	Initials	IV Volume/ Solution	Additives	Flow Rate	Site	Stop Time	Action	Comments
05/02/12 0900	DL	1000 cc Normal Saline	None	100 ml/hr	LAC	05/02/12 1900	None needed	PICC line insertion site intact; no redness, swelling, or drainage
05/02/12 1900	AS	1000 cc Normal Saline	None	100 ml/hr	LAC	05/03/12 0500	T	PICC line insertion site intact; no redness, swelling, or drainage
05/03/12 0500	WM	1000 cc D5W	20mEq KCL	100 ml/hr	LAC	05/03/12	C, D	PICC line insertion site intact; no redness, swelling, or drainage

Figure 9-1:
An example of an IV therapy flow sheet.

Illustration by Wiley, Composition Services Graphics

The insertion of a peripheral VAD

The insertion of the VAD is one of the most important aspects of infusion therapy. Complications that may arise due to poor insertion techniques include hematoma, infection, infiltration, and thrombophlebitis (see Chapter 12 for details). Using the correct insertion technique each time reduces the risk of complications. If, however, your patient does develop a complication during IV therapy, your documentation should demonstrate that you followed the standard of care throughout all phases of the infusion, starting with the insertion.

When documenting the insertion of a peripheral VAD, include the following details:

- ✔ Site preparation, including the infection-prevention techniques and safety precautions you used
- ✔ Type and gauge of VAD
- ✔ Anatomical location of the insertion site and the vein accessed
- ✔ Use of a local anesthetic (if one was used) and the method of administration
- ✔ Date and time of insertion
- ✔ Number of attempts made, the location of each attempt, and the vein attempted
- ✔ Stabilization technique (for example, tape or other stabilization device)
- ✔ Type of dressing
- ✔ How the device functioned after the insertion (for example, whether it flushed easily and whether you got a blood return)
- ✔ What, if any, complications occurred and the steps you took to intervene
- ✔ Your patient's response to treatment
- ✔ Education offered to the patient and/or the primary caregiver and his understanding of what you taught him

Always clearly label the dressing on the catheter insertion site with your initials, the date, and the time of the insertion.

The administration of the infusion

You'll most likely administer IV therapy after you insert your VAD, unless a saline lock has been ordered. Here are some suggestions of what to include in your documentation of IV therapy administration:

- Type of drug, dose, and rate of administration
- Method of administration (for example, primary and secondary continuous infusion or primary intermittent infusion)
- Which drug or solution is going in which pathway (when multiple drips are hanging simultaneously or the patient has more than one VAD)
- Laboratory results pertinent to the infusion
- What, if any, complications occurred and the steps you took to intervene
- Your patient's response to treatment
- Education offered to the patient and/or the primary caregiver and his understanding of what you taught him

The ongoing monitoring of the site

The insertion of the VAD is often the most difficult part of IV therapy. But equally important is the ongoing monitoring of the IV site and your documentation showing that you're keeping a close eye on it. When documenting your monitoring of the IV site, be sure to include the following information:

- The reason for the continuing need for the device
- The condition of the site, dressing, and/or stabilization device
- Whether or not you performed a dressing change and what steps you took to perform it
- Any site care that you did
- Tubing or solution changes that you made
- What, if any, complications occurred and the steps you took to intervene
- Your patient's response to treatment
- Education offered to the patient and/or the primary caregiver and his understanding of what you taught him

The removal of the device

Documenting removal of a peripheral or central line is an essential part of completing the procedure. After you receive the required doctor's order to remove a VAD or CVAD, remove the device according to facility protocol or INS standards and include the following information in your documentation:

- Date and time of the removal
- Position of patient (if removing a CVAD)
- Location of the site
- Condition of the site
- Integrity of the device (that is, was it intact?)
- Reason for the removal of the device (such as discontinuation of therapy, infiltration, phlebitis, or infection)
- Interventions applied during the removal (such as applying pressure to stop bleeding)
- Type of dressing (such as gauze or pressure dressing)
- What, if any, complications occurred and the steps you took to intervene
- Your patient's response to the procedure
- Education you provided to the patient and/or caregiver and his understanding of what you taught him

Chapter 10

Calculation Central: Figuring Drug Dosages, Drips, and Flow Rates

In This Chapter

▶ Getting to know different calculation methods

▶ Calculating drip rates, flow rates, infusion times, and total volumes

*M*ention the word *math* and many nurses turn on their heels and run. But math is an integral part of healthcare, and one of its most critical uses is in calculating medication and fluid dosages in IV therapy.

Fortunately, you can use the same simple math principles you use to get a patient's heart rate (by counting the patient's pulse for 15 seconds and multiplying by 4) to solve seemingly complex dosage calculations. To help you get started, this chapter reviews the metric system and some basic math computation skills. Then it introduces you to two different calculation methods for dosing — the formula method and the ratio-proportion method. Finally, it shows you how to calculate drips and flow rates and provides you with real-life dosing scenarios to help you put all your new skills to work.

Calculating Correct Drug Dosages

Calculating drug dosages correctly is one of the most critical steps in preparing medications for administration because correct calculations help prevent medication errors. After all, calculation mistakes account for most drug errors.

To minimize calculation errors, you must possess the basic math skills of addition, subtraction, multiplication, and long division. In addition, you need to know how to do simple unit conversions and how to use two different methods for calculating dosages. Lucky for you, this section covers the types of conversions and calculation methods you'll use most in your healthcare career.

Understanding the metric system

In the healthcare field, doctors and nurses use metric measurements much more often than standard American units. Consistency is one reason; ease of use is another. The metric system is based on units of ten, which makes doing math calculations fairly simple.

The metric system also uses Latin prefixes that help make its units easy to remember. For example, in the metric system, the Latin prefix *kilo-* always means 1,000. Whether you're measuring 1,000 kilograms (kg) of weight or 1,000 kilometers (km) of distance, kilo- means 1,000. Similarly, the prefix *milli-* means one-thousandth. If you're measuring volume in milliliters (mL), milli- means one-thousandth of a liter (L); if you're measuring weight in milligrams (mg), milli- means one-thousandth of a gram (g).

You need to be very familiar with metric prefixes when doing calculations in IV therapy because you use *kilo*grams to measure patient weight and *milli*liters to measure IV fluids and medications. Table 10-1 lists a few commonly used metric prefixes in IV therapy.

Table 10-1	Common Metric Prefixes in IV Therapy	
Metric Prefix	*Numerical Value*	*In Words*
Kilo-	1,000	One thousand
Deci-	0.1	One-tenth
Centi-	0.01	One-hundredth
Milli-	0.001	One-thousandth
Micro-	0.000001	One-millionth

Because almost all healthcare facilities use the metric system but many Americans still rely on the American system in daily use, nurses and IV therapists frequently have to convert American standard units to metric units, especially when dealing with patient weights.

To convert adult and infant patient weights from American units to their metric equivalents, use the conversion factors listed in Table 10-2 to go from American pounds (lb) to metric grams (g).

Table 10-2	American-to-Metric Conversions
American Standard Measurement	*Metric Measurement*
1 pound	454 grams
1 pound	0.454 kilograms
2.2 pounds	1 kilogram
0.035 ounces	1 gram

Nurses frequently also have to do metric-to-metric conversions to calculate drug doses in IV therapy. Table 10-3 lists the most common conversions you need to know.

Table 10-3	Metric-to-Metric Conversions
Metric Measurement and Abbreviation	*Metric Equivalent and Abbreviation*
1 kilogram (kg)	1,000 grams (g)
1 gram (g)	1,000 milligrams (mg)
1 milligram (mg)	1,000 micrograms (mcg)
1 gram (g)	1 milliliter (mL)
1 cubic centimeter (cc)	1 milliliter (mL)
1 liter (L)	1,000 milliliters (mL)

Using different calculation methods

Calculating medication dosages is one of the most important responsibilities of IV nurses. In this section, we focus on two of the most frequently used calculation methods: the formula method and the ratio-proportion method. Most healthcare professionals routinely use whichever method works best for them. We recommend that you become familiar with both methods so you can decide which one you're more comfortable using. You may find that one method works well in certain situations while the second method works better in other situations.

The formula method

Because of its easy-to-use format, the *formula method* (also called the *equation method*) is the preferred calculation method of many nurses. You can use this method whenever you have three pieces of a puzzle and you're searching for a fourth piece — in many cases, the correct dose. In terms of IV therapy, the formula method enables nurses to calculate doses by using the amount of the prescribed medication and the dose that's available for use.

To use the formula method, set up the following equation:

D (dose) = O (ordered) $\times$ Q (quantity) $\div$ H (have on hand)

Here's a quick look at what the variables in this equation mean:

- ✔ **D (dose):** The desired dose
- ✔ **O (ordered):** The dose ordered by the doctor
- ✔ **Q (quantity):** The quantity listed on the medication label
- ✔ **H (have on hand):** The dose per unit you have on hand, as listed on the medication label

Use the formula method to calculate dosing in the following clinical example:

> Your elderly pneumonia patient spikes a fever and the physician orders cephaloxin (Keflex) 200 mg IV every 6 hours. The drug concentration supplied by the pharmacy is 125 mg per 5 mL. What volume, in mL, do you administer?

To calculate the correct dosage by using the formula method, follow these steps:

1. Set up the following equation:

   D mL = 200 mg (ordered) $\times$ 5 mL (quantity) $\div$ 125 mg (have on hand)

2. Multiply.

   $200 \times 5 = 1{,}000$

3. Divide and solve.

   $1{,}000 \div 125 = 8$ mL

   The mg cancel out, so you're left with mL. The answer is 8 mL. You must administer 8 mL every 6 hours.

The ratio-proportion method

As the name indicates, the *ratio-proportion method* involves two elements: a ratio and a proportion. A *ratio* describes one number as compared to another number, and a *proportion* is an equation that compares two ratios. Together, these two elements form a calculation method that you can use to determine how much medication you need to administer to achieve the dose ordered by the physician.

Like the formula method, the ratio-proportion method is only useful when you have three known pieces of information from the physician's order and one unknown piece — often, the correct dose. Here's what the ratio-proportion structure looks like:

$$\frac{\text{Known equivalent}}{\text{Known equivalent}} = \frac{\text{Known equivalent}}{\text{Unknown equivalent}}$$

The following example can help you practice calculating the correct dosage by using the ratio-proportion method:

> Your pregnant patient is admitted with hypertension and preeclampsia. To prevent seizures, the physician orders magnesium sulfate 2 g IV. Your medication label shows 40 g of magnesium sulfate per 1,000 mL of IV fluid. What volume of fluid, in mL, delivers 2 g?

To solve this problem by using the ratio-proportion method, follow these steps:

1. **Set up the following ratio-proportion:**

   $$\frac{40 \text{ g}}{1,000 \text{ mL}} = \frac{2 \text{ g}}{x \text{ mL}}$$

2. **Cross-multiply.**

   $40x = 2,000$

3. **Divide and solve.**

   $2,000 \div 40 = 50 \text{ mL}$

   The g cancel out, so you're left with mL. The answer is 50 mL. You give 50 mL of fluid to deliver a 2 g dose.

If you're not big on math and you'd rather take a shortcut, you can use a free online calculator, such as the one at www.manuelsweb.com/nrs_calculators.htm.

Practicing dosing calculations

After you know how to use the formula method and ratio-proportion method to do dosage calculations, you have everything you need math wise, at least, to administer medications in a variety of clinical settings ranging from every-day medical-surgical units to critical-care units and emergency rooms. The following sections offer you more practice in both.

Calculating everyday doses

You can use either the ratio-proportion method or the formula method to calculate everyday doses. The following example uses the formula method:

> Your patient's laboratory report shows low potassium and the physician orders potassium chloride (KCl) 25 milliequivalents (mEq) IV piggyback (through a smaller, secondary infusion bag hung at least 6 inches higher than the primary infusion bag). The medication label indicates that 10 mL equal 40 mEq of potassium chloride. How many mL should you put in the piggyback?

To solve this problem, follow these steps:

1. **Set up the following equation:**

   D mL = 25 mEq (ordered) $\times$ 10 mL (quantity) $\div$ 40 mEq (have on hand)

2. **Multiply.**

   $25 \times 10 = 250$

3. **Divide and solve.**

   $250 \div 40 = 6.25$ mL

The mEq cancel out, so you're left with mL. The answer is 6.25 mL. You give 6.25 mL of potassium chloride in the piggyback.

Calculating critical-care doses

Although you can also use the formula method to find the correct dosage in critical-care situations, we use the ratio-proportion method in the following example:

> Your patient is admitted to critical care with congestive heart failure, and the physician orders furosemide (Lasix) 40 mg IV stat. The drug label reads 10 mg/mL. How many mL do you administer?

To solve this common critical-care problem, follow these steps:

1. **Set up the following ratio-proportion:**

   $$\frac{10 \text{ mg}}{1 \text{ mL}} = \frac{40 \text{ mg}}{x \text{ mL}}$$

2. **Cross-multiply.**

   $10x = 40$

3. **Divide and solve.**

   40 ÷ 10 = 4 mL

   The mg cancel out, so you're left with mL. The answer is 4 mL. You administer 4 mL of furosemide.

Going with the Flow: Calculating Drip Rates, Flow Rates, and Infusion Times

Working in healthcare presents many challenges, but few of them are as critical to patient care as calculating the correct drip and flow rates for IV medications and fluids. Fortunately, calculating flow rates is easier to do with help from pharmacies and infusion pumps. However, when the pharmacy is closed and the infusion pumps are all in use, you're responsible for calculating the correct drip and flow rates.

Using drop factors to calculate drip rate

The *drip rate* is a measurement of flow in drops per minute (abbreviated gtt/min or dpm).The drip rate depends on the *drop factor,* which is the number of drops in 1 mL used in IV fluid administration, and the drop factor depends on the size of the IV tubing and drip chamber being used. Drop factors are larger in macrodrip tubing sets than in microdrip tubing sets (see Chapter 3 for details on the differences between these two sets):

- **Macrodrip tubing:** The drop factor in macro IV sets is approximately 10 to 20 gtt/mL; they're used for IV fluid being administered in amounts greater than 100 mL per hour.

- **Microdrip tubing:** The drop factor in micro IV sets is 60 gtt/mL; they're used for fluid deliveries that are less than 100 mL per hour. Microdrips are delivered through a small microdripper tube that's inserted at the top of the drip chamber.

You don't see drop factors and drip rates as frequently in modern healthcare as you used to because infusion pumps help nurses program rates and flows. But knowing how to manually calculate rates is still important; after all, you need to know how to meet your patient's IV needs when pumps aren't available.

To manually calculate drip rate, use this equation:

Drip rate (gtt/min) = Fluid amount (mL) × Drop factor (gtt/mL) ÷ Infusion time (min)

Here's an example to help you practice calculating drip rates:

You have to administer 1,000 mL of fluid at 20 gtt/min over 12 hours. What's the drip rate in gtt/min?

Follow these steps to solve this problem:

1. **Set up the following equation:**

   Drip rate (gtt/min) = 1,000 mL × 20 gtt/mL ÷ 720 min

   Notice that you have to convert the total infusion time from hours to minutes so that all your units match up: 12 hr × 60 min/hr = 720 min.

2. **Multiply, divide, and solve.**

   1,000 mL × 20 gtt/mL ÷ 720 min = 27.78 gtt/min

   Note that mL drop out of the equation. So the drip rate is 27.78 gtt/min.

Using two different methods to calculate flow rates

Flow rate is the amount of IV fluid that you deliver to a patient over a specified period of time. Physician's orders sometimes prescribe specific flow rates, but frequently you have to calculate them yourself. The following sections introduce you to the basic flow-rate formula and show you how to use the ratio-proportion method as an easy alternative.

Understanding the basic flow-rate formula

To calculate flow rate, you can simply use the following formula:

Flow rate (mL/hr) = Total volume (mL) ÷ Specified time (hr)

To put this formula to the test, try out this example problem:

Your patient's culture report comes back from the laboratory showing sensitivity to the antibiotic levofloxacin (Levaquin), so the physician orders levofloxacin 750 mg in 150 mL of dextrose 5 percent in water over 90 minutes. The medication label shows 750 mg/mL. What's the flow rate in mL/hr?

To calculate the flow rate, follow these steps:

1. **Set up the following equation:**

   Flow rate (mL/hr) = 150 mL ÷ 1.5 hr

   Remember to convert the total infusion time from minutes to hours so that all your units match up: 90 min ÷ 60 min/hr = 1.5 hr.

2. **Divide and solve.**

   150 mL ÷ 1.5 hr = 100 mL/hr

   The flow rate is 100 mL/hr.

Using the ratio-proportion method

You can also use the ratio-proportion method to calculate flow rate. Here's an example:

> Your patient is a marathon runner who's admitted to the emergency department with symptoms of heat exhaustion and dehydration. The physician orders 500 mL of 0.9 percent sodium chloride delivered IV over 2 hours. What's the flow rate in mL/hr?

To calculate the flow rate by using the ratio-proportion method, follow these steps:

1. **Set up the following ratio-proportion:**

   $$\frac{2 \text{ hr}}{500 \text{ mL}} = \frac{1 \text{ hr}}{x \text{ mL}}$$

2. **Cross-multiply.**

   $2x = 500$

3. **Divide and solve.**

   500 ÷ 2 = 250 mL

   The hr cancel out, so you're left with mL. The answer is 250 mL/hr for 2 hours.

Using the flow-rate formula to calculate infusion time and total volume

Perhaps the best part about the flow-rate formula that we describe in the section "Understanding the basic flow-rate formula" is its versatility. Not only can you use it to calculate flow rate, but you can also use it to calculate the other two pieces of the equation: infusion time and total volume. All you have to do is move a few things around:

Flow rate (mL/hr) = Total volume (mL) ÷ Infusion time (hr)

Infusion time (hr) = Total volume (mL) ÷ Flow rate (mL/hr)

Total volume (mL) = Flow rate (mL/hr) × Infusion time (hr)

To practice calculating infusion times, consider this example:

> Your patient is being prepped for surgery. The physician orders prophy-
> lactic IV cefazolin (Ancef) 250 mL piggyback to be administered at 60 mL/
> hr immediately preceding surgery. What's the infusion time?

To calculate infusion time, follow these steps:

1. **Set up the following equation:**

   Infusion time (hr) = 250 mL ÷ 60 mL/hr

2. **Divide and solve.**

   250 mL ÷ 60 mL/hr = 4.16 hr

The infusion time is 4.16 hours. Therefore, you must start the infusion
at least 4 hours prior to surgery to administer the prescribed dosage in
time.

Ready to try your hand at a total volume problem? Consider this example:

> Your patient is admitted to the emergency room with heatstroke and
> dehydration, and you need to administer 0.9 percent saline at 125 mL/hr
> over 2 hours. What's the total volume to be infused?

Follow these steps to find the total volume:

1. **Set up the following equation:**

   Total volume (mL) = 125 mL/hr × 2 hr

2. **Multiply and solve.**

   125 mL/hr × 2 hr = 250 mL

The total volume is 250 mL.

Chapter 11

Gravity, Pumps, and Syringes: The Many Ways to Deliver IV Therapy

....

....

*W*hen it comes to intravenous (IV) therapy, one size doesn't fit all. IV therapists rely on several different methods of delivery and several different types of equipment to administer today's increasingly sophisticated medication regimens to their patients. This chapter introduces you to the methods, modes, and machines most commonly used in administering modern IV therapy.

Flowing with an Invisible Force: Gravity-Fed Infusions

Sir Isaac Newton discovered *gravity* three centuries ago when he identified the invisible force that causes apples to fall from trees. When you fast-forward to contemporary medicine, although electronic infusion pumps are the more common choice today (see the next section for details), Newton's invisible force is still at work in some facilities, infusing medications and fluids and saving lives one drop at a time.

But even though gravity-fed infusions are still used today, they're the least accurate method of infusion. The accuracy of flow rates and medication dosages with gravity-fed infusions depends on many factors, including the elasticity and reliability of IV tubings, the sensitivity of adjustable roller clamps, limb position, the size of the vein, venous pressure, the height of the fluid bag, and the number of adjustments needed to maintain flow rates. To improve accuracy rates and reduce the need for frequent roller clamp adjustment, you can use several types of mechanical regulators to maintain constant infusion flow rates. Two of the most common regulators are

- ✔ **Independent flow regulators:** Independent flow regulators attach externally to IV tubing, allowing nurses to adjust flow rate by narrowing or enlarging the flow channel within the regulator. A couple of examples are a flow control screw clamp (which clamps onto the tubing while a screw compresses the tubing to adjust the flow) and a flow regulator (which is a dial that clamps onto the tubing and closes down the tubing as the dial spins to the corresponding number to adjust the flow rate).

- ✔ **Inline flow regulators:** Inline flow regulators are integrated into IV tubing sets; they have external regulator dials to set and adjust flow rates. Some examples are the Rate Flow Regulators (B. Braun USA) and the Exadrop (B. Braun Melsungen AG).

Flow regulators help improve accuracy rates to some extent, but gravity-fed infusions still require somewhat frequent adjustments by nurses. Significant improvement in flow rate accuracy didn't occur until the introduction of the electronic IV pump (a medical device used to deliver fluids into a patient's body in a controlled manner).

Optimizing Therapy with IV Pumps

The earliest automated infusion pumps were developed in the early 1960s, and since then, electronic IV pumps have continued to improve the accuracy of medication dosage and fluid delivery and to relieve nurses of frequent adjusting and constant monitoring of gravity-fed infusion sets. Another great benefit of electronic IV pumps is that they improve and optimize patient safety by alerting personnel to IV line complications and by decreasing the number of medication errors.

Per INS standards, you shouldn't rely on an electronic infusion device to detect infiltration or extravasation because the pump's safety alarms aren't intended to detect disruption of fluid flow.

In the following sections, we go over the two main types of infusions done with electronic pumps — continuous and intermittent — and we introduce the newest member on the automatic pump block: the smart pump.

Administering by continuous infusion

Administering fluids and medications by *continuous infusion* means that you deliver them at a constant rate, one drop at a time. To administer by continuous infusion, IV pumps use small pulses delivered at periodic intervals to infuse a specific volume of medication or fluid over a designated period of time. Also known as *continuous-rate infusions,* continuous infusions with an IV pump achieve steady-state concentrations of medication, ensure constant exposure to the drug over a prolonged time, and provide a continuous infusion of IV fluids. (In case you're wondering, *steady-state concentration* refers to the pharmacological equilibrium achieved when the rate of administration of a medication is equal to the rate of elimination of the medication.)

One of the main benefits of continuous-rate infusions with an IV pump is that they produce a steady-state level of medication in the bloodstream without the peaks and valleys associated with intermittent drug administration (see the next section). They also give a steady flow of fluids to maintain constant hemodynamics within the body.

Nurses commonly use continuous-rate infusions for a wide variety of IV therapies, including

- ✔ Analgesics and narcotics in pain-control therapy
- ✔ Fluid and electrolyte therapy
- ✔ Insulin or diabetic management therapy
- ✔ Sedation during and after surgery
- ✔ Parenteral nutrition therapy

Delivering intermittent IV therapy

In contrast to continuous therapy, *intermittent infusions* deliver medications or fluids at specific times and at designated intervals during a 24-hour period. Because they deliver a small volume of fluid or dosage of medication over a shorter period of time, they usually do so at a higher flow rate. Nurses commonly use intermittent infusions for delivering medications such as antibiotics that have to be given at certain times and in certain doses and that don't require additional fluid, which could cause fluid overload.

IV pumps that you use for intermittent infusions are programmed to perform the following functions:

- Administer prescribed medication doses at prescribed times.
- Administer doses at increased flow rates and specific intervals.
- Return to low, keep-vein-open flow rates between intermittent doses.

Nurses deliver medications and fluids intermittently in a variety of ways, including by piggyback, saline locks, and volume-control burettes.

Delivering by piggyback

When you first hear the term *piggyback,* you may think of a fun ride on the back or shoulders of a parent or friend. In IV therapy, however, *piggyback* refers to something entirely different — a smaller, secondary infusion bag that hangs on the IV pole at a position at least 6 inches higher than the primary infusion bag. Because the piggyback is in a higher position, gravity infuses the piggyback solution first and then allows the primary infusion to continue.

Piggybacks deliver a small volume of fluid or dosage of medication over a short period of time. They're used to deliver intermittent medications. When a piggyback solution is finished, the primary infusion resumes flow, reducing the possibility for empty-bag air embolism.

Nurses frequently use piggyback infusions, sometimes abbreviated *IVPBs,* for delivering an assortment of IV medications and therapies, which may include

- Lipid emulsions
- Medications such as antibiotics and electrolytes
- Vitamins and hormones

Using saline locks

Another device that nurses use for delivering intermittent infusions is the *saline lock,* a short, indwelling peripheral VAD that's sealed to prevent venous backflow. It contains an injection port that nurses can access for periodic IV drug therapy or fluid therapy and blood draws. Saline locks are extremely beneficial for intermittent drug therapy, enabling the patient to be ambulatory without an infusion bag.

Sometimes called *heparin locks,* saline locks are inserted peripherally, secured with tape or a stabilization device, and flushed routinely to keep the catheter patent. Nurses commonly use them for the following types of IV therapies:

- ✔ Conversion from continuous to intermittent IV therapy
- ✔ Intermittent fluid administration
- ✔ Intermittent, frequent medication administration
- ✔ Keep-vein-open requirements

Delivering small intermittent amounts with a volume-control burette

Nurses sometimes deliver small, intermittent volumes of fluids and doses of medications through a volume-control burette. A *volume-control burette* has its own specialized drip chamber that inserts into the primary infusion tubing and allows for the mixing of small amounts of medications and fluid. A burette also features an independent injection port and a roller clamp. You use the injection port to add medications and diluents into the drip chamber and the roller clamp to stop flow of the primary infusion until the burette medication has been delivered.

Volume-control burettes are designed for delivery at a slower rate than macro- or microdrip chambers and are particularly beneficial in monitoring fluid intake in pediatric and fluid-restricted renal patients.

Infusing through smart pumps

Over the years, infusion pumps have become increasingly more technologically advanced and sophisticated. Case in point: Many hospitals (37 percent in the U.S., to be exact) now use the *smart pump,* a software-driven pump that delivers medications, fluids, and nutrients at precisely controlled rates and dosages.

In addition to being extremely precise in dosing, smart pumps offer the following benefits:

- ✔ They allow hospitals to integrate with electronic medical records, computerized order entry systems, and medication barcode scanning.
- ✔ They deliver complex medication regimens with escalating flow rates, IV pushes (see the later section for details), and tapered dosages that previously required administration by nurses.
- ✔ They help prevent serious medication errors and reduce the number of adverse drug events (ADEs) by alerting nurses about incorrect dosages or rates of infusion, and improper routes of administration.
- ✔ They include safety innovations like alarm systems, bar codes, and drug libraries, which greatly improve patient safety. We cover these three safety innovations in the following sections.

Safety alarms

Many smart pumps include state-of-the-art safety alarm systems that help improve patient safety by alerting nurses to the following particulars:

- Dosage maximums and minimums to provide safety in bolus, intermittent, or timed infusions

- Patient weight limits to provide safety in pediatric fluid and medication dosing

- Body surface area (BSA) limits to make sure dosages don't exceed BSA limits in pediatric or chemotherapy patients

- Infusion rate limits in milliliters per hour for IVs that don't require dosage calculations, such as parenteral nutrition

- Dosing errors or pump settings that conflict with facility protocol (thanks to the integration of dose-error-reduction software, or DERS)

Bar codes

Many smart pumps contain integrated bar-code readers that allow nurses to quickly and easily retrieve information from the pharmacy, the blood bank, and the patient's medical record. Specifically, bar-code readers enable smart pumps to assist nurses with the following practical clinical functions:

- Accessing the blood bank for guidelines in blood administration and protocols for adverse blood reactions

- Accessing facility protocol associated with administration of a specific medication

- Accessing pharmacy guidelines for administration of high-alert medications

- Providing alerts to patient allergies and potential drug interactions with current medications

- Selecting the correct medication, dosage, and concentration

- Verifying patient identification information

In some facilities, IV pump bar-code programs also document the administration of medications, bill accounts receivable, and reorder medications when necessary.

Drug libraries and clinical advisories

Another significant advance in smart pump technology is the integration of drug libraries and clinical advisories into IV pumps. In addition to listing drug names, dosages, and routes of administration, sophisticated drug libraries and clinical advisories that are integrated into smart pumps provide a new dimension of practical applications and resources to clinicians, including the following:

- ✔ Drug libraries enable the selection of drug and dosage based on patient diagnosis, such as by providing the correct dosage of Beta blockers to treat the diagnosis of either congestive heart failure or essential hypertension.

- ✔ Clinical advisories provide practical clinical information (and, in turn, promote patient safety) by alerting nurses to important messages, such as "Administer this medication only through a central line."

- ✔ Clinical advisories promote patient safety by providing administration and monitoring warnings, such as "This administration must be filtered with a 0.22 micron filter."

To make smart pumps even smarter and safer, designers are already planning the following features for next-generation pumps:

- ✔ Capability to update drug libraries and extract data when the pump is in use

- ✔ Comprehensive drug libraries to include all therapies, not just medications, delivered by pumps

- ✔ Default rate settings that require manual override

- ✔ Prevention of bypassing drug libraries and DERS (dose-error-reduction software)

- ✔ Rate settings that default to zero when an infusion is complete

Space-age technology in the form of IV pumps is available in most hospitals in the U.S. But despite technological advances, smart pumps are still involved in adverse drug events that occur each year. One of the primary reasons for errors with smart pumps is that nurses bypass the pump's safety net by manually entering rate and volume parameters. When nurses manually enter these parameters, the DERS isn't in place to prevent potential dosing errors. IV nurses are in a unique position to harness the power of smart pumps to reduce adverse drug events and optimize patient outcomes. By taking time to understand and effectively use all the smart pump's integrated safety features, nurses can play a major role in reducing errors and saving lives.

Giving Infusions a Little IV Push

IV push (or *bolus*) *administration* is used when you administer more concentrated IV medications directly from a syringe into the bloodstream to produce a rapid peak in drug level. IV push medications are usually diluted and administered into the IV injection port slowly over a period of several minutes.

Doctors prescribe IV push administrations for many reasons, including the following:

- ✔ To convert a patient from frequent intramuscular injections to less painful, less tissue-destructive IV injections
- ✔ To deliver frequent, intermittent, or smaller doses of medications
- ✔ To initiate medication therapy with *loading doses* (initial higher doses of a drug that may be given either IV push or bolus at the beginning of a course of treatment prior to the maintenance infusion)
- ✔ To obtain a rapid response to medication during an emergency
- ✔ To prevent drug incompatibility by not mixing medications or solutions into the primary continuous infusion

Going Automatic with Auto-Syringe Pumps

An *auto-syringe pump* is the infusion pump's version of IV push. Auto-syringe pumps enable medication-filled syringes, which are filled by either the pharmacy or the nurse, to be inserted into the pump chamber and automatically compressed to deliver a specific amount of medication at a controlled flow rate. Figure 11-1 shows an example of what an auto-syringe pump looks like.

Auto-syringe pumps deliver very small amounts of fluid at very low rates, sometimes as low as 0.01 milliliters per hour, making them ideal for use with infants and fluid-restricted adults.

Indications for using auto-syringe pumps include the following:

- ✔ Intermittent or frequently administered medications
- ✔ Fluids that require very slow rates of administration
- ✔ Low-concentration medications
- ✔ Medications that require larger volumes or slower infusion rates than IV push drugs
- ✔ Medications that require lower volume than piggyback meds
- ✔ Single-dose medications

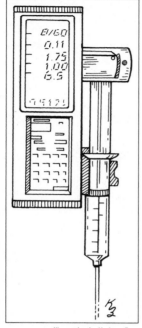

Figure 11-1:
An auto-
syringe
pump.

Illustration by Kathryn Born

In addition to administering medications with auto-syringe pumps, you can use them to perform the following other IV functions:

- ✔ Delivering IV therapy to ambulatory patients
- ✔ Keeping the vein open
- ✔ Maintaining arterial lines

Empowering Patients with PCA Pumps

Patient-controlled analgesia (PCA) is a drug delivery system that enables patients to administer their own pain medications by pressing a control button attached to a continuous IV pump. When they press the PCA button, the pump releases a prescribed amount of analgesic or narcotic into the IV tubing and delivers it by the primary infusion. Figure 11-2 shows you what a PCA pump looks like.

The physician prescribes the drug, dosage amount, dosing interval, and bolus amount, and the nurse programs this info into the pump. Typical dose intervals enable the patient to self-medicate every six to eight minutes, not exceeding total dose intervals, which are usually set at one to four hours.

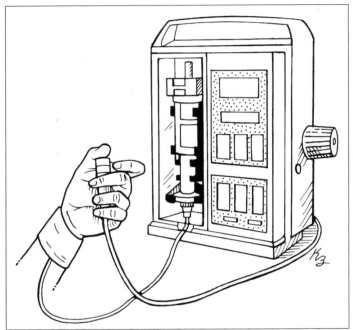

Figure 11-2:
A PCA pump and control button.

Illustration by Kathryn Born

Doctors are prescribing PCA with increasing frequency, often using it in place of standard basal and intermittent pain medications. Advantages of the PCA include

- ✔ Better pain control and management
- ✔ Decreased nursing workload
- ✔ Fewer side effects and less use of narcotic
- ✔ Patient involvement and greater patient satisfaction
- ✔ Steady-state medication concentrations

Chapter 12

Going for the Hand or Arm: Peripheral IV Essentials

*W*orking with peripheral IVs (PIVs) can be a daunting task, especially when you lack opportunities to gain experience and perfect your skills. Lucky for you, we're here to offer you a head start on inserting and maintaining peripheral IVs. From the challenging task of starting an IV to the rewarding task of removing the IV when your patient no longer needs it, this chapter walks you through all the essentials of intravenous (IV) therapy through a peripheral line.

Specifically, this chapter reviews the basic principles of peripheral IV therapy and identifies which IV infusions are appropriate to administer peripherally. Here, you find out how to choose the right vascular access device (VAD) for the right patient and how to start IVs and keep them flowing while monitoring and managing any complications that arise. You also become familiar with the various types of dressings and find out how and when to change them. Finally, you find out when and how to discontinue an IV.

Getting Started with a Few Peripheral IV Basics

To administer peripheral IV solutions into your patient, you use a peripheral IV. *Peripheral IVs* (PIVs) are small, flexible catheters that you insert into a patient's peripheral vein. The over-the-needle catheter (ONC) is the "Gold

Standard" of PIV infusion and has been around since the 1950s. You introduce an ONC into the vein by using a *stylet* (needle), which is subsequently removed, leaving the small catheter in place inside the vein.

PIVs are typically 1 to 3 inches in length and are designed for short periods of use, not exceeding one week. You usually place them on the dorsal surface of the patient's hand or arm, avoiding the underside of the wrist, to provide the patient with more comfort and mobility and to decrease the risk of nerve damage. (See the later section "Gathering Your Equipment: Selecting the Appropriate Peripheral VAD" for more details.)

Medical professionals most commonly use peripheral IVs to administer the following solutions:

- ✔ Fluid and electrolyte replacement
- ✔ IV medications
- ✔ Blood and blood products

PIVs aren't recommended for solutions with a pH greater than 9 or less than 5 or for solutions whose osmolarity is greater than 600 mOsm/L because of the possibility of infiltration and severe tissue damage. Such solutions include chemotherapy, total parenteral nutrition (TPN), vasopressors, and other caustic drugs.

Performing an Initial Vascular Access Assessment

The Infusion Nurses Society (INS) recommends that every IV patient receive an initial vascular access assessment before therapy begins. After all, early assessment is critical to selecting the appropriate VAD and minimizing risk for IV complications. What does this assessment entail? Generally speaking, an *initial vascular access assessment* involves thoroughly evaluating the patient for conditions that may impact or complicate the IV therapy ordered by the physician. Specifically, it involves verifying the physician's order and evaluating the following parameters:

- ✔ Condition of the patient and the patient's veins
- ✔ Patient preferences
- ✔ Type and length of the prescribed IV therapy
- ✔ Type of VAD

The following sections walk you through the initial vascular access assessment in more detail.

Verifying the order

Before you insert or infuse through a peripheral IV, you must obtain a physician's order. The physician's order should include the following details:

- ✔ Type of solution
- ✔ Route of administration
- ✔ Rate of administration
- ✔ Amount to be infused, either hourly or 24-hour volume
- ✔ Duration of administration
- ✔ Physician's signature

If any of these details are missing, you must clarify the order with the prescriber before beginning the infusion.

Preparing your patient

Starting a peripheral IV may become a routine occurrence for you, but for your patient, it may be the most invasive, terrifying experience of his life. When a patient fears a procedure, that fear can trigger an autonomic nervous system reaction, known as *vasovagal response,* causing a decrease in heart rate and blood pressure from vasodilation of blood vessels, and may even cause him to faint.

To avoid vasovagal reactions, you need to prepare your patients mentally and emotionally for IV procedures before you even start preparing them physically. Carefully explain the details of the PIV procedure and ask your patients about previous IV experience or lack of experience. Go over the advantages of peripheral IVs compared to other methods of administration, such as painful, repeated intramuscular injections. Taking a few moments to establish rapport, address specific concerns, and get patient feedback goes a long way toward alleviating patient fears, instilling confidence, and ensuring compliance.

Checking for allergies

One of the most common uses for peripheral IVs is to administer IV medications. Thus, identifying a patient's medication allergies is a critical part of the initial patient assessment. After all, checking a patient's medication allergies is the first line of defense in preventing allergic and adverse drug reactions to IV medications.

To check for medication allergies, review your patient's medical record and ask your patient about his drug allergy history. Explain the most common types of allergic reactions and ask whether he has ever experienced similar symptoms.

In assessing your patient for allergies, be sure to ask him about allergies to iodine and latex. Although these substances aren't medications, they can produce a powerful anaphylactic response, so you must avoid using them around patients with known allergies.

We go over common allergic reactions in more detail in Chapter 14.

Confirming the five rights

More than half of the most serious, life-threatening adverse drug reactions are the result of IV administration, and the vast majority are caused by *medication error* (any wrongful administration of a medication, such as a mistake in dosage or route of administration, failure to prescribe or administer the correct drug or formulation for a particular condition or disease, use of expired drugs, failure to observe the correct time for administration of the drug, or lack of awareness of adverse effects of certain drug combinations).

To prevent errors and adverse drug reactions, confirm the following five "rights" before administering any medication:

- ✔ Right patient
- ✔ Right medication
- ✔ Right dose
- ✔ Right route of administration
- ✔ Right time

When identifying the right patient, consider using the buddy system and have a coworker confirm the patient's identification and allergies with you. We offer more on preventing adverse reactions in Part IV.

Gathering Your Equipment: Selecting the Appropriate Peripheral VAD

Getting your equipment together is a key part of performing a successful peripheral venipuncture procedure. (*Venipuncture* simply means the puncture of a vein.) To select the right VAD, you first need to assess your patient and determine the purpose and type of IV fluids you'll be administering. Your patient's condition and the fluids you plan to administer help you determine which size catheter and which VAD you need to use; we discuss both in the following sections.

To ensure your equipment is in proper working condition, perform the following inspections each time you use it:

- Inspect glass solution containers by holding them up to the light and looking for cracks, clarity, and particulate contamination. Also be sure to check the expiration date.

- Inspect plastic infusion bags by squeezing them to look for pinholes, clarity, and particulate contamination. Also be sure to check the expiration date.

- Inspect administration sets for damage to packaging or tubing and check to see if they're vented or nonvented.

- Inspect the catheter for damage to the packaging, catheter, or needle.

- Inspect the infusion pump and/or IV pole to make sure it's in good mechanical condition.

In addition to the equipment in this list, you also need antiseptic prep solution, paper tape, gauze, and gloves (see Chapter 3 for more on standard IV equipment).

Size does matter: Choosing the correct catheter size

The first thing to consider when choosing the right VAD is catheter size, or *gauge*. The catheter gauge refers to the cannula's inner diameter, also called *lumen* (*cannula* is just a tube for insertion into a vessel). Common gauge sizes range from large-lumen, 14-gauge catheters to small-lumen, 24-gauge catheters.

Which size catheter you use depends on the condition of your patient, the prescribed IV therapy, the length of treatment, the duration of dwell, the vascular integrity, and the patient's preference. For example, if your patient is a trauma victim with massive blood loss, select a large-bore, 14- or 16-gauge catheter to accommodate copious amounts of blood and fluid replacement. If your patient is a frail, elderly woman, select a smaller, 22-gauge catheter to minimize trauma to her fragile veins.

Table 12-1 helps you determine which gauge catheter is recommended for various types of infusions.

Table 12-1	Guide to Selecting the Right Catheter Gauge
Catheter Gauge	*Type of Infusion*
14- to 18-gauge	Large-volume or rapid administrations, including blood or blood products (suggested for trauma and adults)
18- to 24-gauge	Any isotonic solution administration, including blood or blood products (suggested for adults)
22- to 27-gauge	Any isotonic solution administration, including blood or blood products (suggested for pediatric patients and neonates)

Considering the type of device

Approximately 300 million VADs are sold in the U.S. each year. Innovations in catheter technology have resulted in the availability of many different types and sizes of catheters. In the following sections, we outline some of the most important factors you need to consider when selecting which peripheral catheter to use.

Catheter length

Standard peripheral catheters come in 3/4- to 2-inch lengths. The most commonly used length is 1 inch. The peripheral catheter should be of the smallest length and gauge to accommodate the prescribed therapy. (Remember that *gauge* refers to catheter diameter; catheters come in a variety of gauges. Of course, the sizes are in reverse order, meaning that a 27-gauge catheter is the smallest and a 14-gauge catheter is the largest. See the earlier section "Size does matter: Choosing the correct catheter size" for more details.)

To help you decide which size catheter to use, consider the following:

- **Duration of therapy:** Any length or gauge can be used when the IV therapy doesn't extend beyond one week.

- **Site selection:** The infusion site should be a distal area of the upper extremities, not an area of flexion or with valves. The vein should be able to accommodate the gauge and length of the catheter required for the prescribed therapy.

- ✔ **Type of infusate:** PIVs are used to administer everything from fluid and electrolytes to blood and medications. Consider using a larger catheter, such as an 18-gauge or larger, for emergencies. *Note:* Chemotherapy and other irritant or vesicant solutions are recommended to be infused through a central vascular access device (CVAD).

- ✔ **Condition of patient:** Age, diagnosis, comorbidities, vasculature, skin condition at the intended insertion site, and history of previous IV attempts all play a role in which size catheter you use.

Midline catheters are peripheral VADs that are longer than the previously described catheters but not as long as peripherally inserted central catheters (PICCs) or CVADs; see Chapter 13 for details on these. Midline catheters are designed to provide long-term, frequent IV access, usually between one and four weeks, without the risks associated with central venous lines.

Midline catheters are typically between 3 and 10 inches long, with 8 inches being the most commonly used. A midline catheter is inserted in the *antecubital* (or inner elbow area) and extends to the axillary area. Midline catheters should never reach the central venous system, and they shouldn't extend beyond the axillary area into the chest.

Although midline catheters are well-suited for repeat administrations of many antibiotics and fluids, they're not appropriate for use with hyperosmolar or vesicant administrations. For those types of administrations, you should use a CVAD, such as a PICC line, because they reach the central venous circulation where hyperosmolar and chemotherapy agents can be diluted so they don't cause damage to vessels.

When a physician orders a midline catheter, a certified registered nurse or infusion specialist usually inserts it at the patient's bedside under sterile conditions. After insertion, the nurse labels the catheter to make sure no one mistakes it for a CVAD. To secure the catheter, we recommend using a sutureless device, but you can also secure it with small adhesive strips at the insertion site and connector hub.

Don't draw blood or take blood pressure on the arm with a midline catheter. Drawing blood can puncture the catheter, and using a blood pressure cuff can damage it or the vein.

Catheter composition

Peripheral catheter composition may be polyvinylchloride (PVC), polyurethane, or silicone. Advancements in catheter composition have produced the following unique features:

- ✔ Ultrasmooth outer surface

- ✔ Capability to soften within the vessel, making it more comfortable for the patient

These advancements translate into many benefits for the patient, including the following:

- ✔ Reduced risk of mechanical phlebitis because of less trauma to the vessel wall

- ✔ Reduced risk of infiltration, resulting in fewer IV restarts (which can translate to greater sparing of peripheral vein sources)

- ✔ Reduced risk of clot and occlusion thanks to the catheter's less-inflammatory and nonthrombogenic features

Catheter design

Catheter designs have improved greatly with evolving technologies. Here are just a few of the improvements you may see in catheters today:

- ✔ Thin-walled catheters now provide larger gauges for increased infusion flow rates, as well as ease of insertion and increased patient comfort by allowing smaller needles to be used for insertion.

- ✔ Indwelling catheters are designed to be radiopaque or to have a radiopaque strip for detection by X-ray in case they become damaged or lost in circulation.

- ✔ New safety features include active or passive safety needles that protect healthcare workers from accidental needle punctures and closed administration sets that reduce the risk of contamination and air embolus.

Determining the Best Peripheral IV Site

One of the tricks of the trade in selecting the best peripheral IV site is knowing the difference between desirable veins and undesirable veins:

- ✔ *Desirable veins* are smooth and pliable, with adequate distance between valves to allow for easy threading of a catheter. When you use a tourniquet near desirable veins, they become plump and distended and feel spongy when palpated. Avoid areas of flexion like the wrists or elbows.

- ✔ *Undesirable veins* are bumpy, knotty, and thrombosed. They don't distend or plump with a tourniquet, and they appear fixed and attached to the skin. Often, patients who are IV drug users have scarred, hard, and sclerosed veins.

Being able to recognize the difference between desirable and undesirable veins helps you know which IVs you want to start yourself and which ones you want to give to the vascular access specialist.

Before selecting an IV site, read the patient's medical record and become familiar with her medical history, including past surgeries she's had and the medications she's currently taking. If she's had a mastectomy, deep vein thrombosis (DVT), or stroke, avoid starting an IV in her surgical extremity or the extremity affected by the stroke. If she uses a cane or walker to assist with ambulating, avoid inserting an IV in her hands.

Medications also play a role in where you place an IV because medications can cause damage to peripheral veins. Anticoagulants, for example, cause bleeding and bruising in peripheral veins. Knowing that your patient is taking anticoagulants helps you determine that you'll need a larger vein, a smaller needle, and a very gentle touch when you insert the peripheral IV.

Other factors to consider when selecting the best IV site are

- ✔ Patient age, size, and condition
- ✔ Type of infusate
- ✔ Duration of IV therapy (*Note:* As a rule of thumb, choose a vein that can support 72 to 96 hours of therapy)
- ✔ Condition of peripheral veins
- ✔ Your skill level

Areas to avoid when selecting an IV site include

- ✔ Areas that are *distal,* or below, a previous infiltration
- ✔ Areas that are distal to phlebitis or inflammation
- ✔ Extremities with shunts or fistulas for dialysis
- ✔ Areas with bruising or hematoma
- ✔ Areas affected by edema or trauma

Beginning the Insertion Process

After your initial vascular assessment determines that the patient is a good candidate for a peripheral IV and you've selected the best site, you're ready to face the challenging task of inserting the VAD. Take a few minutes to prepare the IV solutions, prime and clamp the tubing, and set the volumetric control device according to physician orders or facility protocol. Assemble all the supplies and equipment you'll need during administration so you're ready to administer the therapy the moment you've successfully inserted the VAD. After you gather your supplies, wash your hands, put on your gloves, and apply the tourniquet. Then keep reading to find out what to do next.

Prepping the site

To prepare the skin, clean the site by using the antimicrobial recommended by facility policy or use one of the following preferred antimicrobials:

- ✔ Chlorhexidine 2 percent (preferred)
- ✔ Iodophor (povidone-iodine)
- ✔ Isopropyl alcohol 70 percent
- ✔ Tincture of iodine 2 percent

Whichever one you use, apply the antimicrobial according to the manufacturer's recommended guidelines. Then allow the site to dry.

Note: INS recommends using a new pair of disposable gloves in conjunction with a no-touch technique; in other words, don't repalpate the site after cleaning it unless you wear sterile gloves.

When preparing the peripheral IV site, don't shave or use a *depilatory* (hair removal) cream on the site. Shaving creates microscopic cuts in the skin that can lead to infection, and depilatory creams run the risk of starting an allergic reaction. When necessary, use scissors or clippers to rid the area of excess hair.

Administering an anesthetic

Anesthetics promote patient comfort and compliance; use them in accordance with a physician's order or facility policy. Here are your main options:

- ✔ When appropriate, you may apply a cream mixture of two local anesthetics — lidocaine 2.5 percent and prilocaine 2.5 percent (brand name EMLA) — to the skin under an occlusive dressing to provide effective anesthesia; however, the cream must stay in place for 45 minutes to be effective, per the manufacturer's guidelines.
- ✔ You can inject 0.1 to 0.2 milliliters (mL) of 1 percent lidocaine with a tuberculin syringe prior to venipuncture.
- ✔ You can use a freeze spray that cools down the insertion site, rendering it numb.
- ✔ You can inject normal saline with preservative the same way you inject the lidocaine to numb the area.

Don't use topical creams or intradermal injections for patients with a known sensitivity to lidocaine or prilocaine.

Inserting the peripheral IV

You typically insert a peripheral VAD by using the direct method or the indirect method. The direct method consists of the following steps:

1. **Tighten the skin to ensure vein immobility by pulling the skin below the intended puncture site.**

2. **Place the needle directly above the vein and insert it, bevel up, usually at a 10- to 20-degree angle, but be sure to check the manufacturer's recommendations.**

3. **Penetrate all layers of the vein in one motion, taking care to avoid puncturing the back wall of the vessel.**

4. **When you feel resistance of the vessel wall, followed by a lack of resistance when the needle enters the interior of the vein, look for blood flashback, indicating the needle tip is in the vein.**

5. **When you see blood flashback, lower the angle of the needle and carefully advance the catheter over the needle and into the vein.**

6. **When the catheter is fully advanced, release the tourniquet while the stylet is still partially in the catheter.**

7. **Occlude the vein at the catheter tip, remove the stylet, and connect the IV administration set or extension set to the catheter hub.**

8. **Secure the catheter without obscuring the view of the insertion site (see the next section for details).**

Figure 12-1 shows the direct method of inserting a peripheral IV.

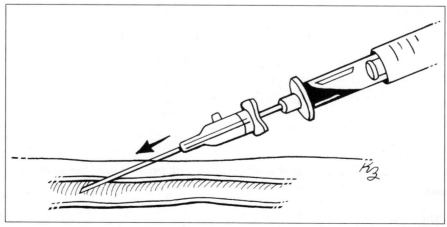

Figure 12-1:
Inserting a peripheral IV via the direct method.

Illustration by Kathryn Born

To insert a VAD by using the indirect approach, follow these steps:

1. **Insert the VAD at about a 10- to 20-degree angle (refer to the manufacturer's recommended guidelines) into the subcutaneous tissue alongside the intended vein.**

2. **Thread the needle through the subcutaneous tissue and enter the vein from the side.**

3. **After you receive blood flashback, advance the catheter over the needle and into the vein in the same manner as in the direct method (see Step 5 in the preceding list).**

4. **Complete the procedure by following Steps 6 through 8 from the direct method.**

INS standards allow for only two IV insertion attempts per nurse on any one patient.

Securing the catheter

You can use several different methods to secure the catheter and prevent accidental removal or other complications. Here are just some of the securing methods you can choose from:

- **Adhesive, transparent dressing method:** You can secure a catheter by placing an adhesive, transparent, semipermeable dressing (TSD) over the insertion site.

- **U or H method:** You can secure a winged IV catheter by applying half-inch adhesive strips in an *H-* or *U-*shaped pattern over the wings, without obstructing the view of the insertion site. This method can also be used to secure nonwinged catheters. *Note:* After you apply the transparent, semipermeable dressing, the adhesive strips should be placed below the tip of the hub with the adhesive side up and then folded down the sides of the catheter so they lie on top of the dressing, not over the catheter or under the dressing, making a *U* or *H* shape. (Refer to Chapter 3 for more on the winged catheter.)

- **Stabilization device:** Stabilization devices, routinely used in securing midline catheters and central venous lines, are becoming increasingly popular in stabilizing peripheral catheters. Medical professionals are using stabilization devices more frequently with peripheral catheters because they're associated with fewer complications and less risk. As of 2011, stabilization devices are now recommended by INS and the Center for Disease Control and Prevention, or CDC. (Turn to Chapter 3 for details on stabilization devices.)

If you use tape to secure a catheter, don't place the tape directly over the insertion. Place it so that you can still observe the insertion for complications, and be sure to leave all injection ports accessible for intermittent administrations. Relieve tension on the catheter by taping a loop of IV tubing to the patient's skin, independent of the catheter dressing (in most facilities, this is the J-loop extension set or pigtail).

Dressing your site

After successfully securing the catheter, you need to dress the insertion site with either of the following:

- Transparent, semipermeable, occlusive, adhesive dressing to be changed when the VAD is changed

- Sterile gauze occlusive dressing with adhesive tape to be changed every 48 hours (not common practice, but may be used if a patient is allergic to the transparent, semipermeable dressing)

Figure 12-2 shows both types of peripheral VAD site dressings.

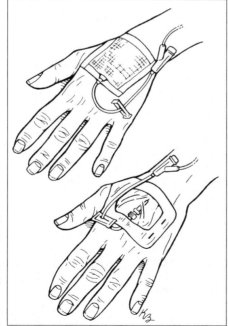

Figure 12-2:
Gauze versus transparent VAD site dressings.

Illustration by Kathryn Born

When you're finished dressing the insertion site, label the dressing with the following information:

- Date and time of insertion
- Gauge size and length of the VAD
- Your initials

Initiating therapy

When the VAD is in place and you've removed the tourniquet, follow these steps to initiate the IV therapy:

1. **Connect the catheter to the prepared IV tubing.**
2. **Open the tubing clamp.**
3. **Set the infusion pump for the prescribed rate.**
4. **Start the flow of solution.**
5. **Monitor the insertion site and patient reaction.**

Check out Chapter 3 for what a typical infusion bag and piggyback set look like.

Labeling the infusion bag and line

Accurate labeling is essential in providing safety and continuity of care to patients who are receiving IV therapy. To ensure effective communication among different nurses, make sure that all infusion and piggyback bag labels include the following details:

- Patient name and ID number or date of birth
- Medication additive
- Date and time started
- Initials of infusion nurse

IV tubings currently have to be labeled with the date of the previous tubing change and the date for the next tubing change, but most nurses agree that all tubings (even piggyback tubings that are rapidly administered) need to include the medication name, as well.

In facilities where syringe pumps are frequently used, the syringes also need to be labeled with the medication name.

Medication labels on IV tubings and syringes provide one additional check-point to ensure that the right medication is going to the right patient at the right time in the right way.

If you're uncertain about what information goes on which label, check your facility's policy and procedure manual or infusion-standards manual.

Verifying and documenting your actions

After you start the IV, you must verify your actions by documenting the fol-lowing details of VAD insertion in the patient's record:

- ✔ Physician's order for VAD insertion
- ✔ Aseptic technique and site preparation
- ✔ Anesthetic type, amount, and route of administration (if used)
- ✔ Date and time of insertion
- ✔ Gauge and length of device
- ✔ Specific name and location of accessed vein
- ✔ Number of attempts for successful IV start (not more than two)
- ✔ Type of solution being infused
- ✔ Type of infusion — by gravity or electronic infusion device (EID)
- ✔ List of add-on devices, if appropriate
- ✔ Type of dressing and label
- ✔ Patient reaction, education, and understanding

Monitoring the Infusion

After you successfully start the IV and document the whole procedure in the patient's record, you have to monitor the site to optimize treatment and mini-mize risks.

Assessing the site for complications

You need to assess all peripheral IV sites for signs of infection or other com-plications at least every eight hours, or as needed if potential complications are suspected.

Use the following guidelines to help you assess an IV site:

✔ Observe the dressing to ensure that it's dry and intact.

✔ Palpate the insertion site through the dressing to note edema or tenderness.

✔ Inspect the insertion site for erythema, phlebitis, or infiltration.

✔ Inspect the catheter for leakage to rule out occlusion or damage.

✔ Inspect the tubing for kinks, closed clamps, damage, or contamination.

✔ Assess the patient for any signs of systemic infection, such as fever, chills, or disorientation.

✔ Check the patient's medical record to verify that the correct infusate is being administered at the correct flow rate.

Flushing the line

Flushing the line is the process of pushing normal saline through the catheter, and it's an important step you need to take to keep your patient's catheter clean and viable. Because most PIVs are basic, open-ended catheters, flushing procedures are usually simple and straightforward.

To flush an open-ended peripheral catheter, follow these steps:

1. **Wash your hands, apply clean gloves, and use an aseptic technique.**

2. **Cleanse the injection port by scrubbing the hub for at least 15 seconds with an appropriate antiseptic solution and then let it dry.**

3. **Insert the syringe of normal saline into the injection port.**

4. **Slowly aspirate to get a blood return and ensure patency.**

5. **Inject the normal saline while assessing for any signs of pain, discomfort, or leakage.**

6. **Remove the syringe and discard in the proper sharps container.**

7. **Document the procedure.**

Flush the line every eight hours and before and after every administration of fluid or medication or in accordance with the facility policy or physician's order. You usually need to flush the line before you administer incompatible medications or fluids and when you're converting the line from a continuous infusion to an intermittent infusion.

Watching for complications

The longer an IV is in use and the more times you access an IV for administration, the greater the risk for complications that can delay the course of a patient's treatment and jeopardize his recovery. Peripheral IVs pose an additional risk for complications because they're set up in extremities that patients use constantly for eating, drinking, and other activities.

To guard against complications that can arise from peripheral IVs, you need to be aware of the most common complications and vigilantly monitor the insertion site and peripheral equipment. Table 12-2 lists some of the most common complications related to peripheral IVs, along with their signs or symptoms, preventive measures, and treatment.

Table 12-2	Complications of Peripheral IV Therapy			
Complication	*Definition/ Cause*	*Signs or Symptoms*	*Preventive Measures*	*Treatment*
Infiltration	Fluid flowing into tissues rather than veins Most commonly caused by needle or cannula punctures on the side wall of the vein	Skin coolness around insertion site Dependent edema at insertion site and extremity Leaking from insertion site	Use the smallest, shortest catheter possible. Avoid entering the vein at a steep angle. Insert VAD with bevel up. Avoid placement in flexion areas, such as the anticubital fossa. Use arm boards in places adjacent to flexion areas. Use stabilization devices to secure the VAD. Avoid hand veins in patients who are active or on walkers or crutches. Start placement as low on the forearm as possible without interfering with patient activity.	Stop infusion. Obtain order to discontinue and start new catheter. Apply compresses, as ordered, and elevate the affected extremity. Use infiltration scale when available and appropriate. Follow extravasation guidelines when available and appropriate.

(continued)

Table 12-2 *(continued)*

Complication	Definition/ Cause	Signs or Symptoms	Preventive Measures	Treatment
Phlebitis	Inflammation of the vein Results from a catheter that gets infected (usually due to improper site cleaning prior to insertion) or the administration of a caustic drug, such as chemotherapy Can also result from the trauma of routine VAD placement	Skin warmth, redness, and/or pain around insertion site Local edema Red streaks along the vein Slow infusion rate	Same measures as for infiltration plus these: Use strict aseptic technique during venipuncture, line access, and line maintenance. Add a buffer to irritating medications or fluids. Change VADs, administration sets, solution containers, and dressings according to protocol. Use larger veins for hypertonic solutions. Carefully monitor fluids/meds associated with high risk for phlebitis, such as potassium chloride, amino acids, dextrose solutions, erythromycin, tetracycline, nafcillin, and vancomycin.	Stop infusion. Obtain order to discontinue and start new catheter. Apply warm compresses, as ordered.
Hematoma	A collection of blood that has seeped into tissues from a vein injury Generally caused by an unsuccessful IV insertion or the removal of a cannula when the IV is discontinued	Bruising or discoloration at insertion area Local edema or tenderness Resistance during catheter flushing	Use indirect method of venipuncture. Apply tourniquet right before venipuncture. Avoid sharp angle of venipuncture. Insert the needle with bevel up. Avoid any site below a recent venipuncture. Apply pressure after removing a VAD.	Stop infusion. Obtain order to discontinue and start new catheter. Apply pressure to insertion area. Elevate extremity.

Complication	Definition/ Cause	Signs or Symptoms	Preventive Measures	Treatment
Thrombosis	A formation of blood that collects at the tip of the catheter in the vein and obstructs the flow of fluids through the catheter	Tenderness around insertion site Hardening, cord-like distention of the vein Sluggish or stopped flow rate Inability to flush catheter	Use volumetric pumps to ensure consistent flow through the catheter. Use keep vein open (KVO) rates 30–50 mL/hr unless otherwise ordered by the physician. Use microdrip sets with gravity flow if rate is below 50 mL/hr. Avoid venipuncture in flexion areas, such as the inner aspect of the elbow and wrist.	Same treatment as for phlebitis plus the following: Assess for circulatory impairment.
Localized infection	Can be caused by skin-dwelling organisms, such as *Coagulase-negative staphylococcus* or *Candida albicans*	Redness and edema at insertion site Evidence of purulent exudate from site Chills or fever Increased white blood cell count	Keep the area clean and dry and covered with a dressing.	Stop infusion. Obtain order to discontinue and start new catheter. Apply sterile dressing, as ordered. Administer antibiotics, as ordered.

(continued)

Table 12-2 *(continued)*

Complication	Definition/ Cause	Signs or Symptoms	Preventive Measures	Treatment
Fluid overload	Can occur when fluids are given at a higher rate or in a larger volume than the system can absorb or excrete	Weight gain Puffy eyelids and generalized edema Increased blood pressure Intake greater than output Rise in central venous pressure (CVP) Shortness of breath Respiratory crackles Distended neck veins	Carefully monitor your patient for input and output of fluids.	Decrease IV rate. Notify physician. Place patient in high Fowler's position. Monitor vital signs. Administer oxygen as needed.

In addition to the complications listed in the table, patients with peripheral IVs are also at risk for septicemia and air embolism. For specific information on these complications, see Chapter 13.

Documenting your actions

If you suspect an IV complication, such as infiltration or phlebitis, your first actions are to stop the infusion, remove the PIV, and assess the site for the degree of complication. Always follow your facility's protocol pertaining to IV complications and when to notify the physician.

After you've treated the patient, you must document your findings and actions. Follow your facility's policies on documenting all pertinent information. Some policies require taking pictures to document the event and help clinicians evaluate the progress and scope of injury.

Refer to the INS's *Infusion Nursing Standards of Practice* for a standardized grading scale that you can use to grade an infiltration. Incorporate the grade and description of other criteria into your documentation.

In general, accurate documentation of all peripheral IV complications and interventions includes the following:

- ✔ Stopping the infusion
- ✔ Discontinuing the catheter
- ✔ Notifying the physician
- ✔ Obtaining orders
- ✔ Restarting the IV
- ✔ Resuming the fluid or medication infusion
- ✔ Applying warm or cold compresses, as ordered
- ✔ Elevating the extremity, as ordered
- ✔ Documenting with pictures, according to policy
- ✔ Measuring and noting arm circumference, according to policy
- ✔ Grading and noting the infiltration
- ✔ Following extravasation policy, if appropriate
- ✔ Monitoring the patient's reaction to complication and intervention
- ✔ Instructing the patient to keep extremity elevated and compresses in place

Including these details in your documentation helps standardize the description of IV complications and enables healthcare professionals to track the course of complications and improve the quality of patient care.

Replacing Peripherals at Regular Intervals

To minimize the risk of complications with peripheral IVs, you have to replace the PIV and its components (administration set, infusion bag, and dressing) at regular intervals, as dictated by your facility's protocol. You may also replace IV peripherals according to industry standards set by professional organizations, such as the INS in their *Infusion Nursing Standards of Practice.*

Although policies and procedures vary from facility to facility, most policies agree to replace IV peripherals according to the following general guidelines:

- ✔ **Peripheral IVs:** Replace and rotate PIVs every 48 to 96 hours (INS recommends when clinically indicated) or according to facility protocol. If you can't replace a PIV within the prescribed time frame, you need to obtain a physician's order to leave the PIV in place for another 24 hours. After that, you have to obtain another order daily until you replace the PIV.

  INS states to replace PIVs that were inserted under emergency conditions or placed in the field by EMS within 24 hours because of a possible break in aseptic technique during emergency treatment.

- ✔ **IV administration sets and tubings, including piggyback tubings:** Change the administration set and tubing every 96 hours or at least every seven days or when you replace the PIV. But don't replace tubings more frequently than at 72-hour intervals unless clinically indicated.

- ✔ **IV administration sets used to infuse blood, blood products, or lipid emulsions:** Replace blood administration sets every 4 hours and administration sets used for lipid emulsions every 24 hours.

- ✔ **Infusion bags:** Replace infusion bags every 24 hours or as needed or according to facility policy.

- ✔ **Catheters with signs of complications:** Stop the infusion immediately and remove the PIV.

- ✔ **Dressings that are transparent, semipermeable, and occlusive:** Replace the dressings when you replace the PIV or as needed when loose, wet, or contaminated.

After you replace the PIV, you must label the new PIV, administration set, infusion bag, and dressing according to the guidelines we go over earlier in the section "Labeling the infusion bag and line." Then document your actions by updating the patient's record with the date and time of the next replacement and the other information we list in the earlier section "Verifying and documenting your actions."

Discontinuing the Peripheral Line

You may have to remove a peripheral line from a patient for the following reasons:

- ✔ Replacement of the PIV at the appointed interval
- ✔ Replacement of the PIV due to complications
- ✔ Removal due to completion of IV therapy

To successfully discontinue and remove a peripheral line, follow facility protocol or INS standards. Take as much care to remove the catheter as you did to insert it to avoid causing a hematoma or other complication.

When a peripheral IV administration is complete, be sure to document the procedure with all the pertinent information, including the date and time of removal, assessment of the sight, disposition of the catheter, type of dressing applied, patient's response to removal, and patient's understanding of education pertaining to the IV removal.

Chapter 13

The ABCs of the CVAD

Central vascular access devices (CVADs) are essential in the care of acutely and chronically ill patients, especially when repeated infusions are required for weeks, months, or even longer. Generally speaking, only doctors, physician assistants (PAs), or nurses with advanced training insert CVADs into patients. But even if you don't receive this advanced training and never have to insert a CVAD, you'll most likely care for patients who have them throughout your career in healthcare.

Having a solid understanding of how to use and maintain CVADs is critical in preventing catastrophic consequences associated with CVAD complications. Also, finding out how to correctly work with CVADs prepares you to care for the most seriously injured and ill patients at a critical time in their lives.

In this chapter, we cover the basics of CVADs, from obtaining an order to discontinuing the CVAD and everything in between. As a bonus, we also explain how to use an implanted port for central venous access.

Starting from Scratch: CVAD Basics

Central vascular access devices (CVADs) are catheters that are placed in large veins of the neck, chest, arm, or groin for long-term, repeated infusions. CVADs allow large amounts of medications to rapidly dilute and move quickly into the patient's bloodstream.

In most clinical situations, appropriate infusions for CVADs include the following:

✔ Long-term infusions (more than five days)

✔ Chemotherapy

✔ Parenteral nutrition

✔ Certain intravenous (IV) medications, such as vesicants or irritants

✔ Fluids for rehydration

✔ Emergency situations when large infusion volumes are needed

✔ Home infusion therapy

For infusions that are appropriate for both CVADs and peripheral IVs, which we discuss in Chapter 12, you determine which device to use based on many factors, including the vascular access need (based on the therapy or treatment), the length of time the device is left to dwell, the viable vasculature, and the amount of skill and knowledge the person taking care of the infusion has.

First Things First: What to Do Before Using the CVAD

Before you infuse through a newly placed CVAD, you need to have the CVAD's tip location confirmed with a chest X-ray and then obtain an order from the physician. This section guides you through both of these steps.

Ordering a chest X-ray

After a doctor, PA, or trained nurse inserts the CVAD into your patient but before you can infuse through the device, you must obtain a chest X-ray to confirm the CVAD's tip location. This X-ray may be ordered by the person inserting the CVAD, but it needs your confirmation before the infusion can begin. Using an X-ray to verify the catheter tip's location prevents complications and ensures that fluids and medications flow freely into the patient's central veins.

The correct anatomic location for a CVAD tip is a controversial subject among clinicians. Most prefer to place the tip in the distal end (bottom one-third) of the superior vena cava, using the carina as one of the landmarks, while some prefer to place it in the right atrium of the heart. The Food and Drug Administration (FDA), Centers for Disease Control (CDC), Infusion Nurses Society (INS), Association for Vascular Acces (AVA), most clinicians, and CVAD manufacturers recommend placing the tip in the superior vena cava, especially because reports of heart arrhythmias have been associated with placement in the atrium. But regardless of the location choice, your job is to obtain a chest X-ray to verify the location of the catheter's tip and document the location in the patient's medical record before starting any infusions.

To achieve proper tip placement, the doctor, PA, or specially trained nurse usually inserts the CVAD through the chest (subclavian approach), a neck vein (internal jugular approach), or the groin (femoral approach), though he can also use an upper extremity (used for PICC placement). If the doctor chooses the femoral vein, you use the chest X-ray to confirm that the tip is correctly placed in the inferior vena cava prior to use.

Obtaining an order to infuse

After you verify the correct tip location, depending on your facility's protocol, you likely also have to obtain a physician's order to infuse through the CVAD. All infusions administered through a central venous catheter (another name for a CVAD) should go through an infusion pump to ensure that the proper dose and amount of fluids are infused.

Remember: Before you start an infusion, be sure to verify the physician's order, the five rights of medication administration, and the CVAD's tip location and to assess the catheter insertion site.

Gathering the Supplies You Need to Infuse through a CVAD

After you verify that the tip location is correct and you have received the doctor's order to infuse through a CVAD, you need to get your supplies and equipment together.

You need most of the same equipment you use for a peripheral IV (refer to Chapter 12) when you're infusing through a CVAD, plus the following additions:

- ✔ Infusion pump
- ✔ Flushing solutions (such as normal saline)
- ✔ Heparin and locking solutions for open-ended catheters (if your facility protocol specifies)
- ✔ Large-diameter syringes (greater than 5 cc) for flushing, locking, and blood aspiration
- ✔ Medication or fluids that will be infused

See Chapter 3 for details on the standard equipment needed for IV administration and tips on how to set up your equipment.

Choosing the right infusion device

In the past, doctors used central venous catheters only for short periods of time for critical patients. Today the use of CVADs has expanded to both short- and long-term infusions in patients to treat a broad range of conditions from trauma injuries to malnutrition.

To administer a wide variety of fluids and medications over short- and long-term durations, central venous catheters have evolved from a simple single *lumen* (the interior space of the tubular device) to multiple types of single-, double-, and triple-lumen catheters. Most catheters fall into the following four categories:

- ✔ **Non-tunneled central catheters:** *Non-tunneled central catheters* are inserted into the subclavian, internal jugular, or femoral vein, threaded through the vein to the superior vena cava, and sutured in place at the insertion site. These catheters are designed for short-term use, and a large portion of the catheter remains outside the skin.

- ✔ **Tunneled central catheters:** *Tunneled central catheters* are placed in the chest but tunneled into the subclavian or jugular vein; a majority of the catheter is tunneled beneath the skin to help prevent infection and provide stability. These catheters are designed for long-term use, and only a small portion of the catheter and its attachments are visible externally. They sometimes have a Dacron (ingrowth) cuff, positioned 2 to 3 centimeters from the skin exit, which promotes tissue growth over the cuff to secure the catheter and minimize the risk for infection.

- ✔ **Peripherally inserted central catheters (PICCs):** PICCs are non-tunneled central catheters that are inserted into a large vein in the arm and threaded centrally to the superior vena cava. PICCs are used for short- to intermediate-term therapies and are usually smaller than other CVADs.

- ✔ **Implanted ports:** Implanted ports are surgically implanted by a physician into a pocket under the skin with the catheter inserted into a vein such as the subclavian or jugular. The tip of the catheter typically ends in the superior vena cava. Implanted ports are typically used for long-term treatment and can last for many years with proper care and maintenance. You access the ports with a non-coring needle. Find out more about imported ports later in this chapter in the section "Using an Implanted Port Instead."

Each type of catheter is designed for optimal use in certain clinical settings for the administration of specified fluids and medications, and each one has distinct advantages and disadvantages. Table 13-1 identifies the pros and cons of each catheter type. Check out Chapter 3 for even more on CVADs.

Table 13-1   Advantages and Disadvantages of Catheter Types

Catheter Type	Advantages	Disadvantages
Non-tunneled	Ease of insertion, exchange, and removal	Limited to short-term use
	Can be used for all medication infusions, including TPN, chemotherapy, and vesicants or irritants	Higher risk for infection
	Some catheters can be used for dialysis and hemodynamic monitoring	
	No requirements for surgery	
Tunneled	Appropriate for long-term use	Require surgical procedures for insertion, replacement, and removal
	Can be used for all medication infusions, including TPN, chemotherapy, and vesicants or irritants	
	Some catheters can be used for dialysis and hemodynamic monitoring	
	Lower risk for infection	
Peripherally inserted central catheter (PICC)	Ease of insertion and removal	Risk of deep vein thrombosis (DVT)
	Can be used for all medication infusions, including TPN, chemotherapy, and vesicants or irritants	Restricts patient from being able to swim and requires covering the dressing when showering
	Some catheters can be used for hemodynamic monitoring	
	Lower risk of infection	
Implanted ports	Can last for years when properly maintained	Discomfort from a needle stick each time the port is accessed
	Lowest risk of infection because ports are completely buried beneath the skin	Difficult self-access to administer medications
	Allow patients to perform care and maintenance on their own port	Require surgery to implant and remove the port
	High patient mobility (such as taking showers and going swimming)	Unavailability of triple lumens

Surveying the different types of CVADs

Central venous catheters come in a wide variety, although the most common types are open ended or valved:

- **Open-ended catheter:** Open-ended catheters have no occlusive devices and must be clamped closed when not in use to prevent air from entering the catheter at the external end. Clamping also prevents blood from refluxing into the catheter at the internal tip end. Open-ended catheters are clamped during tubing changes and may be locked with heparin after each intermittent use. We offer details about using heparin with CVADs later in the section "Locking the line."

- **Valved catheter:** These catheters guard against air entry into the tubing and blood entry into the catheter by means of a valve at either end of the catheter. The valve automatically opens during flushing and fluid administrations and during blood withdrawal or aspiration. When the catheter isn't in use for administration or aspiration, the valve automatically remains shut. These catheters don't need heparin locks.

Preparing the Line and Starting the Infusion

To minimize the risk of infection and other serious complications that can arise with CVADs, you must closely follow all institutional protocols and manufacturers' instructions and perform all CVAD care and maintenance procedures, starting with IV line and tubing preparation and continuing through every step of the infusion process until the CVAD is removed.

Use the following guidelines as you prepare the line and start the infusion:

- Double-check the order for correct infusate, medications, and flow rate.

- Double-check the patient's identification and allergies.

- Use the appropriate sterile priming solution and prime the IV tubing to remove all air; then seal the tubing by clamping.

- Add filter or peripheral devices, as ordered.

- Apply gloves and follow institutional protocol to initiate the infusion.

- Properly disinfect the end cap or injection port for 10 to 15 seconds.

- Check for blood return by aspirating the CVAD. (To aspirate, attach the appropriate flushing solution to the CVAD hub and pull back on the plunger, checking for blood return.)

✔ After checking for blood return, flush the line and ensure that the catheter is unobstructed by observing ease of flow.

✔ Attach the primed IV tubing to the designated catheter lumen.

✔ Insert the tubing into the infusion pump, set the desired flow rate, and start the pump just before opening the clamp.

✔ Monitor the patient for any signs of adverse reactions or problems.

To refresh your memory on infusion pumps, check out Chapters 3 and 11.

To protect yourself, you patients, and your medical team, take a proactive approach to documenting your actions and interactions with the patient. Accurate, complete documentation includes noting all your actions and observations during the CVAD procedure. Include the following specifics in your documentation:

✔ Document the use of universal precautions and the date and time of the procedure.

✔ Document the blood return.

✔ Document whether the catheter flushes easily.

✔ Document the heparin lock if you perform one.

✔ Document the ease or difficulty of flushing and aspirating and the functionality of the catheter device.

✔ Document the type, amount, and flow rate of the infusate.

✔ Document the appearance of the CVAD and the insertion site and the type of dressing.

✔ Document any adverse incidences.

✔ Document the CVAD type.

✔ Measure and document the external catheter length from its insertion site.

✔ Document the patient's response to the procedure, the patient education you gave, and the patient's understanding of your teachings.

Documenting your efforts to follow protocols and minimize patient risk provides a public record of your attempts to prevent potentially serious complications through nursing diligence.

Monitoring the Line

Because CVAD infusions go directly to the central venous system, you must frequently monitor the line to clear any obstructions that may impede the flow of fluid and lead to clotting and infection. Monitoring the line for stabilization is also critical, particularly because the INS currently recommends manufactured catheter stabilization devices to provide secure stabilization of a CVAD. Refer to your facility's guidelines for a list of approved stabilization devices. We offer more details on stabilization devices in Chapter 3.

The following sections walk you through the different steps involved in monitoring the line.

Checking out the surroundings

Each time you enter a CVAD patient's room, make the following steps part of your routine:

✔ Observe the infusion equipment and supplies. Observe the IV tubing to make sure no kinks are impeding infusion and all clamps are released to allow uninterrupted administration. Inspect the IV connections, injection ports, and access caps for signs of blood or other contamination.

✔ Inspect any administration sets or piggyback sets for damage, leakage, or contamination.

✔ Monitor infusion pumps for flow-rate accuracy and proper mechanical function.

✔ Check out your patient by asking about any unusual pain or complaints. Chest discomfort/EKG changes may be a sign that the catheter tip has *migrated* (or moved) from its original position. Neck pain or chest discomfort with CVADs or redness, swelling, or pain in the PICC arm may be associated with vein thrombosis or clotting. Other indications of vein thrombosis include engorgement or bulging superficial veins of the chest wall or neck. ***Remember:*** Immediately report any symptoms of thrombosis to the physician and be sure to document the incident.

Assessing the site

When you assess your patient's CVAD insertion site, per the CDC 2011 guidelines, carefully palpate through the dressing around the insertion site. As you inspect and palpate the surrounding area, look for the following symptoms:

✔ Erythema or redness

✔ Edema or swelling

✔ Tenderness or warmth

Patient complaints of tenderness or discomfort during palpation may indicate a thrombus or infection. Remove the dressing and visually inspect the site right away. If you suspect a thrombus or infection, notify the doctor, get orders for treatment, and document your findings.

If the patient complains of hearing a running water sound or gurgling noises on the side of the catheter insertion, the catheter tip may have migrated out of the vena cava and into the jugular vein. Report these complaints to the physician immediately.

Flushing the line

Flushing the central venous line accomplishes many goals, but its main objective is to ensure that the line stays open (or *patent*). Proper technique for flushing is to flush using a push/pause technique. Per INS, flushing the CVAD consists of flushing the catheter with 0.9 percent of preservative-free normal saline (NS). If the medication that was infusing is incompatible with NS, then you can use 5 percent dextrose followed by the NS and/or a heparin lock solution.

Flushing the line accomplishes several objectives for each step of the infusion process:

- ✔ **After you prepare the line but before you start the infusion:** To make sure the line is open and free-flowing and to remove any residual medication or blood in the line

- ✔ **After administration of the medication:** To push the medication through the IV tubing and ensure that all the medication has been delivered and the line is clear

- ✔ **Between medications:** To help keep incompatible drugs separated from each other, thus preventing adverse drug interactions or drug incompatibility issues

- ✔ **At the end of a medication administration:** To infuse NS/heparin lock into the line to keep it free from clots and to keep the catheter open (see the next section for more about this IV flush, which is also called *locking the line*)

When flushing a line, never force the solution administration. If you feel resistance and continue to force the administration, you risk rupturing the catheter and causing embolism (see the later section "Checking for and preventing common complications" for details on this condition).

Instead of forcing the flush, stop and look for the following possible issues:

- ✔ A closed clamp or kink in the tubing
- ✔ A clogged inline filter or injection cap that needs replacing
- ✔ A stabilization device that needs adjusting
- ✔ A positional problem that you may be able to alleviate by having the patient change positions

If infusion resistance remains after you check for these problems, you may be dealing with a more serious situation, such as an occlusion or thrombus, in which case you need to immediately notify your supervisor or the patient's physician.

 INS recommends that you use single-dose flush solution syringes and vials for flushing CVAD lines because these syringes reduce the risk for contamination and infection. Higher infection rates are associated with multiple-dose vials and large-volume fluid bags. To further reduce the risk for contamination, use single-dose flushing solutions and dedicate each one to a single patient.

Understanding the goals of flushing CVAD lines helps you recognize the need to adhere to every step of the flushing protocol even when patient loads are heavy and time is short.

Locking the line

Locking the line refers to the IV flush you do after the CVAD administration when the administration is intermittent and the line needs to remain open for repeated infusions. Locking the line generally involves flushing with saline or heparin-lock solution and allowing it to stay in the line to keep the line free from clots or other obstructions even when it's not in use. You don't have to lock the line when you use the CVAD for continuous infusions.

CVAD lines are most frequently locked by flushing with heparin solution or 0.9 percent preservative-free normal saline. The standard in most facilities is to use 10 units/milliliter (mL) of heparin in 5 mL vials or 10 mL of normal saline (20 mL of normal saline, if after a blood draw or blood infusion).

To ensure that all internal surface areas receive adequate turbulence and flushing, manufacturers recommend that the volume of locking solution be equal to at least twice the volume of the capacity of the catheter and add-on devices.

Although locking the line is essential when you're using it intermittently, the use of heparin is controversial because of the potential for heparin-induced *thrombocytopenia,* a decrease in platelets in the blood. Many heparin-lock solutions now contain warnings about the potential for thrombocytopenia. Manufacturers of CVAD-related products and healthcare facilities recognize this potential reaction and have produced alternative products that use only normal saline for locking.

Checking for and preventing common complications

Doctors, PAs, and specially trained nurses insert more than 7 million CVADs each year in the U.S. Today these central venous lines are remaining in place longer and are being used for a broader range of medication and nutrition infusions than they used to. This increased use and the longer periods of treatment translate into a potential increased risk for complications. In this section, you find out about the most common and most serious complications associated with CVADs.

Infection

One of the most serious and life-threatening complications related to the CVAD is bloodstream infection (BSI), also known as catheter-related bloodstream infection (CRBSI), which can lead to *septicemia,* or systemic infection. Each year, in the U.S., CRBSIs occur in approximately 80,000 ICU patients with central venous lines. When you count patients outside of the ICU, central venous lines are linked to more than 250,000 bloodstream infections each year and associated with a 12 to 25 percent mortality rate.

The risk for CRBSI begins the moment the doctor, PA, or trained nurse penetrates the patient's skin to insert the central catheter and continues for the duration of the catheter placement because of the skin's own microflora that dwells on the skin's surface and within the sebaceous glands. Cleansing with chlorhexidine or iodophor solution helps disinfect the surface, but neither solution can penetrate to the deeper glandular areas. When the needle and eventually the catheter pass through these glands, the microbes attach to their surface and are carried into the entry site and the bloodstream.

Following are some of the other common causes of CVAD-related infection that can lead to septicemia:

- Contamination of the insertion site during the insertion procedure
- Contamination of the vascular access device
- Vessel wall injury during catheter insertion, causing inflammation or phlebitis
- Contamination through improper hand hygiene
- Contamination through improper cleansing of the insertion site or improper aseptic technique during care, maintenance, or infusion of the CVAD

Risk of infection increases when contamination enables bacteria to adhere to surfaces at the insertion site and form a slimy, glue-like substance called *biofilm*. Biofilm binds to all types of materials, including plastics, implant catheters, and tissues.

When biofilm forms at the insertion site of CVADs, it can grow retrograde along the central catheter pathway and enter the central circulatory system, resulting in septicemia. Biofilm infections are extremely difficult to treat because they frequently consist of several different types of bacteria that are resistant to most antibiotics.

In addition to causing septicemia from the insertion site, biofilm also causes septicemia from the indwelling central venous catheter. When biofilm forms on a central venous catheter, fibrin and other clotting products build up to cover and protect the biofilm. When the buildup becomes thick enough, it breaks off and can cause an embolism and lead to septicemia. The longer the catheter remains in place, the greater the risk that biofilm will build up on the catheter.

Symptoms associated with CVAD systemic infections (septicemia) include the following:

✔ Fevers, chills, tachycardia, hypotension, shock, and hyperventilation

✔ Impaired kidney function and decreased urine output

✔ Altered mental status

For symptoms associated with insertion-site infections, check out the section "Assessing the site" earlier in this chapter.

As the use of CVADs increases, the risk for infection also increases. In recent years, the Institute for Healthcare Improvement (IHI) has recognized this increased risk and implemented a *care bundle campaign* to improve patient outcomes and prevent central line infections. The *central line care bundle* is a group of evidenced-based interventions designed to reduce risk for complications in patients with central venous catheters. When the interventions are implemented together, the result is a better patient outcome than when the interventions are implemented separately. The central line care bundle has the following five key components:

✔ Hand hygiene

✔ Maximum barrier protection for insertion

✔ Chlorhexidine skin antisepsis

✔ Optimal catheter site location (avoiding the femoral line in adults)

✔ Daily review of the necessity for a central line

When implemented as a group, the central line care bundle has been effective in reducing CVAD-related infections.

Air embolism

Air embolism is when a bolus of air enters the venous or arterial bloodstream and lodges in the heart, lungs, or brain. If the air bolus is large enough, air embolism can cause brain damage, stroke, or even death.

CVADs bring with them an increase in the risk of air embolism because their long, hollow tubes create a pathway into the bloodstream. If air enters the central venous system through a CVAD, it travels through the pathway of the central catheter and goes directly to the right side of the heart, resulting in catastrophic consequences.

Typical nonvalved or valved CVAD-related causes of air embolism include the following:

- **A hole in the catheter or tubing (valved or nonvalved):** You risk damaging the tubing when you use scissors, clamps, or other objects around a central line, and damage to the tubing can allow the influx of air.

- **Improper priming (valved or nonvalved):** When you don't completely remove all the air from the IV tubing during the priming procedure, the air remaining in the tubing between the pump and catheter gets pushed into the venous system by the central line pump.

- **Improper closure of injection ports (nonvalved):** When you fail to properly close these sites (for example, stopcocks, ports, or extension tubing), air can enter the central line.

- **Improper changing of infusion bags (nonvalved):** When you allow infusion bags to become empty, air can be pulled from the bag into the central line.

- **Improper removal of a central line (valved or nonvalved):** Removal of a central line creates an opening into the vein, and unless you take precautions like the Valsalva maneuver (which requires the patient to take a deep breath and hold it or bear down while the catheter is being removed), air can enter the central circulatory system and cause air embolism. This maneuver is usually used for the removal of internal jugular (IJ) catheters and catheters located in the subclavian veins; it decreases the potential of an air embolus.

To prevent an air embolism, follow these safety tips:

- Ensure clamps, ports, and vents are closed during tubing changes.

- Adhere strictly to institutional guidelines or manufacturer's instructions when priming IV tubing.

- ✔ Change infusion bags before they're completely empty.
- ✔ Check frequently for damaged tubing, access caps, and injection ports.
- ✔ Check frequently to make sure all infusion-related devices, such as piggybacks, stopcocks, and vents, are securely closed.
- ✔ Instruct patients to lie flat and still and perform the Valsalva maneuver when removing an IJ- or subclavian-located central line.
- ✔ Use air-eliminating filters when appropriate.

Catheter-related embolism

Catheter-related embolism occurs when the actual catheter ruptures and catheter remnants flow into the bloodstream. Catheter rupture can occur when you meet resistance during an attempt to flush the catheter and you force the flushing solution through the catheter anyway or when you use a syringe smaller than recommended.

You can prevent flushing-induced embolism by never forcing fluid against resistance in a central catheter. If the flushing solution doesn't flow easily into the catheter, notify the patient's doctor or refer to institutional protocol for directions on what to do next.

Catheter-related embolism can also occur because of the following:

- ✔ **Catheter pinch-off syndrome:** This syndrome happens when the central catheter is caught between the juncture of the first rib and clavicle, pinching and obstructing the catheter to the point of rupture.
- ✔ **Manufacturing or material defects:** Manufacturing defects in the catheter lumens or material defects in the silicone or polyurethane catheters can cause loss of wall integrity and risk of rupture.

You can prevent catheter-related embolism by not forcing the flushing and by using the appropriate, recommended size syringe for flushing. You can also carefully inspect the packaging and the central venous catheter before insertion.

Catheter-related venous thrombosis

Thrombosis is the formation, development, or presence of a blood clot (called a *thrombus*) within a vessel. *Catheter-related thrombosis* can occur when the vessel wall suffers an injury from the catheter or when the vessel wall reacts to the insertion of a catheter or to medications administered through the catheter. As a result of injury, thrombosis forms at the catheter tip and begins to block the flow of blood and fluid through the catheter.

Catheter-related thrombosis can occur quickly or slowly, and it can cause a partial or complete obstruction of the central venous catheter. Thrombotic occlusions (or obstructions) have a significant impact on the function of a CVAD, preventing the patient from receiving medications and fluids that are administered through the central access device and limiting the performance of procedures that are routinely done through a central venous catheter.

Following are some of the CVAD procedures that thrombosis limits:

- ✔ Administering fluids
- ✔ Administering medications or parenteral solutions
- ✔ Flushing or locking the catheter
- ✔ Aspirating or withdrawing blood
- ✔ Performing hemodynamic monitoring

Catheter-related thrombosis is associated with 58 percent of all occlusions that occur in central venous catheters, but you can decrease the risk of catheter-related thrombosis by taking preventive measures like these:

- ✔ Maintain positive pressure during flushing and locking procedures.
- ✔ Frequently assess infusion delivery systems for damage, kinks in the tubing, mechanical defects, and loose connection points.
- ✔ Use clamps when changing administration sets or add-on devices.
- ✔ Review medications for incompatibility when you're infusing multiple drugs.
- ✔ Educate the patient to observe the dressing for leaks or dampness.

If you suspect that a catheter is being blocked because it's pressing against the vessel wall, try to change the catheter position by having the patient change physical positions. For example, have the patient raise his arms above his head, cough, or lie down. You can also try a gentle flush with 10 mL of normal saline, taking care not to force the fluid and risk dislodging the clot.

If these methods don't work and you suspect thrombosis, notify the provider and obtain an order to administer a fibrinolytic agent to dissolve the clot. After the clot dissolves, you can gently aspirate it to restore patency or openness to the catheter.

Pulmonary embolism

Pulmonary embolism (PE) is the blockage of the lung's pulmonary artery or one of its branches by a substance, usually a blood clot. Pulmonary embolism causes increased pressure on the right ventricle of the heart, decreases the exchange of oxygen and carbon dioxide, and results in serious complications or death.

Pulmonary embolism is often associated with CVADs because of the risk for clot formation around the central catheter and the close proximity of the catheter to the right ventricle of the heart.

Maintaining CVADs

Everything about CVAD maintenance, including regularly replacing IV tubing, access caps, and site dressings, is designed to prevent catheter-related infections. The following sections cover the key components of CVAD maintenance.

Changing ports, access caps, and IV tubing

When you're dealing with CVADs, you have to change injection ports, access caps, and IV tubing on a regular basis according to facility protocol. Although different institutions follow different protocols, the general consensus recommends changing injection ports and access caps when you change the IV tubing, usually every 96 hours. The CDC recommends that you change needleless components during IV tubing changes but no more frequently than every 72 hours, and INS recommends that you change them every 96 hours. Check your facility's protocol for more specifics.

For certain types of infusions, you have to replace IV tubing more frequently. For example, when administering blood or blood products, INS states to change the tubing every 4 hours and when administering fat emulsions, the CDC recommends changing IV tubing within 24 hours after initiating the infusion. For propofol infusions, you should change IV tubing every 6 to 12 hours, or when the propofol vial is changed, according to manufacturer's instructions.

Because most injection ports are incorporated into IV tubing, the ports are automatically changed when the IV tubing is changed. Access caps are replaced after each removal or when contamination is noted.

Routine changing of IV tubing is critical in minimizing risk for infection, but it also adds an element of risk of its own. If air enters the IV tubing during a tubing change, it can cause air embolism, a potentially fatal complication associated with central venous lines (see the earlier section on common complications for details). To guard against air embolism when changing IV tubing, make sure all the air is out of the tubing and all clamps are shut before connecting to the catheter hub. Also, be sure to properly disinfect all injection ports for 15 seconds prior to connecting to the catheter hub.

To ensure a complete, accurate medical record, note the following information every time you change a tubing, port, or access cap:

✔ Date and time of tubing, injection port, and access cap change

✔ Ease or difficulty of the change

✔ Patient tolerance to the procedure

✔ Resumption of infusate type and flow rate

✔ Any pertinent patient education and patient's understanding

Performing site care and dressing changes

From the moment the central catheter penetrates the skin, the patient's first line of defense is broken, and a perfect pathway opens up for the entry of bacteria. To prevent bacteria from traveling up the central venous catheter and causing a bloodstream infection, you must change the insertion site dressing at regularly scheduled intervals or as needed and keep it clean and dry.

Although protocol on changing site dressings varies slightly from institution to institution, most agree that you should change transparent dressings every seven days and gauze dressings every 48 hours. However, if you see any evidence of redness, swelling, or drainage near the insertion site, you need to change the dressings immediately. You should also change the dressings as needed when they become soiled, wet, or loose.

The recommended dressing type for use on a central venous catheter is a transparent semipermeable dressing because a transparent dressing allows you to monitor for signs of infection or leakage.

When you're caring for a central venous access device and especially when you're changing the dressing, the two most important things to remember are adherence to institutional protocol and use of strict aseptic technique. Your goal when changing the dressing is to prevent serious bloodstream infections. You can do so by following these 12 steps:

1. **Thoroughly wash your hands with soap and water or an alcohol-based hand sanitizer, identify yourself to the patient, verify the patient's identity, and explain the dressing change procedure.**

2. **Position the patient comfortably in the bed or chair, rewash your hands, and apply non-sterile gloves.**

3. **Remove the old dressing by releasing the transparent film from the outside to the inside to avoid pulling on the catheter and insertion site (see Figure 13-1).**

   Never pull the dressing away from the insertion site; if you do, you risk dislodging the catheter.

4. **Observe the insertion site for any drainage, swelling, redness, or other signs of possible infection and inspect the dressing for drainage, blood, discoloration, or wetness.**

5. **Inspect the catheter to ensure that the external catheter hasn't advanced beyond its original insertion point or come out; confirm that the catheter and hub are in good condition.**

   You also need to change the sutureless securement device, if used.

6. **Prepare a sterile field that includes a disinfectant (chlorhexidine or iodophor), a transparent occlusive dressing, sterile gloves, small sterile drape or sterile towel, and gauze and place it at the patient's bedside.**

   You can also use a prepackaged sterile kit.

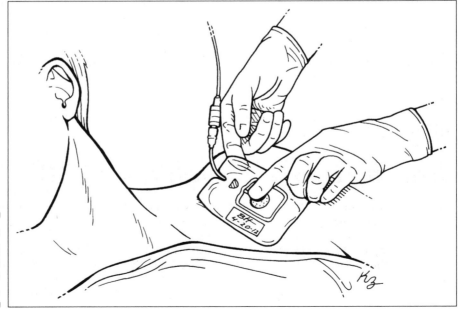

Figure 13-1:
Removing
an old
central line
dressing.

Illustration by Kathryn Born

7. Apply your mask, rewash your hands, and apply sterile gloves.

8. Clean the insertion site thoroughly with 2 percent chlorhexidine (scrub for 30 seconds) and allow the site to dry completely (about 30 seconds).

9. Apply an occlusive, transparent, semipermeable dressing over the catheter securement hub per institution protocol and allow the end of the line with the hub to hang out for access.

10. Inspect the catheter hub to ensure that the tubing is locked and tape a loop of tubing to the patient's skin to minimize tugging at the catheter insertion site.

11. Write the type, size, and length of the catheter and the date and time of the dressing change on the label, sign it, and apply it to the dressing.

12. Document the dressing change and any abnormal findings in the appropriate section of the patient's chart (see next section) and notify the physician if needed.

Documenting your actions

Just like all other CVAD procedures, you have to document your dressing change and site assessment in the patient's medical record. Be sure to include the following details in your documentation:

✔ Infusate, rate, medications, flow, and CVAD

✔ Condition of the catheter, insertion site, and dressing

✔ External length of the catheter from the insertion point

✔ Any problems or interventions

✔ Patient's response, patient education, and patient's understanding

Drawing Blood through the CVAD

Drawing blood through the CVAD isn't recommended because doing so increases the risk for infection, clots, and other systemic complications. But when a patient's peripheral veins are inaccessible due to sclerosis or collapse, the CVAD is the best option. The following sections walk you through the process of drawing blood through a CVAD.

Drawing blood from CVADs may alter laboratory results because of flushing and infusing solutions or medications. As a result, you shouldn't draw blood for clotting tests like prothrombin time (PT) and partial thromboplastin time (PTT) through CVADs because of the impact heparin, if used, can have on the laboratory values.

Obtaining an order

As with all access entries into central venous lines, you have to obtain an order from the physician or provider before you can access the line and draw blood. After you obtain the order, document the date, time, and details of the order in the patient's medical record.

Withdrawing the blood

When drawing blood from the CVAD, you must use strict aseptic technique and adhere to institutional protocol. The following steps walk you through the basic procedure:

1. **Place the patient in a supine position and apply a mask or have the patient turn away from the insertion site.**

2. **Turn off the infusion when you enter the room and begin to prepare for the procedure before withdrawing blood.**

   You need to turn off the infusion at least one minute before withdrawing blood.

   According to INS standards, choose the largest lumen for blood draws. For multiple staggered lumen catheters, use the proximal lumen (highest in the superior vena cava) and draw from the lumen that isn't being used for drug infusions.

3. **Wash your hands thoroughly and apply sterile or non-sterile gloves (follow facility protocol).**

4. **Remove the access cap.**

   Never draw blood through the needleless connector because residual blood can be left in it and can cause infection. If, for some reason, you do, you must change the needleless connector by following your facility's protocol or flush it with at least 20 mL of 0.9 percent normal saline.

5. **Clean the catheter hub with alcohol or other acceptable antiseptic for 15 seconds.**

6. **Attach the syringe directly to the catheter hub.**

7. **Using a 10-mL syringe, withdraw 5 mL of blood and discard the syringe.**

8. **Use a new syringe to withdraw the required amount of blood for testing and transfer the blood to an appropriately labeled vacutainer tube.**

    Withdraw the blood slowly to prevent damage to or collapse of the catheter or blood vessel.

9. **After you withdraw the amount needed for testing, flush the line with at least 20 mL of normal saline and infuse heparin into the port according to institution protocol.**

10. **Replace the access cap with a new, sterile cap.**

11. **Document the procedure, any difficulties encountered, and patient tolerance in the patient's medical record.**

Discontinuing and Removing the CVAD

To prevent risk for infection, clots, or other complications, the INS standards state that central venous catheters should be removed immediately when therapy is discontinued, contamination is suspected, or complications are unresolved. As soon as you observe any of these situations, notify the patient's physician or provider so that she can issue an order for catheter discontinuation and removal as soon as possible. After all, central venous catheters provide an entry point and pathway for bacteria to cause systemic infection and must be removed quickly (see the earlier section "Checking for and preventing common complications" for details on bloodstream infections). In the following sections, we explain the procedure for removing CVADs, including who can remove them, and we cover what you have to do after removal takes place.

Following the right procedure

Nurses with documented competency in the procedure can remove percutaneously inserted CVADs such as PICCs and non-tunneled subclavian or jugular CVADs. Double-check the physician's order and check out your facility's policy and your state's scope of practice to avoid issues with liability. Keep in mind that nurses aren't allowed to remove tunneled catheters because they're embedded beneath the skin and must be removed by an MD, PA, or ARNP.

After you check with facility protocol and scope-of-practice regulations to determine which types of central venous catheters you can remove, follow these guidelines to remove them:

1. **Place the patient in a supine position, keeping the insertion site at or below the level of the heart, to reduce risk for air embolism (see the earlier section "Air embolism" for details).**

   When removing an IJ or subclavian central line, have the patient perform a Valsalva maneuver to prevent air embolism.

2. **Discontinue the IV flow.**

3. **Apply non-sterile gloves and use aseptic technique to remove the dressing and catheter stabilization device.**

4. **Use short, gentle strokes to slowly withdraw the catheter.**

   Don't force the withdrawal if you encounter resistance when withdrawing the catheter. The resistance could be caused by kinking or knotting of the catheter or a muscle spasm in the vessel wall. If kinking or knotting of the catheter is causing the resistance, forcefully removing it can fracture the catheter and cause fragment embolus. Resecure the catheter, contact the provider, and document the incident.

   When removing a PICC, if you continue to feel resistance after a few minutes and you think a muscle spasm may be the cause, have the patient relax and take deep breaths to relieve the spasm or place a warm compress around the patient's arm.

5. **If the physician orders the catheter tip to be cultured, as the catheter clears the vein and skin, don't let it become contaminated by touching the patient's skin or clothing; trim the tip off into a sterile container, label it, and send it to the lab.**

6. **Apply a sterile dressing to the site and use digital pressure to stop the bleeding.**

7. **Place antiseptic ointment and a sterile dressing over the insertion site.**

   The ointment will help seal the puncture wound at the insertion site. If you observe bleeding from the insertion site, apply more digital pressure until the bleeding stops.

8. **Instruct the patient to leave the dressing in place for at least 24 hours until the site has closed.**

Inspecting the catheter

After the catheter has been removed, inspect it for any internal structural damage that may have caused leakage of fluid and medication into the chest. Observe the external portion of the catheter to ensure catheter integrity and the absence of any damage.

If you observe any damage to the catheter, notify the provider and follow institutional protocol for follow-up procedures.

Documenting your actions after the removal

Accurate documentation provides proof that you followed protocols, minimized risk, and maximized safety for your patient. This documentation includes noting all your actions and observations during the removal procedure, as well as your adherence to institutional protocol. Include the following specifics in your post-removal documentation:

- The reason for removal (such as discontinued therapy, infection, embolus, or occlusion)
- The use of aseptic technique and the date and time of the removal procedure
- The supine position of the patient and the discontinuance of the IV solution
- The ease or difficulty of catheter removal
- The type of dressing applied to the insertion site
- The placing of immediate pressure on the insertion site
- The prevention of contamination of the catheter and tip, the sterile collection of the catheter and tip, and the transfer to the laboratory
- The appearance of the injection site and the application of antiseptic ointment, sterile gauze, and a labeled, transparent, semipermeable dressing over the insertion site
- The instruction to the patient to leave the dressing in place for 24 hours and the patient's understanding of the instruction
- The full length of the catheter prior to the tip removal
- The patient's response to the procedure
- Notification of any adverse events to the provider

Using an Implanted Port Instead

Implanted central venous ports offer another avenue for direct access to the central circulatory system, particularly when continuous infusion isn't necessary but frequent venous access is required, such as with the intermittent administration of chemotherapy drugs. Implanted ports consist of a central venous catheter attached to a self-sealing septum buried within a pocket of subcutaneous tissue (see Figure 13-2). Licensed nurses use these ports to administer medications, fluids, and blood products and to collect blood specimens as ordered by physicians or providers. They're a mainstay of treatment for long-term delivery of medications because they're safe and easy to implant and they improve the patient's quality of life.

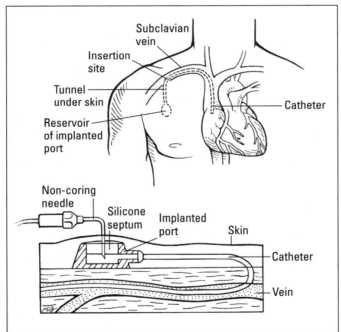

Figure 13-2: Implanted venous port for central vein access.

Illustration by Kathryn Born

Applying a local anesthetic

To minimize patient discomfort when accessing a port, you may apply local anesthesia in the form of a transdermal anesthetic cream or aerosol freeze spray each time the port is accessed. For maximum effectiveness, be sure to apply the cream one hour before the scheduled port access. Check with your facility's policy. Note that the anesthetic cream usually requires a physician's order.

Other techniques you can use to minimize discomfort include using the smallest gauge, shortest needle possible and rotating the needle insertions to different sides of the port, thus allowing the skin to rest and heal between treatments.

Gaining access with a non-coring needle

To access an implanted port, you must use sterile technique and a safety infusion set with a special non-coring needle, like the one shown in Figure 13-3, to pierce the port's *septum* (a silicone plug where the non-coring needle is placed) and infuse through the central venous catheter. The safety infusion set features a *non-coring needle* with an angled or deflected point that enters the septum as it penetrates the implanted port. It's recommended for accessing all implanted ports because it doesn't core or disrupt the self-sealing feature of the septum. Standard needles can core the septum and cause a loss of leak-tight integrity.

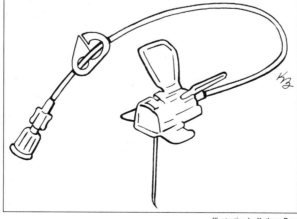

Figure 13-3:
Safety infusion set with a non-coring needle for implanted port access.

Illustration by Kathryn Born

When using a safety infusion set and non-coring needle with an implanted port, follow these guidelines:

- ✔ Correctly position the needle inside the port chamber and feel the bottom of the port chamber before starting the infusion.
- ✔ Don't tilt or rock the needle after it enters the port chamber.
- ✔ Change the needle every seven days or as needed to maintain integrity and document the date you change it.

Administering therapy through the port

Ports may appear safer than CVADs because they have no external catheter or injection ports, but they provide the same central pathogenic pathway to the bloodstream and pose the same risk for serious complications of infection. For this reason, you need to use the same strict aseptic technique that you use in caring for and accessing central venous catheters when you're caring for and accessing implanted ports.

To maintain proper aseptic technique when accessing an implanted port, follow institutional protocol and use the following steps as guidelines:

1. **Place the patient in a comfortable supine or semi-Fowler's position.**

2. **Wash your hands and apply non-sterile gloves, according to protocol.**

3. **Palpate the implanted port, locating the outer port perimeter and the center of the septum.**

4. **Wipe away all the anesthetic cream that you applied an hour before the scheduled port access (see the earlier section "Applying a local anesthetic").**

   If you're not using a central line kit, also take some time to saturate the gauze with chlorhexidine or another approved antiseptic.

5. **Create a sterile field by using a central line dressing drape or sterile glove wrapper.**

6. Wash your hands again and then apply sterile gloves and thoroughly scrub the port and surround site with the chlorhexidine or other approved antiseptic; allow the antiseptic to dry completely.

7. Maintaining sterility, remove the cap from the non-coring needle tubing and connect the needleless injection plug.

8. Using a sterile 10-mL syringe, prime the tubing and non-coring needle with 1 to 2 mL of 0.9 percent normal saline, expel the air, and close the tubing clamp.

Whether you're administering infusions or collecting samples through an implanted port, use a syringe that's no smaller than 10 mL to minimize pressure inside the catheter, prevent rupture, and avoid embolization from ruptured catheter remnants.

9. With your nondominant hand, grasp the port with your thumb and forefinger to stabilize the port, locate the port septum center, and insert the non-coring needle through the skin and septum until you feel the bottom of the port chamber.

10. Aspirate for blood return to ensure proper placement, flush with saline, and administer the infusion.

If you meet resistance when flushing, don't forcefully inject the saline, because you risk dislodging a clot or rupturing the catheter. Verify the needle position, and if resistance remains, call for further orders. If you successfully flush the port but can't get a blood return, instruct the patient to change positions, cough, take deep breaths, or perform the Valsalva maneuver.

11. Flush with the remaining saline and apply an antimicrobial dressing.

Communicating with your patient

Patient communication is a central part of accessing and infusing through an implanted port. So be sure to ask questions and elicit comments from the patient and family before you start any infusion procedure. Doing so helps allay fears and frequently allows you to uncover invaluable information, especially if the patient is a long-term implant patient.

Keep in mind that an implanted port has a long, usable life, and many patients have their implanted ports indefinitely if they maintain them properly. Thus, a long-term patient can provide invaluable information about the amount of time she's had the port, the needle size that worked best in the past, and any complications she has experienced. Some patients and family even have manufacturer's literature on the implanted device. So be sure to keep those lines of communication open!

Part IV
Administering IV Therapy

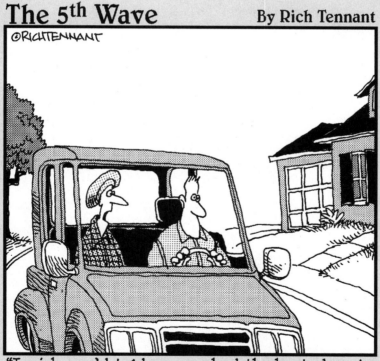

The 5th Wave   By Rich Tennant

"I wish you'd told me you had the heated seats on. I thought I was having another side effect from the chemo."

In this part . . .

*P*art IV covers the practical, how-to aspects of administering and monitoring common types of IV therapy. It picks up where Part II leaves off by describing the everyday, practical aspects of administering and monitoring IV medications and detailing the verification, administration, and documentation procedures associated with blood transfusions. It also covers the dangers and precautions related to working with hazardous, life-saving chemotherapy drugs and describes the process of administering fluids and electrolytes. It finishes up by explaining how to administer IV nutrition to patients in a clinical setting.

Chapter 14

Practical Pharmacological IV Administration

· ·

In This Chapter

▶ Evaluating five critical safety issues during your patient assessment

▶ Safely initiating, monitoring, and discontinuing IV medications

▶ Identifying and managing adverse drug reactions

▶ Protecting yourself when handling and disposing of pharmacological agents

· ·

*I*nfusing medications through pharmacological infusion (IV) therapy is one of the quickest and most effective ways to deliver drugs directly into a patient's bloodstream. But it's also one of the fastest ways to induce severe adverse reactions.

This chapter takes you through the practical aspects of safely administering IV medications, from assessing your patient and initiating therapy to discarding pharmacological agents. Here, you find out how to assess your patient for five critical issues central to the safe administration of IV medications, and you gain a new understanding of the differences between allergic, adverse, and crossover reactions and the techniques you can use to manage them. Thanks to this chapter, you can be confident that the medication you're adding to a piggyback or pushing through an IV tubing is healing, not harming, your patient.

Assessing Your Pharma Patient

When you're dealing with pharmacological IV therapy, the first step in ensuring patient safety is familiarizing yourself with the patient's medical record, diagnosis, medical and surgical history, and treatment plan. The next step is performing a physical assessment when you enter the patient's room. You start by introducing yourself and then evaluate the patient's general physical condition, handicaps, or other circumstances that may complicate treatment via IV therapy.

In addition to the physical assessment, you need to find out more about your patient's history with IV medications. A thorough patient assessment provides the first opportunity for you to determine your patient's possible responses to the anticipated treatment. After all, the most important goal of patient assessment is to ensure a positive patient experience with IV therapy. In the following sections, we show you how to reach that goal by assessing your patient's condition and asking the right questions as you do so.

Considering five critical safety issues

When you're administering medications intravenously, the margin of safety is narrow, and the potential for severe consequences, including death, is associated with every infusion. Many of the most serious safety concerns revolve around the following five critical issues, which all have to do with drug reactions and which you can address during your patient assessment:

✔ Medication allergies

✔ Adverse drug events (ADEs)

✔ Drug-to-drug interactions

✔ Crossover reactions

✔ Reactions with over-the-counter drugs, such as herbal and nutritional supplements

Medication allergies

Identifying medication allergies is the first line of defense in preventing allergic and other adverse drug reactions to IV medications. In terms of pharmacology, an *allergic reaction* is when your immune system reacts abnormally to a medication. The most common signs are hives, rash, and/or fever. True allergic reactions involve the activation of the immune system by the drug. (See the next section for details on adverse drug reactions.)

To verify your patient's allergy history, ask your patient about her drug allergies and then repeat her answers. Specifically, ask your patient what medications she has taken in the past or is currently taking. Note whether she has had any mild or major allergic reactions, including the following:

✔ Confusion or anxiety

✔ Difficulty breathing

✔ Dizziness

✔ Fatigue

✔ Nausea, vomiting, or diarrhea

✔ Skin rash, redness, irritation, or itching

✔ Stuffy, swollen, or runny nasal passages

✔ Swelling or tightening of the throat

To ensure that the answers you receive from your patient about her medication allergies are accurate and complete, check the patient's medical record, the medication reconciliation form (MRA), and the physician's initial admission note for any discrepancies.

If you uncover any new or previously unrecorded medication allergies, document them immediately on the patient's medical record and identification bracelet.

Adverse drug events

Adverse drug reactions or side effects are unexpected and undesired consequences of drug administration. Unlike allergic reactions, which are caused by a local or systemic immune response, adverse drug reactions are caused by events that aren't usually associated with the immune system. Because most drugs are taken by mouth, loss of appetite, nausea, vomiting, constipation, and diarrhea are common adverse drug reactions. The events that cause adverse drug reactions are cleverly called *adverse drug events,* or ADEs, and include the following:

✔ Administration of a newly approved drug

✔ Overreaction or severe reaction to a known drug

✔ Reaction to a medication error in prescribing, dosing, or administering

Knowing the difference between allergic and adverse drug reactions allows you to more clearly communicate symptoms with the patient's physician and speeds up effective treatment.

When a patient says that a medication causes nausea, that nausea may be a side effect, not an allergic reaction. Many medications, such as antibiotics and narcotics, cause gastric distress as a side effect or adverse reaction, which explains why these meds are best taken with food.

Drug-to-drug interactions

Most hospitalized patients take at least one medication on a daily basis, and many take more. When physicians add new medications to the mix, the risk for a *toxic drug combination,* or severe drug-to-drug interaction, skyrockets.

After all, the more medications a patient takes, the more likely the patient is to experience drug-to-drug interactions.

Of the more than 1,100 known toxic drug combinations, the following drugs, when used in combination with other medications, are among the most high-risk offenders:

- ✔ Angiotensin-converting enzyme (ACE) inhibitor antihypertensives, such as lisinopril
- ✔ Digoxin heart medications, such as Lanoxin
- ✔ Theophylline respiratory drugs, such as Theolair
- ✔ Warfarin anticoagulant, commonly known as Coumadin

Being aware of common medications that produce severe drug interactions is central to preventing toxic drug combinations in your patients. If your patient is currently taking any of these drugs, contact the prescribing physician and pharmacy for alternative therapies that may be compatible.

You can also prevent dangerous interactions by using electronic medication delivery systems, infusion pumps with drug libraries, and drug reference books to identify potential toxic combinations. See Chapter 4 for more details about preventing drug-to-drug interactions.

Crossover reactions

Patients who have a known allergy to one drug are at risk of having an allergic reaction to a different drug with a similar chemical structure. This type of allergic reaction is called a *crossover reaction,* and it's caused by the immune system's ability to recognize similarities between allergens found in different medications.

Here's a simple example to help you understand crossover reactions: A person with an allergy to shrimp is likely to have a crossover allergy to other shellfish, such as lobster and clams.

In the field of IV therapy medications, a person with an allergy to penicillin may also have an allergy to cephalosporin antibiotics, such as cephalexin (Keflex). Following are some other drugs that can cause crossover reactions:

- ✔ Barbiturates and the antiseizure medication phenytoin (Dilantin)
- ✔ Opiates and the antibiotic levofloxacin (Levaquin)
- ✔ Oxycodone and the narcotic hydromorphone (Dilaudid)
- ✔ Sulfonamide antibiotics and the diuretic hydrochlorothiazide (HCTZ)

To guard against crossover reactions, notify the physician and clarify the order if you suspect the potential for cross-reactivity.

Reactions with over-the-counter medications

More than 3,200 over-the-counter (OTC) drugs, 300 dietary supplements, and 600 herbal products are currently available in the U.S., and many of them produce severe drug-to-drug interactions when taken in combination with prescribed meds.

From common headache remedies to antiyeast vaginal creams, OTCs interact with prescription medications in several ways, including the following:

✔ Decreasing or increasing (or *potentiating*) the drug's potency

✔ Decreasing kidney or liver elimination and clearance of the drug

✔ Reacting chemically to the drug to produce cardiac, respiratory, or other symptoms

To prevent drug interactions between OTCs and IV meds, ask your patient about all OTC medications she's taking, including pain relievers, herbal products, or nutritional supplements, and report them to the physician. Even seemingly harmless supplements, such as St. John's Wort, are linked to adverse interactions with commonly prescribed medications, such as antibiotics and blood thinners.

OTC medications aren't the only potentiators of prescription medications. *Furanocoumarin,* the active ingredient in grapefruit juice, is a strong potentiator of Beta blockers. Drinking as little as 4 ounces of grapefruit juice while on these heart medications has been associated with adverse reactions, ranging from slow heart rate to cardiac arrest and death.

The following classifications of medications have an increased risk for potentiating drug effects, and Table 14-1 lists a few of the most common IV medication potentiators:

✔ Antibiotics

✔ Anti-inflammatories

✔ Antihistamines

✔ Cardiac and blood pressure medications

✔ Central nervous system depressants

✔ Diuretics

✔ Pain relievers and opioid products

Table 14-1	Common Potentiators of IV Medications	
IV Medication	*Medication Potentiator*	*Possible Effects*
erythromycin (E-Mycin)	amlodipine (Norvasc)	Increased low blood pressure effects
warfarin (Coumadin)	amiodarone (Cordarone)	Increased anticoagulant effects
morphine (MS-Contin)	imipramine (Tofranil)	Increased sedation and narcotic effects
fentanyl (Sublimaze)	promethazine (Phenergan)	Increased central nervous system and respiratory depressive effects

Asking patients about their problems

Studying a patient's medical record helps you identify symptoms, medications, and prognosis, but you also need to get the patient's version of what's going on. Asking questions and learning about the patient's assessment of her current problems and medication history can help you understand the critical role that IV medications may play in the patient's treatment plan and recovery (and how the patient feels about that role).

Asking the right questions helps you elicit a genuine self-assessment from your patient and uncover any preconceived ideas or fears of treatment with IV medications. Addressing these preconceived ideas upfront helps relieve the patient's fears and promotes better compliance for future treatment.

Here's a series of questions you can ask to get the patient's self-assessment:

- What symptoms are you currently having?
- Would you rate your symptoms as mild, moderate, or severe?
- What medications have you taken for these symptoms?
- Did the medications help relieve your symptoms?
- Have you received IV medications before?
- Did they help relieve your symptoms?
- Did you have any allergic or other type of reaction to the IV medications?
- Did you feel that IV medications were the best treatment?

✔ Was there a downside to IV medications?

✔ Would you take IV medications if your doctor recommended them?

✔ What is your understanding of your current treatment plan?

Understanding your patient's interpretation of her current illness and expectation of treatment makes you a valuable member of the medical team and a more responsible advocate for your patient.

Knowing your patient's medication history from past to present

Delivering successful IV therapy requires you to know your patient's current and past medications. Your patient's medical record is the first place to look for a list of current medications, but you should also personally ask the patient about any medications she's currently taking or has previously taken. After confirming medications with the patient, check the medical record to ensure that all medications are listed and that the record is up-to-date. This is called *medication reconciliation,* or identifying the most accurate list of all medications that the patient is taking.

If you identify prescriptions that have recently been discontinued, altered, or renewed, refer to the patient's medical record to uncover any possibility of interaction between the patient's recently discontinued meds, newly prescribed meds, and the IV meds that may be part of the patient's treatment plan.

Initiating Pharmacological IV Treatment

The first step in safely administering IV drugs is becoming familiar with the medication you're infusing and all the equipment or supplies you have to use to administer it. The next step is properly preparing the med for the infusion. Then, of course, you have to actually administer the medication and closely monitor the infusion to make sure the patient isn't experiencing any side effects or adverse reactions. We explain all this in the following sections.

Note: Many states consider hold the nurse primarily responsible for being familiar with the medication, its side effects, and the management of adverse reactions, even when a physician administers the drug.

Before you begin: Getting ready for the infusion

Before you start any pharmacological IV, you need to do the following:

- ✔ Read the manufacturer's instructions regarding the correct diluent, possible side effects, and management of adverse reactions.

- ✔ Check the physician's order and verify the recommended safe-dosing concentration, dosage, and route of administration. Refer to your drug reference guide or the pharmacy if you have any questions or if you notice any discrepancies between the manufacturer's instructions and the physician's order.

- ✔ Inspect the infusion pump to make sure it's working properly and verify that the dose error reduction software (DERS) is in place and hasn't been bypassed.

- ✔ Familiarize yourself with IV access ports, particularly on multiple-lumen catheters. Ensure that the port you're accessing for medication delivery is either dedicated for medications only or designated for multiple uses including medications.

- ✔ For added safety, flush the line before (and after) each use, according to facility protocol.

In addition to doing these things, you must also take a few extra steps to protect yourself as well as your patient whenever you're preparing pharmacological agents for IV therapy. (*Pharmacological agents* are biologically active substances that produce a therapeutic response in the body; see Chapter 4 for details.) Following safe drug preparation techniques (as well as disposal techniques, which we talk about later in this chapter) reduces exposure to toxic agents and risks for subsequent health complications.

Use the following guidelines to protect yourself and your fellow nurses from risks of exposure to IV medication mixtures:

- ✔ Read the medication package insert and any other guidance documents for specifics on the drugs you're preparing.

- ✔ Consistently wear recommended personal protective equipment (PPE), such as gloves, gowns, and face and respiratory protectors.

- ✔ Remove protective gear and wash hands thoroughly after drug preparation.

- ✔ Follow your facility's recommended guidelines for safe transport of drugs.

✔ Clean up medication spills immediately according to recommended procedures.

✔ Follow institutional procedures for reporting and following up on accidental exposure to hazardous drugs.

Use the following guidelines to protect your patient:

✔ Ensure a clean work area for preparing the drug.

✔ Complete an accurate medication label.

✔ Follow medication instructions for reconstitution (see Chapter 4 for details).

✔ Adhere to strict aseptic technique.

✔ Swab vials, ampoules, and IV ports with alcohol before use.

✔ Double-check the physician's order, dosages, and labels before administering the drug.

✔ Ensure the use of the five rights of drug administration: right patient, right drug, right dose, right route, and right time.

Starting IV medication therapy

Starting IV therapy with medications is a lot like starting any other IV therapy. It starts with either a peripheral vascular access device (VAD), as discussed in Chapter 12, or a central VAD, as discussed in Chapter 13. Here are a few basic guidelines you need to follow to initiate IV medication therapy in both peripheral and central infusions:

✔ **Check the infusion bag for damage, prime the tubing, and disinfect the injection port.**

✔ **Use strict aseptic technique to inject the medication into the bag.**

✔ **After the injection, gently mix the drug into the bag by inverting the bag a couple of times and observe the fluid for cloudiness, precipitation, or color changes.**

✔ **Attach tubing to the VAD and open the roller clamp to start the infusion and set the correct flow rate.**

✔ **Label the infusion container with the following information:**

- Medication name and dosage

- Date and time of addition and expiration

- Route of administration and nurse's initials

When you're administering high-risk medications, such as chemotherapy agents or narcotics, two nurses should verify the physician's order, dosage, and route of administration. For a list of some of the most common high-risk medications, turn to Chapter 4.

Monitoring the infusion

Frequent monitoring is especially important right after you initiate IV medication to a patient because untoward side effects or serious adverse reactions usually occur during the first few minutes after initiating an infusion. As you monitor your patient, be sure to do the following:

✔ Observe the patient for local symptoms of pain at the injection site, generalized symptoms of rash and itching, or systemic symptoms of breathing difficulties.

✔ Monitor the injection site for inflammation, swelling, or signs of extravasation.

✔ Check the IV dressing for dampness, discoloration, or other signs of leakage.

✔ For gravity-fed infusions, check the drip chamber for slowing or sluggish flow rates, indicating possible occlusion by clot or crimped catheter.

If you notice slow rates, the first step to fixing the problem is to check for blood return. If you can't obtain blood return, reposition the IV tubing or the patient's extremity to resolve a crimped catheter issue. If the sluggish flow rates persist and you suspect a clot or thrombus, notify the physician or follow facility protocol to manage the occlusion and reestablish the desired flow rate.

Turn to Chapter 12 for more details on monitoring IVs in general. If you notice symptoms that suggest the patient is having an adverse reaction to the drug, keep reading.

Recognizing and Managing Adverse Drug Events (ADEs)

Adverse reactions to IV medications fall into the following two major categories:

✔ **Allergic reactions:** When the immune system mistakenly responds to a drug by creating an immune response, such as rash, hives, itching, fever, facial swelling, shortness of breath, or anaphylaxis (a life-threatening reaction)

✔ **Nonallergic reactions:** When events that aren't usually associated with the immune system, such as loss of appetite, nausea, vomiting, constipation, and diarrhea, occur

Both types of reactions can be either acute or delayed response.

Allergic adverse reactions are triggered by the immune system and may be as mild as a skin rash or as severe as an anaphylactic reaction. Nonallergic adverse reactions can be triggered by a number of causes, including drug interactions, chemical toxicity to a drug component, or medication error (see the earlier section "Considering five critical safety issues" for more details on adverse drug reactions).

For both allergic and nonallergic reactions, the first steps in treatment are stopping the infusion stat, keeping the vein open, and notifying the physician. In cases of mild allergic reactions, the physician will likely order antihistamines and supportive care. For more severe reactions, such as anaphylactic shock, treatment depends on the patient's condition and the physician's orders.

In cases of nonallergic reactions, you may need to administer antidotes or other medications, and treatment depends on the severity of the patient's symptoms.

Discontinuing IV Medications

After verifying the physician's order to discontinue IV therapy, check the medication record to ensure that all doses of ordered IV medications have been administered, and use these steps as guidelines for discontinuing IV medications through peripheral IVs (see Chapter 13 for details on discontinuing IV meds through CVADs):

1. **Close the roller clamp to stop the infusion.**

2. **Loosen the dressing and tape by pulling toward the insertion site, taking care not to accidentally dislodge the catheter.**

3. **Stabilize the catheter and press gauze or a cotton ball over the insertion site.**

4. **Gently pull the catheter straight back and out of the insertion site.**

5. **Apply pressure immediately for 30 to 60 seconds to obtain *hemostasis* (that is, to make the bleeding stop).**

6. **Assess the insertion site for bleeding and apply a clean dressing.**

7. **Inspect the catheter to ensure that it's not damaged.**

8. **Document your actions with the following details:**

   • Date and time of removal and discontinuation of infusion

   • Ease or difficulty of removal

   • Achievement of hemostasis

   • Application of dressing

   • Condition of catheter

9. **Educate the patient about the benefits of treatment, particularly the positive outcomes of improved symptoms and a restored sense of wellness.**

   Ensure that your patient has a positive experience with IV medication therapy by discussing how his compliance with treatment resulted in an improved outcome and shorter hospital stay. Educating patients about the benefits of pharmacological IV therapy can help improve patient attitudes about future IV therapy.

Staying Safe: Disposing of Pharmacological Agents

Following the proper techniques for medication disposal is a central part of safely handling pharmacological agents. Improper or inadequate disposal of drugs leads to unnecessary risk exposure to both healthcare personnel and patients.

Make sure you're familiar with all facility protocol regarding the disposal of pharmacological agents and follow these basic guidelines:

✔ Wear proper PPE, such as gowns, gloves, and masks, as recommended by the drug manufacturer and your facility's protocols for disposal of IV therapy equipment.

✔ Dispose of all medications, sharps, IV bags, IV tubing, and other IV peripherals in designated, properly labeled containers, and follow institutional instructions for specific drug disposals.

✔ Place potentially contaminated disposables in a plastic bag before placing them in the designated container.

✔ Never overfill or pack designated waste containers.

Chapter 15

Transfusing Blood Components

. . . .

In This Chapter

▶ Getting ready to do a blood transfusion

▶ Starting the transfusion

▶ Identifying and managing transfusion reactions

▶ Stopping the transfusion and safely disposing of all blood products

. . . .

Transfusions provide vital blood components for illnesses such as leukemia and hemophilia and for emergencies such as hemorrhagic shock. In 2006, more than 5 million people received blood transfusions in the U.S., and this number continues to be high today. So you're bound to have to start, monitor, and discontinue transfusions often in your career as a medical professional.

This chapter gives you an overall picture of the nurse's role in safely delivering blood components via transfusions. Here you find out about the precautionary steps you need to take prior to a transfusion, and you identify the types of equipment you use to safely administer blood components. Finally, you discover how to monitor a transfusion, recognize and manage adverse events, discontinue treatment, and safely dispose of all blood products afterward.

Preparing for a Blood Transfusion

Although blood transfusions are considered to be far safer today than they were even 20 years ago thanks to better donor screening and improved processing techniques, patients still suffer from adverse reactions to transfusions and some even die because of them.

Ensuring that the right blood type goes to the right patient prevents many of the adverse reactions that were common in the past, especially life-threatening hemolytic reactions. So this section starts off by giving you the tools you need to verify donor blood compatibility with the recipient's blood type. It then walks you through the process of preparing your equipment and your patient for the transfusion, obtaining informed consent, and administering any pretransfusion medications that may be necessary.

Verifying the physician's order and the patient's blood type

Despite efforts to prevent transfusion errors, many life-threatening reactions still occur because nurses give the wrong blood to the wrong patient. Because nurses administer most transfusions, they're responsible for correctly matching the patient's blood type to the type being transfused and preventing blood incompatibilities.

The first step in preventing incompatibilities is verifying the physician's order by checking the following details:

- ✔ Verify the physician's order, noting the indication, rate of infusion, and any premedication orders.
- ✔ Verify the product (such as whole blood, fresh frozen plasma [FFP], or platelets) and number of units to be administered.
- ✔ Verify any special orders.

The second step is verifying the patient's information in the following ways:

- ✔ Recheck the physician's order.
- ✔ With another qualified staff member, verify the patient and blood product identification.
- ✔ Verify the patient name and medical record number on the identification wristband.
- ✔ Verify the number of units cross-matched and available via the blood bank.

Preparing your equipment

Before you start transfusing blood or blood components, you need to prepare the equipment you'll use for the infusion. You usually transfuse blood by using a blood administration set with a Y-type tubing that leads into a single drip chamber. The Y tubing has two spikes, one for 0.9 percent normal saline (NS) and one for the unit of blood.

Be sure to do the following as you prepare your transfusion equipment:

✔ Check the insertion site to ensure the line is patent and working properly.

✔ Inspect the blood administration tubing to make sure it doesn't have any kinks or defects.

✔ Check the infusion pump to verify that it's working properly.

✔ *Prime* (fill completely with fluid) one spike of the blood administration set with 0.9 percent normal saline.

✔ Follow facility protocol to ensure that the proper blood filter is attached and make sure it's primed.

You may need to use leukocyte-reduction filters for transfusions every once in a while, but blood is often leukocyte-filtered by the supplier. In addition, blood components, such as platelets and albumin, may require specialty filters. In many situations, specialty filters are supplied by the manufacturer or pharmacy. Check your facility's guidelines on which filters are needed to infuse specific blood components.

✔ Make sure you have access to pressure infusers and blood warmers. You may need them in emergency situations for the rapid administration or transfusion of multiple units.

Turn to Chapter 3 for more on infusion equipment in general and Chapter 5 for details on specialty equipment needed for infusing blood components.

Preparing your patient

Receiving blood for the first time is a fearful prospect for many patients. By carefully explaining the risks and benefits of transfusions, you can go a long way toward allaying your patient's fears.

To emotionally prepare your patient for a blood transfusion, first describe the details of the procedure and then answer any questions she has. Offer additional patient education materials from the local blood bank or FDA's Circular of Information and reassure your patient that you monitor the procedure throughout the entire transfusion to make sure everything goes smoothly.

To physically prepare your patient, take her baseline vitals and assess her for rashes, wheezing, chills, fever, or nausea prior to the transfusion. Notify the physician if you identify any clinical symptoms that need to be addressed before the transfusion can begin.

Obtaining informed consent

Before you can administer any blood products (except in emergency transfusion situations), a qualified professional who can explain the risks, benefits, and alternatives of transfusion — this may very well be you — must obtain informed consent from the patient. Obtain your patient's consent as early as possible before the procedure to make sure the patient fully understands the transfusion and doesn't have any unanswered questions.

A single consent usually covers multiple transfusions, especially if they're part of a single course of treatment. You may need additional consents if your patient's status changes or if she's transferred to another unit in the hospital. Be sure to check your facility's policies and procedures for details on blood administration and consent.

If the patient refuses a transfusion, follow your facility's protocol on managing and documenting transfusion refusals. You may need to use a Patient's Release Form for Refusal of Blood or Treatment, which you can see an example of at www.hospital-forms.com/443.pdf.

Administering pretransfusion medications

Sometimes doctors order certain medications to be administered before transfusions to reduce the incidence and severity of the most common reactions to blood transfusions, such as nonhemolytic febrile reaction (fever) and allergic reactions. The pretransfusion medication that doctors use most often to reduce fever is acetaminophen (Tylenol) 325 milligrams (mg), and the medication they use most often to reduce allergic reaction is diphenhydramine (Benadryl) 25 mg.

In some cases, doctors prescribe acetaminophen before a transfusion when the patient has experienced previous fever episodes after transfusion or when the patient has a fever prior to transfusion. Doctors may also give diphenhydramine pre- or posttransfusion if the patient has experienced rash-like symptoms (such as skin welts or raised, red, itchy bumps) either previously or during the transfusion.

If a doctor prescribes a pretransfusion medication for one of your patients, verify the physician's order, administer the medication as prescribed, and follow your facility's protocol for obtaining vital signs before and after you administer pretransfusion medications.

Clinicians disagree about the efficacy and safety of using pretransfusion medications, so it's not recognized as a standardized practice. Follow your physician's orders or check your facility's protocol for policy guidelines on pretransfusion medications.

Initiating Treatment

After you take your patient's pretransfusion baseline vital signs and observe for any preexisting allergic symptoms, such as skin rashes or swelling, you need to check for patency of the vascular access device (VAD), presence of appropriate blood administration sets with filters, and easily accessible emergency equipment, such as a hypersensitivity kit and oxygen, in case the patient experiences a transfusion reaction. Then you can take the steps we outline in the following sections to initiate treatment.

Verifying blood at the bedside

The major cause of transfusion-related death is hemolytic incompatibility, which occurs when a patient receives the wrong type of blood. To help prevent this life-threatening mistake, nurses must verify that the patient's blood type matches the blood being transfused before they can officially initiate treatment. Bedside verification of the patient's blood type with the blood bag labels is the last chance you have to identify a possible mismatch and prevent a catastrophe.

Before every blood transfusion, two qualified professionals must perform bedside verification, during which they check the blood bag and patient for the following details:

- ✔ The patient's name and medical record number on the blood bag label match the patient's identification bracelet and medical record or bar code.

- ✔ The blood type and Rh factor are the same on the blood bag label, the blood tag label, and the patient's medical record or bar code.

- ✔ The blood component type and number on the blood bank label matches the blood supplier label or bar code.

- ✔ The expiration date and time are after the current date and time.

Figure 15-1 shows what a typical blood transfusion bag looks like, along with a close-up cutaway of the blood bag label. The label displays essential information regarding the blood type, patient, blood bank, and hospital.

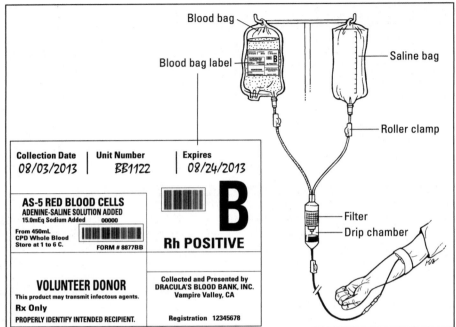

Blood bag

Blood bag label

Saline bag

Roller clamp

Collection Date	Unit Number	Expires
08/03/2013	BB1122	08/24/2013

AS-5 RED BLOOD CELLS
ADENINE-SALINE SOLUTION ADDED
15.0mEq Sodium Added   00000
From 450mL
CPD Whole Blood
Store at 1 to 6 C.   FORM # 8877BB

B

Rh POSITIVE

VOLUNTEER DONOR
This product may transmit infectous agents.
Rx Only
PROPERLY IDENTIFY INTENDED RECIPIENT.

Collected and Presented by
DRACULA'S BLOOD BANK, INC.
Vampire Valley, CA

Registration 12345678

Filter

Drip chamber

Figure 15-1:
An example
of a blood
transfusion
bag and
label.

Illustration by Kathryn Born

As final verification, ask the patient to state his name and date of birth and verify what he says with what's listed in his medical record. Before spiking the blood bag, check the blood's appearance for evidence of the following:

✔ Clots, clumps, or cloudiness

✔ Damage or defects in the bag's integrity

If the blood passes inspection and you don't find any discrepancy between the blood and patient information, slowly start the transfusion (see the next section for details).

If you find a discrepancy between the patient and blood bag information, *don't* initiate the transfusion. Report the discrepancy to the blood bank and physician immediately and follow facility protocol for possible blood type mismatches.

Going with the flow: Starting a blood transfusion

After you verify the patient's blood type with the blood bag, double-check the blood bag for any damage, and get a baseline set of vital signs, you're ready to start the transfusion. To do so, follow these steps:

1. **Mix the blood gently by inverting the bag several times.**

2. **Connect (spike) the blood bag to the Y tubing of the primed blood administration kit.**

   Remember that you should've already spiked the Y tubing with the 0.9 percent normal saline and primed the tubing. (See the earlier section "Preparing your equipment" for details on how to prime your administration kit.)

3. **Slowly initiate the transfusion by opening the roller clamps on the tubing or setting the infusion pump and beginning the infusion.**

Slow rates of infusion are recommended for the first 5 to 15 minutes of every blood transfusion so you can recognize any adverse reactions that occur. After monitoring the patient for 15 minutes without evidence of reaction, you can adjust the flow rate according to the physician's orders or facility protocol. Flow rates are typically based on the type of blood component and the age of the patient. Table 15-1 lists some recommended flow rates. (See the next section for more on monitoring patients during blood transfusions.)

Table 15-1	Recommended Flow Rates for Nonemergent Blood Transfusions		
Patient	*Blood Component*	*Flow Rate*	*Duration*
Adult	Platelets, plasma, or cryoprecipitate	4 to 10 mL/min	30 minutes to 1 hour
Adult	Whole blood or red blood cells	2 mL/min for the first 15 minutes If no adverse reactions are observed, increase the rate to 4 mL/min	1.5 to 2 hours is recommended; maximum infusion time period for a single unit of blood is 4 hours
Pediatric	All blood products	Calculated per age and weight	Based on total volume to be transfused

Monitoring the transfusion

Like any other infusion, blood transfusions require careful monitoring throughout the entire procedure. Here are the key things you need to do as you monitor each transfusion patient:

✔ Monitor your patient very closely during the first 5 to 15 minutes of the transfusion for rashes, fever, chills, or difficulty breathing. This initial period is when most transfusion reactions occur.

✔ At the end of 15 minutes, take your patient's vital signs and compare them with the baseline vitals. If no adverse reactions are apparent, adjust the infusion rate to match the time specified by the physician's orders.

✔ Throughout the transfusion, monitor your patient's vital signs at 30-minute intervals, or according to facility protocol, until the transfusion is complete.

✔ After the transfusion, take your patient's vitals and continue to monitor the patient for delayed transfusion reaction for at least one hour.

You must start administering blood components within 30 minutes after they leave the blood bank refrigerator (because glucose may become depleted and bacteria may begin to grow after this time period). You must complete the transfusion within four hours (because the longer the blood hangs, the warmer it gets and the more bacteria will begin to grow).

Recognizing and Managing Adverse Reactions

In the U.S., approximately 14 million blood transfusions are administered each year to several million patients, and adverse reactions occur in as many as 6 percent of patients who receive blood components. Although blood components are washed, filtered, spun, and packed to make them safer, each transfusion carries both the potential reward of saving a patient's life and the risk of causing an adverse reaction or even death.

Whether you transfuse one unit of blood a day or one unit of blood a year, you must be able to recognize and manage transfusion reactions. Lucky for you, this section provides the information you need to know.

Identifying the type of reaction

Transfusion reactions range from mild to severe and can occur within minutes of the start of the transfusion as *acute reactions* or within 2 to 30 days as *delayed reactions.* Types of acute transfusion reactions include the following:

- ✔ Acute hemolytic reaction, also called immune-mediated reaction
- ✔ Allergic reaction
- ✔ Nonhemolytic febrile reaction
- ✔ Non-immune-mediated reaction

We cover these four acute reactions in the following sections, along with the most common delayed reaction — graft versus host reaction.

Acute hemolytic reaction

Acute hemolytic reaction, also called *ABO incompatibility* or *immune-mediated reaction,* is the most serious transfusion reaction and usually results when a patient receives an incompatible blood type. Acute hemolytic reaction triggers a violent immune response that causes rapid hemolysis, or destruction of red blood cells. As the patient's red blood cells break down, they release their chemical contents into the patient's bloodstream, damaging the liver, kidney, and other organs.

Outward symptoms include back pain, bloody urine, chills, fainting or dizziness, fever, flank pain, and flushing of the skin. Even after the transfusion is stopped, symptoms continue to cascade into potentially fatal events, such as disseminated intravascular coagulopathy (DIC) and circulatory collapse.

Managing acute hemolytic reaction involves discontinuing the blood immediately and providing systemic support as directed by the physician and the patient's condition (see the later section "Managing blood transfusion reactions" for what this systemic support may entail). Early recognition and treatment is critical and may save the patient's life.

Acute hemolytic reaction is preventable as long as everyone associated with the transfusion takes the time to verify (and reverify) the patient's blood type with the blood type of the blood being transfused *before* initiating the transfusion (see the earlier sections "Verifying the physician's order and the patient's blood type" and "Verifying blood at the bedside" for details).

Note: Hemolytic reactions can also be delayed, with *febrile* (feverish) symptoms not appearing for several weeks. Delayed reactions are usually much milder than acute hemolytic reactions and frequently don't require treatment. Even so, educating your patient about the signs and symptoms (and instructing her to notify her physician if symptoms are present) and documenting your education are very important steps in the transfusion process.

Allergic reaction

Allergic transfusion reactions are usually the result of the patient's sensitivity to proteins in the blood or blood components. Allergic reactions typically manifest in the form of skin rashes, hives, or facial swelling. More serious allergic reactions can cause symptoms of respiratory distress and anaphylaxis.

Nonhemolytic febrile reaction

The most common type of transfusion reaction is *nonhemolytic febrile reaction,* which manifests as fever and is sometimes accompanied by chills. Nonhemolytic febrile reactions occur in approximately 7 percent of all blood transfusions and are usually self-limiting when treated with *antipyretics* (fever reducers). However, fever may indicate a more serious hemolytic reaction. Notify the physician if you notice any febrile reactions to a transfusion. You'll likely need to take blood samples to rule out hemolysis. After that, the doctor may have you treat the patient with antipyretics.

Non-immune-mediated hemolytic reaction

Non-immune-mediated hemolytic reaction is the hemolysis or destruction of red blood cells caused by physical or chemical events (rather than an immune response, as is the case in acute hemolytic reaction; see the previous section).

The following physical circumstances can lead to the physical destruction of red blood cells:

- ✔ Temperatures that are too cold during storage
- ✔ Temperatures that are too hot from blood warmers
- ✔ Infusion pumps with pressures that are too high

The infusion of incompatible medications or IV solutions causes the chemical destruction of red blood cells, especially if the incompatible meds are infused immediately before, during, or after transfusion.

Prevention is the key element in avoiding physical and chemical hemolysis. Here are just a few of the steps you can take to help prevent non-immune-mediated hemolytic reaction:

- ✔ Follow facility protocol when using blood warmers and infusion pumps.
- ✔ Use normal saline exclusively to prime and flush blood administration tubings.
- ✔ Never mix medications with blood components.

Graft versus host reaction

Although most transfusion reactions are acute and occur within the first 15 minutes to 1 hour of transfusion, delayed reactions also occur. *Graft versus host reactions,* which occur in immune-compromised patients, may not manifest until 2 to 30 days after the transfusion. Symptoms include rash, coughing, abdominal pain, vomiting, profuse diarrhea, and *red man syndrome* (an inflammatory skin disease with erythema and scaling that affects nearly the entire cutaneous surface). Providing your patients with proper education on these signs and symptoms and instructions for when to notify their physician is an essential part of your nursing plan.

Using leukocyte-depleted products (blood components with decreased white blood cells) and irradiated products (blood components that have been exposed to radiation) decreases the risk of graft versus host reactions.

Managing blood transfusion reactions

No matter what type of blood transfusion reaction occurs, the first critical actions are

- ✔ Stop the infusion stat.
- ✔ Change the tubing to a fresh administration set.

After you stop the transfusion, treatment depends on the severity and type of reaction, the physician's orders, and facility protocol. Table 15-2 provides an overview of the different types of transfusion reactions and the critical actions you need to take if you suspect them.

Table 15-2	Managing Blood Transfusion Reactions	
Type of Reaction	*Clinical Symptoms*	*Nursing Actions*
Acute hemolytic reaction	Fever, chills, headache, dyspnea, cyanosis, chest pain, tachycardia, hypotension	Keep the vein open with normal saline and take a blood and urine sample, as per protocol. Notify the physician immediately, provide support, and monitor vital signs, intake, and output.
Allergic reaction (mild)	Flushing, itching, hives, rash, wheezing, dyspnea	Give antihistamines as ordered, notify the physician, keep the vein open, and monitor vital signs.
Allergic reaction (severe)	Flushing, dyspnea, chest pain, circulatory collapse, cardiac arrest	Keep the vein open, notify the physician immediately, follow the physician's orders, give oxygen and prescribed drugs, and provide cardiopulmonary resuscitation per agency protocol.
Nonhemolytic febrile reaction	Fever, chills, flushed skin, headache, anxiety, muscle pain	Notify the physician, give antipyretics as ordered, keep the vein open, and monitor vital signs.
Non-immune-mediated hemolytic reaction	*Hemoglobinemia* (presence of excessive hemoglobin in the blood plasma) and *hemoglobinuria* (abnormal presence of hemoglobin in the urine) but usually no other symptoms	Monitor the patient for significant hemolysis; you may need to give IV fluids, vasopressors, or diuretics.
Graft versus host reaction	Fever, skin rash, diarrhea, hepatic dysfunction, and *bone marrow aplasia* (when bone marrow greatly decreases or stops production of blood cells)	Monitor the patient if she's an in-patient; for discharged patients, instruct them on signs and symptoms to report to the doctor.

As soon as you recognize a transfusion reaction — no matter what kind it is — and stop the transfusion, notify the attending or on-call physician immediately to report the symptoms and obtain orders for treatment. Then notify the blood bank, return the blood bag and tubing to the blood bank as directed, and follow facility protocol for additional procedures.

In most facilities, standard protocol also requires you to collect blood and/ or urine samples and send them to the laboratory following a transfusion reaction. Follow facility policy or the physician's orders to obtain the correct samples.

Discontinuing the Transfusion

When a transfusion is complete, follow these steps to discontinue the transfusion:

1. **Remove the blood bag and change the IV tubing or flush the tubing with 0.9 percent normal saline until clear.**

2. **Obtain patient vital signs.**

3. **Take posttransfusion blood samples, if ordered by the physician or facility protocol, and send them to the lab.**

   Most posttransfusion blood samples are tested for the following:

   - Bleeding time
   - Hematocrit
   - Hemoglobin
   - Serial platelet count

4. **Document the procedure, including the date, the time, the volume of infusion, and the patient's tolerance to the transfusion.**

In most cases, discontinuing an uneventful transfusion requires discarding the blood bag into an appropriate hazardous waste receptacle rather than returning the blood bag to the blood bank (as you do after transfusion reactions). But be sure to check with your facility's policy for proper blood bag disposal.

If your patient has three or more transfusions, you'll likely need to administer calcium gluconate, a common calcium replacement. When you transfuse blood, you're essentially putting calcium-free blood into your patient's body because the citrate added to the blood to keep it from clotting binds with calcium, making the transfused blood low in calcium. So be sure to notify the physician to obtain an order when you're infusing multiple units.

Safely Handling and Disposing of All Blood Products

Blood and blood products carry the potential risk for blood-borne pathogens, so you must take care to safely handle and dispose of them in order to protect the patient, yourself, and your work environment.

To safely discard blood waste products, follow facility protocol, which likely includes these guidelines:

- ✔ Place all contaminated and potentially contaminated materials in a designated hazardous waste container.

- ✔ Discard IV bags, attached IV tubing sets, and filters in the proper waste container.

- ✔ Discard contaminated sharps and vials in a designated sharps container.

- ✔ Decontaminate the medication room and transfusion preparation area by doing the following:

    - Cleanse all affected areas with an appropriate disinfectant, according to facility guidelines.

    - Disinfect the patient's bedside area, including the bedside table, bed railing, and IV standards.

    - Discard all cleansing agents and supplies into an appropriate hazardous waste container.

Chapter 16

Infusing Chemotherapy with Caution

*H*ealthcare professionals administer more than 100,000 doses of chemotherapy every day around the world. Chemotherapy (*chemo,* for short) drugs are among the most toxic medications you'll encounter in your career, so you need to know how to handle, administer, and dispose of them in the safest ways possible. That's where this chapter comes in.

Here, you get to know all the supplies necessary for safe administration, as well as the protective equipment you must use to prevent serious long-lasting health problems. You also find out about the most dreaded complications of chemotherapy and discover how to minimize risk and manage any complications that do occur. In doing so, you develop a firm understanding of how to keep yourself and your patient safe while giving this toxic, yet life-saving, therapy.

An excellent resource for cancer and chemotherapy information is www. thecancerjourney.org/treatment.

Preparing for Chemotherapy

The same powerful chemotherapy drugs that save thousands of lives each year are known to be hazardous to the health of both medical personnel and their patients if they're not handled correctly. In fact, the Occupational Safety and Health Association (OSHA) puts chemotherapy agents in the same category of hazardous drugs as formaldehyde and asbestos.

Nurses are almost always the ones administering chemotherapy, which means they're at ground zero for exposure to biohazardous agents. Following safety protocols from start to finish, even when time is short and workloads are heavy, creates a safer environment for healthcare workers and patients and minimizes the risk for serious health consequences now and later in life. This section guides you through the steps necessary to protect yourself and your patient as you prepare both your patient and the prescribed chemo drugs for administration. We talk about safely administering and disposing of chemotherapy drugs later in this chapter.

Protecting yourself

Although many chemotherapy drugs are prepared in the pharmacy, nurses frequently have to prepare and handle hazardous chemo drugs that can cause cancer, miscarriages, birth defects, or other serious health consequences. By understanding the risks of working with toxic agents and taking precautions to maximize safety, you can protect yourself from the potentially devastating effects of long-term exposure to hazardous drugs.

Personal protective equipment (PPE) is your best defense against chronic, daily exposure to hazardous drugs. So whenever you're handling chemotherapy agents, use the following PPE, recommended by the National Institute of Occupational Safety and Health (NIOSH), to ensure maximum safety:

- ✔ **Gowns:** Use disposable gowns made of fabric that has low permeability to the agents being handled. The best gown options have closed fronts and cuffs and are intended for single use only.

- ✔ **Gloves:** Wear powder-free gloves made of latex, nitrile, or neoprene that have been labeled and tested for use with chemotherapy agents.

- ✔ **Face and eye shield:** Wear a face and eye shield, especially when splashing is possible.

- ✔ **Respirator:** Use a NIOSH-approved respirator when you're at risk of inhaling aerosols, such as during spill clean-up.

In many industries that deal with hazardous materials, OSHA mandates that PPE is available to all employees and routinely used. Employers who disobey this rule are fined. In hospitals, however, using PPE is voluntary. Medical personnel can make their own decision to use protective gear, not use protective gear, or use partial protective gear. In other words, it's up to each healthcare worker to practice safe drug handling, minimize the risk of dealing with biohazards, and promote a safer workplace environment for everyone.

TIP

Taking the confusion out of chemotherapy infusion

Chemotherapy drugs have long, complicated names that sound similar and share the same suffixes and prefixes. Even so, to make the infusion environment a safer place, you have to be able to differentiate between various look-alike and sound-alike drug names. Some of the most frequently confused drugs include

✔ Cisplatin and carboplatin

✔ Vincristine and vinblastine

✔ Taxol and Taxotere

✔ Doxorubicin and doxorubicin liposomal

✔ Leucovorin and Leukeran

✔ Myleran and Alkeran

✔ Mitoxantrone and mitomycin

One way to differentiate between similar drug names is to use capital lettering to distinguish and set the drugs apart from each other. For example, use CISplatin to set it apart from CARBOplatin, and vinBLASTine to set it apart from vinCRISTine. Use the capital lettering system to differentiate between similar drugs when you're transcribing physician's orders.

Warning: Never take a verbal order for chemotherapy drugs. The risks for confusion and inaccurate interpretation are too great, and easy access to electronic communication makes verbal orders unnecessary. Verbal orders are only accepted for placing chemo on hold or stopping it.

Unlike major toxic spills that cause immediate nausea, vomiting, and headache, tiny spills that occur every day cause no symptoms and often go unnoticed. As a matter of fact, studies done in cancer centers that don't require the use of PPE have shown chemotherapy residue on nursing stations, countertops, patient charts, and furnishings.

Underscoring the importance of using PPE, a recent study documented chromosomal abnormalities in healthy nurses and pharmacists who worked directly with chemotherapy agents. These chromosome markers are associated with higher risk for therapy-related leukemia and bone marrow disease. Other studies show that 17 percent of chemotherapy nurses, sometime during their career, report exposure to toxic drugs on their skin or in their eyes during preparation or administration.

Protecting your patient

Cancer patients face the prospect of chemotherapy at one of the most stressful and vulnerable periods in their lives. Many fear that they'll lose their jobs, their families, or worst of all, their lives. As a healthcare worker, you need to do everything you can to ensure that every patient is safe from harm during the uncharted course through chemotherapy.

Preventing medication errors is the most important thing you can do to protect your patient during chemotherapy administration. The same medication errors that occur with standard IV therapy also occur with chemotherapy drugs:

- ✔ Incorrect patient
- ✔ Incorrect route, rate, and/or time of administration
- ✔ Overdosing and underdosing

To minimize the risk for medication errors, follow these guidelines, which apply specifically to chemotherapy administration:

- ✔ Ensure competency of all IV specialists, including you, through training and certification.
- ✔ Use a dose-verification process with independent checkpoints.
- ✔ Use a detailed checklist for protocols related to prescribing, transcribing, dispensing, and administering chemo.
- ✔ Calculate doses independently. (In other words, the physician, pharmacist, and nurse should each calculate doses on their own.)
- ✔ Use dosage limit guidelines and question any dose that exceeds those limits.
- ✔ Have two nurses double-check the preparation and administration of drugs and the patient's identification information. Be sure to check the patient's body surface area (BSA), weight, medication, dose, concentration, route, and calculation.
- ✔ Provide care for each patient with the same one or two nurses.
- ✔ Question any aspect of an order that's unclear or contrary to customary practice or that deviates from previous procedures for the patient.
- ✔ Use approved protocols for patient identification and drug administration.

Educating your patient

Few patients are at ease before receiving chemotherapy. After all, knowing that your body is being infused with a poison that can destroy not only the cancer but also your heart, kidneys, and other vital organs is scary. To help your patients through this difficult procedure, start by allaying their fears with empathy and education.

If your patient is receiving chemotherapy for the first time, plan to spend a little more time with her to explain the procedure and answer her questions. During that time, be sure to do the following:

✔ Customize your explanation to fit her specific situation.

✔ Explain the infusion procedure and tell her to inform you immediately if she feels pain, stinging, or burning at the infusion site.

✔ Inform her about the risks and side effects of chemotherapy, but also remind her of the benefits of destroying remaining cancer cells.

If your patient is a veteran at receiving chemotherapy, ask her what side effects she usually experiences and what, if anything, works to relieve them. Tell her what other patients are doing to minimize their side effects.

No matter how many times your patient has gone through the chemo procedure, spend a little time with each patient before you start administering therapy. A few extra moments at the beginning of treatment goes a long way toward making the next few hours more bearable for your patient.

Preparing the chemotherapy agent

If you work in oncology, you're probably exposed to hazardous drugs multiple times every day. Preparing chemotherapy drugs is one of the most critical periods of high risk for exposure. Although most chemotherapy drugs are prepared in the pharmacy, you may have to reconstitute a chemo drug or dilute a chemo admixture for therapy.

To ensure maximum safety when preparing chemotherapy medications, follow your facility's policies and procedures and take the following precautions:

✔ Read the drug manufacturer's Material Safety Data Sheet (MSDS) for details on handling each specific medication.

✔ Prepare each agent in a ducted, biosafety cabinet or isolation chamber.

✔ Prepare every medication over plastic-backed, absorbent, disposable pads and below eye level.

✔ Wear chemotherapy gloves or double gloves of surgical quality, a non-permeable gown, and a face shield designed for use with chemotherapy.

✔ Use syringes that connect, such as a Luer-Lok system, to minimize inadvertent disconnections and wipe them with an alcohol pad to decontaminate them before use.

✔ Transport all chemo drugs in hazardous transport containment bags.

✔ Discard chemo drugs with IV sets attached and place all contaminated materials in a hazardous waste container.

✔ Have a spill kit ready in case you need it and make sure the room where you're working has hazardous containers for disposables and sharps.

✔ Carefully remove your gown and gloves and wash your hands after preparation.

Handling the chemotherapy agent

Safely handling toxic agents involves the same precautions we outline in the preceding section on preparing chemo drugs, plus the following guidelines for labeling, storing, and transporting:

✔ Use warning labels to clearly mark drug containers as *cytotoxics* that must be disposed of properly after use.

✔ Clearly label yellow hazardous material bags and containers as designated containers for hazardous waste.

✔ Store drugs only in areas clearly marked for cytotoxic drug storage.

✔ Transport drugs in clearly marked hazardous transport containment bags or in resealable plastic bags if you don't have transport bags readily available.

Administering Chemotherapy

Chemotherapy can be administered in a variety of ways, including orally, intra-arterially, intra-peritoneally, and by direct injection into the tumor, but the most common method is through IV administration. This section offers a cautionary look at how to safely start and monitor IV chemotherapy.

Before you begin

Whether you're administering chemotherapy through a peripheral IV, a central line, or a port, the first two steps in administration are

1. **Have two nurses double-check the agent to ensure that it's the right agent with the right dilution and infusion rate for the right patient.**

   Be sure to double-check the patient's BSA, weight, and the calculation for dosing, as well.

2. **Get a blood return to ensure that the patient's vein is patent and free-flowing.**

   Follow institutional protocol to obtain blood return before, during, and after IV chemotherapy administration.

See Chapters 12 and 13 for details on these steps for peripheral and central IVs.

Initiating the infusion

After you double-check that the infusion is for the right patient and you establish a blood return, follow these guidelines to safely initiate chemotherapy:

✔ Gently flush the line with normal saline prior to starting the infusion and in between infusions if you're administering multiple agents.

✔ Ensure that the catheter is secure and the insertion site is easy to see. *Note:* Per the Infusion Nurses Society (INS) standards, peripheral IV access should not be used for continuous infusion (more than 48 hours) of vesicants such as chemo.

✔ Spike the infusion, insert the male spike on the IV tubing into the female spike area of the bag, or access the tubing's Y-connector below eye level. *Note:* Per INS standards, administration sets should be attached and primed within a biological cabinet prior to the addition of chemo. If this process is done at the patient's bedside, the administration set should be primed with non-drug-containing fluid prior to adding chemo.

✔ Start the infusion slowly and monitor the patient's reaction (see the next section for details). An infusion pump is the instrument of choice for the infusion.

See Chapter 12 for a lot more information about administering through a peripheral IV and Chapter 13 for details on administering through a central line or port.

Monitoring chemotherapy

Throughout every chemotherapy infusion you administer, you must vigilantly and continuously monitor the infusion site for infiltration and other complications. During this monitoring, be sure to do the following:

✔ Verify patency of the peripheral vein or central line continuously during the procedure by following facility protocol to verify vein patency. This procedure may include verifying patency by aspiration or by occluding the infusion and lowering the bag to get a blood return.

✔ Communicate with the patient to make sure he doesn't have any local symptoms of pain, stinging, or burning at the infusion site or any systemic symptoms of headache, nausea, or dizziness.

Terminate the infusion immediately and notify the physician if the patient has signs of infiltration or systemic symptoms.

We explain how to manage adverse reactions in the next section and how to deal with common chemo side effects in the later section "Managing Common Side Effects."

Reacting to Adverse Reactions

A key part of protecting your patient during chemotherapy is knowing how to react to and treat adverse reactions. After all, chemotherapy drugs are potent, caustic agents that bring with them a high risk for adverse events like the following:

✔ **Nausea and vomiting:** Feeling sick to your stomach, possibly followed by throwing up

✔ **Extravasation:** Experiencing irritation, pain, inflammation, warmth, erythema, or tenderness at the IV insertion site

✔ **Tightening of chest:** Feeling pressure, heaviness, squeezing, or aching across the chest

✔ **Flushing:** Becoming noticeably red in the face and often other areas of the skin

✔ **Changes in heart rate:** Experiencing an irregular beating of the heart

✔ **Low blood pressure:** Experiencing lightheadedness, dizziness, fainting, and often seizures

Adverse reactions can occur within the first few minutes of the first infusion of a new drug, but they aren't limited to this time frame. To minimize risk, start every drug infusion slowly and gradually increase it to the desired rate.

Note: Although adverse reactions can occur within the first few minutes of initiating treatment, some agents, such as cisplatin and carboplatin, can cause reactions after repeated exposure and can occur after four or five treatments.

Taking action as soon as you identify a reaction

Infusing chemotherapy drugs slowly and monitoring your patient closely during the critical first few minutes of each administration leads to early recognition, intervention, and treatment of adverse drug reactions. But what do you do when you identify an adverse reaction in your patient? Acting with speed and safety is key.

To react quickly and safely to an adverse event, follow your facility's protocol and use the following guidelines:

✔ Stop the infusion immediately, call for help, and notify the physician.

✔ Maintain an open IV line with normal saline.

✔ Obtain emergency drugs and administer them according to institution protocol or the physician's orders.

✔ Place the patient in a supine position.

✔ Monitor vital signs every 2 minutes until stable. Then monitor them every 5 minutes for 30 minutes and every 15 minutes after that until the patient has returned to baseline.

✔ Document the incident and the patient's reaction in the patient's medical record.

✔ Keep a record of the drug that caused the adverse reaction, along with the diluent, lot number, and other drug factors for the pharmaceutical company.

During critical adverse events, reassure the patient and his family that physicians and nurses are trained specifically to handle adverse drug reactions and that treatment plans and protocols are in place to reverse the event and restore the patient's health.

In addition to knowing how to recognize symptoms of adverse reactions and implement treatment, you also need to be aware of the drugs that are most commonly associated with adverse reactions. A few of the most common offenders are asparaginase, paclitaxel, and monoclonal antibodies such as rituximab.

Dealing with vesicant extravasation

Chemotherapy drugs fall into one of two categories, depending on their toxicity and the damage they can cause if they infiltrate outside the vein:

✔ **Irritant:** An irritant is less toxic than a vesicant and causes pain, stinging, or inflammation at the injection site if it infiltrates. Examples of irritants include

- Carmustine

- Cyclophosphamide

- Etoposide

- Fluorouracil

✔ **Vesicant:** A vesicant is very toxic and causes blistering, ulceration, or severe damage if it infiltrates and *extravasates* (or leaks) into surrounding tissues. Examples of vesicants are

- Dactinomycin

- Doxorubicin

- Vinblastine

- Vincristine

When a vesicant chemotherapy drug leaks into the area surrounding the vein, it starts rapidly destroying tissues. This infiltration is called *extravasation,* and it's one of the most dreaded and difficult-to-treat complications of chemotherapy.

The number one way to prevent vesicant extravasation is by strictly adhering to established safety guidelines for vesicant administration. But if this complication occurs, you must identify it immediately and intervene as soon as possible to minimize tissue damage.

To identify early signs of extravasation, look for these symptoms as you monitor your patient:

✔ Bleb or blister formation at the infusion site

✔ Burning, stinging, or pain at the infusion site

✔ Swelling or inflammation at the infusion site

Initial treatment for vesicant extravasation is immediate discontinuation of the infusion. Additional treatment varies among different institutions, but the most common treatments include

✔ Aspirating the remaining vesicant by using a 1-cc to 3-cc syringe and notifying the physician

✔ Applying topical cooling and initiating appropriate management measures in accordance with your facility's policy

✔ Marking and photographing the extravasation area according to protocol

Keep extravasation kits available for emergencies. These kits usually contain sterile gloves, syringes, catheters, gauze, cold/hot packs, and approved medications.

Like everything else in IV therapy, vesicant extravasation requires complete documentation. Be sure to include the following details:

- ✔ Intervention and notification of the physician
- ✔ Treatment and pain management, as ordered
- ✔ Extravasation photographing
- ✔ Completion of incident reports according to protocol
- ✔ Observation of patient response

Managing Common Side Effects

When your patients are feeling nauseous, losing their hair, and thinking their mouths taste like a metal pipe, they may have a hard time remembering that chemotherapy is designed to cure, not kill, them. The downside to chemotherapy is the debilitating array of side effects that becomes worse as treatment progresses. Chemotherapy is, after all, a systemic toxin that can't distinguish between healthy cells and malignant cells. As more healthy cells are killed, more devastating side effects emerge.

Dealing with nausea, vomiting, and other GI disturbances

Nausea, vomiting, and other gastrointestinal (GI) symptoms are the first to appear and the most persistent throughout the course of chemotherapy. Fortunately, antiemetic and gastric-acid-inhibitor medications are helpful in preventing and treating nausea, so doctors frequently use them as part of their patients' chemo treatment plan.

Dietary changes are also helpful in relieving GI symptoms. Nutritionists and chemotherapy patients recommend the following changes:

- ✔ Eat small, frequent meals that are easier to digest and less likely to cause nausea and vomiting.
- ✔ Avoid spicy or fried foods because they cause more gastric acid and increase the risk for nausea.

✔ Drink liquids between meals rather than with meals to avoid diluting gastric digestive juices and rest after eating to promote more effective digestion and decrease the risk for nausea.

✔ If your patient can't eat, recommend that she get a prescription for anti-emetic oral dissolving tablets or suppositories to ease the nausea until she can tolerate oral medications. Suggest starting a clear liquid diet and advancing to solid foods as tolerated.

✔ If your patient has diarrhea, advise her to get recommendations for antidiarrhea medications from her oncologist. Tell her to avoid foods that exacerbate diarrhea, such as cabbage, beans, dairy, and raw foods.

✔ If your patient is constipated, tell her to talk with the oncologist about laxatives and stool softeners. Advise her to increase her intake of dietary fiber and fluid and to get some exercise. Remind her that constipation, left untreated, can lead to fecal impactions that require manual removal.

✔ If your patient's mucous membranes become dry and cracked, resulting in sores or lesions, advise her to prevent oral complications by practicing good oral hygiene, avoiding alcohol-containing mouthwash, and eliminating dry foods from her diet.

✔ If food doesn't taste good to your patient anymore (because of a loss of taste, a change in taste, or a chronic metallic taste), advise your patient to use hard candies, mints, and chewing gum to counteract the taste.

Facing hair loss and fatigue

As chemotherapy drugs attack both cancer cells and normal cells, hair loss and fatigue are two of the most common side effects. In fact, they're almost inevitable. Coping with these side effects is daunting, but patients can manage them with a little knowledge and experimentation. This section offers suggestions to help your patients deal with these debilitating side effects.

Coping with alopecia

Alopecia, or hair loss, is one of the most distressing side effects of chemotherapy. Advise your patients to cope with this side effect by wearing wigs, caps, and scarves to make themselves look and feel better during therapy. Reassure them that hair loss is temporary and that normal hair growth will return when chemotherapy is stopped.

Fighting fatigue

Fatigue is one of the first side effects to appear and the last to go away. Patients often refer to it as a "whole-body fatigue" that starts with the first treatment and lasts as long as a year after chemotherapy ends.

The American Cancer Society advises patients to talk with their oncologist to rule out treatable medical reasons for fatigue, such as anemia or low blood oxygen levels. If your patient has no underlying medical condition, advise her to get as much sleep at night as possible and to pace herself and stop rushing. Recommend that she avoid caffeine, alcohol, hot showers, and exposure to cold, because these factors alter metabolism and increase the body's energy requirements, leading to additional stress and fatigue.

Watching for bone marrow suppression

Most chemotherapy agents suppress bone marrow to some degree, resulting in symptoms that range from fatigue to chronic infections. Left untreated, bone marrow suppression, which can occur up to seven to ten days after treatment, places the patient at risk for dire consequences, including overwhelming infection, sepsis leading to cardiac or respiratory arrest, and even death.

You monitor bone marrow suppression via complete blood counts (CBCs) and other laboratory tests that identify the type of blood cell impacted by chemotherapy and the type of treatment needed to fix the problem. The following blood abnormalities occur in chemo-induced bone marrow suppression:

- **Anemia:** A decrease in red blood cells (RBCs) and hemoglobin and an early sign of bone marrow suppression

- **Leukopenia:** A decrease in white blood cells (WBCs), which suggests an impaired ability to fight infection

- **Neutropenia:** A decrease in WBC neutrophils, which impairs the body's ability to fight bacterial and fungal infections

- **Thrombocytopenia:** A decrease in platelets, which impairs the body's ability to form clots and prevent bleeding

Discontinuing Chemotherapy

When the infusion is complete, follow these steps to discontinue chemotherapy:

1. **Check for blood return and flush the line with 10 milliliters of normal saline or flushing solution.**

2. **Remove the needle or needleless connector carefully and avoid dripping vesicant fluid or IV solution on the patient's skin or bed linens.**

3. Observe the patient for any signs of adverse reaction and ensure that the insertion site and dressing are dry and intact.

4. Observe the insertion site for signs of redness, irritation, or infiltration, and notify the physician if you notice any signs of inflammation.

For more details on discontinuing IV medications, check out Chapter 14.

Safely Disposing of Chemotherapy Waste

Safely handling hazardous chemo agents begins with the drug's preparation (see the earlier section) and ends with the safe disposal and decontamination of the drug's trace and bulk waste.

Follow your facility's protocol and these guidelines to safely dispose of and decontaminate chemotherapy waste:

✔ Place all contaminated and potentially contaminated materials in plastic bags before disposing of them in a designated hazardous waste container.

✔ Discard IV bags and attached IV tubing sets, PPE, and other chemotherapy peripherals in the proper waste container.

✔ Discard sharps and vials in a designated sharps container.

✔ Decontaminate the medication room and bedside after each use.

Chapter 17

A Balancing Act: Administering Fluids and Electrolytes

*T*he human body must keep fluid in the cells, between the cells, and in the bloodstream to maintain body functions and sustain life. Balancing this fluid among the extracellular and intracellular spaces and in the bloodstream is one of the main jobs of electrolytes. When fluid and electrolytes don't work in perfect harmony, the heart beats irregularly, the kidneys shut down, and the circulatory system collapses. We discuss the critical role that IV therapy plays in replacing fluid and electrolytes and restoring life-sustaining equilibrium in Chapter 7. In this chapter, we focus on the how-to info you need to know to administer this type of IV therapy.

Here, you realize the importance of patient assessment in identifying fluid and electrolyte imbalance as a potential underlying cause for patient symptoms. You discover the clinical signs that point to fluid and electrolyte imbalance and the vital signs that verify the presence of electrolyte disturbances. You find out how to use lab results to identify blood and urine abnormalities associated with electrolyte imbalance, and you discover how to administer, monitor, and discontinue electrolyte replacement therapy. Finally, you get a handful of practical tips on how to identify, manage, and prevent adverse reactions.

Focusing on Fluids and Electrolytes As You Assess Your Patient

When patients are admitted to the hospital, they're usually admitted with a diagnosis such as cardiac arrhythmia, heatstroke, altered level of consciousness, and so on. The words *electrolyte imbalance* typically don't appear in the admitting diagnosis. A definitive diagnosis of electrolyte imbalance comes later, after you and the doctor take a thorough patient history, interpret the patient's vital and clinical signs, and review all the required laboratory results.

Taking a complete patient history

One of the first parts of any patient assessment is getting a full patient history. Completing a thorough history can help you identify existing medications and diseases as potential causes for fluid and electrolyte imbalance. As you consider your patient's history, keep in mind that the following conditions may contribute to fluid and electrolyte imbalance:

- **Physiologic:** Physiologic causes of electrolyte imbalance include kidney disease, gastrointestinal (GI) losses from vomiting and/or diarrhea, fistulas, and ulcerative GI diseases.
- **Metabolic:** Diabetes, liver disorders, and hormonal disturbances are frequently associated with fluid and electrolyte imbalances.
- **Traumatic:** Major trauma is associated with fluid and electrolyte loss, including loss through hemorrhage, surgery, weeping burns, or wounds.
- **Environmental:** Extreme heat is linked to fluid and electrolyte imbalance, especially in elderly and pediatric patients because of their poor temperature and sweat mechanism regulation systems. Athletes with prolonged heat exposure are also at risk for dehydration and electrolyte imbalance.
- **Medicinal:** Medications such as antihypertensives, hormones, and diuretics are notorious for causing fluid and electrolyte imbalance.
- **Pyschosocial:** Emotional disorders, mental illness, and eating disorders, such as anorexia and bulimia, are all known contributors to fluid and electrolyte imbalances.

Obtaining baseline assessments

Interpreting baseline vital signs and symptoms is another key component of assessing your patient for fluid or electrolyte issues. To help you identify potential fluid and electrolyte imbalances, be sure to check your patient for the abnormalities listed in Table 17-1.

Table 17-1	Vital Signs and Clinical Symptoms That May Represent Fluid and Electrolyte Imbalance
Sign or Symptom	*Possible Fluid/Electrolyte Imbalance*
Vital Sign	
Bounding pulse	Fluid overload
Elevated temperature	Dehydration
Decreased temperature	Hypovolemia
Increased heart and respiratory rate	Fluid volume deficit
Irregular heart rate	Potassium or calcium abnormality
Postural changes in blood pressure	Fluid volume deficit
Clinical Symptom	
Altered level of consciousness	Fluid volume deficit
Changes in skin turgor and capillary refill	Dehydration
Edema	Fluid retention and fluid volume excess
Flushed, dry skin	Fluid volume deficit
Jugular vein distention	Fluid volume excess
Twitches and muscle spasms	Overall electrolyte disturbances

Reviewing lab results

Evaluating laboratory results for fluid status and electrolyte abnormalities is an essential part of completing a thorough patient assessment. When you identify signs, symptoms, and laboratory findings that indicate possible fluid and electrolyte imbalance, notify the physician to obtain orders for intervention and treatment.

Determining fluid status levels

Table 17-2 lists some of the most common tests used to evaluate fluid status. (In the table, mOsm/kg represents milliosmoles/kilogram, mg/dL represents milligrams/deciliter, mmol/L represents millimoles per liter, and mEq/L represents milliequivalents/liter; see the later section "Starting therapy" for an explanation of mEq/L as it relates to replacement therapy.)

Table 17-2	Tests That Evaluate Fluid Status	
Laboratory Test	*What the Test Does*	*Normal Laboratory Value*
Blood (serum) osmolarity	Measures the balance between water and chemicals dissolved in blood. Determines whether severe dehydration or overhydration is present.	280–300 mOsm/kg
Hematocrit (Hct)	Represents the proportion of the blood that consists of red blood cells. Dehydration produces a falsely high hematocrit.	42%–54% in males; 38%–46% in females
Blood urea nitrogen (BUN)	Measures the amount of nitrogen in the blood that comes from the waste product urea. Dehydration can raise BUN level.	6 to 20 mg/dL or 2.1–7.1 mmol/L
Urine osmolality (typical)	Measures the concentration of particles in urine. Greater-than-normal measurements may indicate dehydration.	24-hour urine osmolality is 450–900 mOsm/kg; random urine osmolality is 50–1,200 mOsm/kg
Urine specific gravity	Measures the kidney's ability to concentrate or dilute and is a measurement of the density of urine compared to pure water. A high urine specific gravity indicates dehydration.	1.001–1.030
Urine sodium	Measures the concentration of sodium in the urine. Determines hydration status and the kidney's ability to conserve or remove sodium from the urine.	135–145 mEq/L

Evaluating electrolyte status with the BMP

The most frequently ordered laboratory test used to evaluate electrolyte status is the *basic metabolic panel* (BMP). The BMP provides information about the status of kidney function, blood sugar, and electrolyte balance. Table 17-3 outlines the tests included in the BMP, along with the normal values associated with different age groups. (Turn to the later section "Starting therapy" for a quick look at mEq/L and its place in replacement therapy.)

Table 17-3	**Basic Metabolic Panel (BMP)**	
Test	*Age Group*	*Normal Range*
Calcium	1 month to adult	8.9–10.1 mg/dL
Chloride	1 month to adult	96–106 mmol/L
Carbon dioxide	15 years to adult	22–29 mmol/L
Creatinine	Male adult Female adult	0.75–1.20 mg/dL 0.65–1.00 mg/dL
Glucose	Adult fasting Adult non-fasting	60–99 mg/dL 60–200 mg/dL
Potassium	1 month to adult	3.5–5.5 mmol/L
Sodium	Adult	135–145 mmol/L
Blood urea nitrogen (BUN)	15 years to adult	6–20 mg/dL or 2.1–7.1 mmol/L

Table 17-4 lists the most common electrolyte abnormalities, along with their laboratory values and the clinical conditions that often accompany them. These labs give doctors important information about the current status of the kidneys, blood sugar, and electrolyte and acid/base balance so they can formulate the treatment plan that best suits the imbalance.

Table 17-4	Electrolyte Abnormalities and Their Associated Clinical Conditions		
Imbalance	*Medical Term*	*Lab Value*	*Clinical Condition*
Low potassium	Hypokalemia	< 3.5 mEq/L	Endocrine disorders, gastrointestinal loss
High potassium	Hyperkalemia	> 5.5 mEq/L	Renal failure, cardiac arrest
Low sodium	Hyponatremia	< 135 mEq/L	Endocrine disorders, dehydration, congestive heart failure, psychiatric conditions
High sodium	Hypernatremia	> 145 mEq/L	Renal disease, dehydration
Low calcium	Hypocalcemia	< 8 mEq/L	Malabsorption disorder, acute pancreatitis
High calcium	Hypercalcemia	> 10.2 mEq/L	Renal disease, cancer

For more details on these and other laboratory values related to fluid and electrolyte imbalance, check out Chapter 7.

Administering IV Replacement Therapy

Treatment for an electrolyte imbalance depends on the underlying cause and the severity of the electrolyte abnormality. After the physician identifies the particular electrolyte imbalance, he usually orders replacement therapy. This therapy can include using IV fluids (such a normal saline), IV fluids that contain electrolytes (such as ½ normal saline with 20 mEq of potassium), specific electrolytes (such as 40 mEq of potassium), or any combination of the three. (See Chapter 7 for details on the different types of fluids used in IV replacement therapy.)

The fundamental aspects of electrolyte replacement infusions, including how to administer and monitor them, are similar to infusions for other IV medications. Refer to Chapter 14 for the basics. The following sections outline issues that are specific to administering fluids and electrolytes.

Starting therapy

Many times, pharmacies prepare IV solutions with electrolytes and other fluids, and nurses administer them as IV piggybacks. They use infusion pumps to slowly and cautiously infuse the piggyback preparation through either central or peripheral IV lines.

When patients have existing IV lines, piggyback IVs are an ideal method of replacing electrolytes because electrolytes are usually ordered by the physician as individual doses. Nurses can easily deliver the dose via piggyback and then discontinue the piggyback when the dose is complete. Doctors don't usually order follow-up doses until they recheck electrolyte levels and determine that additional electrolytes are necessary. When a doctor does order follow-up doses, the nurse adds another piggyback IV and then discontinues the piggyback when the dose is complete.

To start replacing electrolytes through an IV piggyback (IVPB), hang the piggyback at least 6 inches higher than the primary infusion, insert the piggyback tubing into an injection port, and release the roller clamp to allow the piggyback infusion to begin. Gravity infuses the piggyback first and allows the primary infusion to continue when the piggyback infusion is complete. For more details on piggybacks, see Chapter 11.

Note: To implement replacement therapy orders, nurses usually administer fluids containing electrolytes, such as lactated Ringer's solution (often used to treat fluid volume deficit) and Normosol-R (used for replacement in acute fluid and electrolyte depletion), by the liter. Specific electrolytes, when ordered as single or intermittent dosings, are usually administered by milliequivalents or by millimoles. A *milliequivalent* (mEq) is one-thousandth (0.001) of the gram equivalent of an ion. A *millimole* (mmol or mM) is one-thousandth (0.001) of the gram equivalent of a substance. You use both units, mEq/L and mmol/L, in dosing electrolytes and understanding lab values. For example, normal laboratory values for sodium are 135 to145 mEq/L and 135 to 145 mmol/L.

Each electrolyte has a maximum daily dosage range. You can use the following guidelines for infusing electrolytes within safe dosing ranges and flow rates:

- ✔ **Central lines:** The safe dosing range for electrolytes infused through a central line is 10 to 20 mEq at a flow rate that spreads the infusion over a period of 1 to 3 hours.

- ✔ **Peripheral lines:** The safe dosing range for electrolytes infused through a peripheral line is 10 mEq at a flow rate that spreads the infusion over a period of 1 to 6 hours.

Go to `www.hosp.uky.edu/Pharmacy/formulary/criteria/` `electrolyte.htm` for more insight on dosage and flow rates of electrolytes.

To avoid potassium overdose when a patient requires both potassium and phosphorus replacements, subtract the mEq of potassium in potassium phosphate from the total amount of potassium required to arrive at the correct amount of total potassium to be administered. If you have any questions, check with the pharmacy.

Monitoring the infusion

Standard monitoring used in administering IV medications also applies to fluid and electrolyte replacement. This monitoring includes observing the patient for adverse reactions such as hypersensitivity (rash or itching) or anaphylactic reactions (throat and facial swelling), verifying flow rate, and checking the insertion site for redness, swelling, or pain, which may indicate infiltration or extravasation.

In addition to following these standard IV monitoring procedures, you need to do more frequent monitoring with electrolyte replacement therapy because electrolytes are powerful substances that help conduct electrical impulses that are critical to maintaining body functions. Frequent monitoring is particularly important in potassium replacement because potassium helps regulate cardiac activity. Too much or too little potassium can cause cardiac arrhythmias or cardiac arrest. That's why some facility protocols require continuous electrocardiogram monitoring when you're administering IV potassium through either peripheral or central venous lines. Potassium is usually administered at 10 to 20 mEq per hour, and levels are rechecked two hours after the infusion is complete.

Additional monitoring is also recommended when you're replacing electrolytes in patients with underlying conditions, such as renal disease, acute pancreatitis, and liver disorders, because an electrolyte imbalance impairs the organs' ability to process and eliminate waste products, leading to further deterioration of function and possible organ failure. This additional monitoring includes obtaining an order to recheck serum (that is, blood) electrolyte levels after infusion. If the infusion hasn't corrected serum levels, notify the physician and obtain orders for additional electrolyte replacement or further treatment.

Recognizing and Managing Adverse Reactions

In most instances, fluid and electrolyte replacement provides a welcome relief of symptoms and a prompt improvement in lab values. Occasionally, however, excessive or deficient amounts of fluid and electrolytes cause undesirable side effects and severe adverse reactions. The following sections provide tips on how to avoid these side effects and adverse reactions, as well as how to recognize and manage them when they do occur.

Avoiding common pitfalls

Fortunately, by avoiding some common mistakes associated with replacement therapy, you can prevent many of the undesired consequences of electrolyte administration. The following list provides tips on avoiding the most common traps and pitfalls:

✔ When administering *albumin* (a blood transfusion product and one of the most frequently used colloid solutions), use the same precautions and guidelines used for safe administration of blood products. (We cover blood administration in detail in Chapter 15, and we explain colloid solutions in Chapter 7.)

✔ Clarify physician's orders that rely solely on solutions of 5 percent dextrose in water (D5W) to treat dehydration because they dilute plasma electrolytes. Generally, doctors don't recommend using D5W solutions for treatment in early postoperative periods and cardiopulmonary resuscitation events.

✔ Intensely monitor hypertonic solutions containing high amounts of sodium chloride, such as 45 percent sodium chloride, for proper flow rates and adverse reactions. Ensure that the physician's order states the specific name of the solution, total volume to be infused, flow rate, and length of infusion time. (See Chapter 7 for more on hypertonic solutions and sodium chloride.)

✔ Minimize the risk for converting hypovolemia into hypervolemia with overinfusion by assessing baseline vital signs and edema status and monitoring for changes during and after completion of infusion. (We cover both hypovolemia and hypervolemia in Chapter 7.)

To monitor for *pitting edema* (caused by a systemic disease, such as congestive heart failure, or local conditions, such as cellulitis, involving just the affected extremities), press your thumb firmly for five seconds over the dorsum of each foot. Pitting edema is present when your thumb leaves a pitting depression in the foot. Pitting edema is graded on a 4-point scale, with +4 being the most severe grade of edema.

✔ When infusing solutions containing electrolytes, such as lactated Ringer's and Normosol-R, use caution when administering additional electrolytes. To avoid potential electrolyte overdose, clarify the physician's order before administering more.

Identifying adverse reactions with some common symptoms

Patients with serious underlying conditions, such as renal, liver, or heart disease, are at greatest risk for adverse reactions from fluid and electrolyte administration, but any patient can experience them. Most reactions manifest in the form of exacerbation of existing symptoms; however, additional symptoms may reflect excessive or deficient dosing. Table 17-5 helps you identify the most common symptoms associated with excessive or deficient dosing.

Table 17-5   Common Symptoms of Excessive or Deficient Dosing

Dosing Excess or Deficit	Symptoms
Sodium excess (hypernatremia)	Edema, seizures, or coma
Potassium excess (hyperkalemia)	Cardiac irregularities and ECG changes
Magnesium excess (hypermagnesemia)	Muscle weakness, ECG changes, sedation, or confusion
Calcium deficit (hypocalcemia)	Muscular paresthesia, cramps, laryngospasm, tetany, or seizures
Magnesium deficit (hypomagnesemia)	Neuromuscular dysfunction, hyperirritability, psychosis, tachycardia, or hypertension
Potassium deficit (hypokalemia)	Impaired neuromuscular function, weakness, or paralysis

Knowing the symptoms associated with over- and underdosing electrolytes is the first step in minimizing undesired consequences. When you notice any of these symptoms, notify the physician and obtain orders for additional treatment and frequent monitoring of blood levels.

Responding to adverse reactions

Whether the reaction is caused by over- or underdosing fluid and electrolytes, stop the infusion as soon as you notice the first signs of adverse reactions. Keep the vein open with normal saline to maintain access for any emergency IV medications or reversal agents and notify the physician immediately for additional orders.

Laboratory findings usually play a major role in the doctor's choice of treatment. The patient's symptoms and condition also influence the doctor's decision to provide additional medical support, such as dialysis treatments for patients with kidney disease and a worsening electrolyte imbalance.

Discontinuing the Replacement Infusion

Discontinuing the electrolyte infusion is a lot like discontinuing IV medications; see Chapter 14 for the basics. To discontinue the electrolyte infusion, use the following steps as a general guideline:

1. **Remove the piggyback and allow the primary infusion to continue.**

2. **If the patient doesn't have a primary infusion, close the roller clamp, remove the dressing, and remove the catheter from its insertion site if no IV is needed.**

3. **Apply pressure for 30 to 60 seconds and attach new dressing.**

4. **Document your actions and the patient's response to treatment.**

For information on safely disposing of IV waste and supplies, check out Chapter 14.

Chapter 18

Making Every Calorie Count: Parenteral Nutrition

. . . .

In This Chapter

▶ Assessing your patient's baseline nutritional status

▶ Initiating parenteral therapy and monitoring the infusion's progress

▶ Watching for complications and knowing how to deal with them

▶ Discontinuing therapy and safely disposing of parenteral products

. . . .

*P*arenteral nutrition (PN) provides nutrients and energy to patients who can't absorb or tolerate nutrients through enteral or tube feedings. Depending on each patient's nutritional needs, parenteral nutrition may consist of a simple protein and sugar mixture administered by infusion (IV) once a day or a complex total parenteral nutrition mixture containing amino acids, dextrose, lipids, and vitamins, administered continuously by IV.

PN is an emerging IV therapy that's proving to help surgical wounds heal more quickly and shorten hospital stays of patients with chronic illness. The benefits and use of PN in various clinical settings mean you'll undoubtedly deal with some form of IV nutritional support in your healthcare career. That's where this chapter comes in.

Here, you find out all about the patient assessment you have to do to obtain a baseline nutritional status, as well as the ins and outs of initiating parenteral therapy and monitoring the infusion. You discover the most common complications associated with PN and find out how to manage them if they occur. Finally, you discover how to keep yourself and your patient safe while administering life-extending nutrients.

Planning around Your Patient's Baseline Nutritional Status

The key to successfully administering nutritional support through parenteral nutrition (PN) is getting the right parenteral product in the right concentrations to the right patient. To determine what the appropriate parenteral product and concentration are for a given patient, you have to do a *baseline nutritional assessment,* which you can use to calculate the patient's baseline nutritional status. The assessment begins with a complete medical and surgical history, including recent or chronic illnesses, past surgeries, medications, and medication allergies, and continues with blood work and a physical assessment.

The goals of the baseline nutritional assessment are to

- ✔ Establish a patient's baseline nutritional status.
- ✔ Identify patients who require aggressive nutritional support.
- ✔ Restore or maintain a patient's nutritional status through specifically prepared nutritional therapies.
- ✔ Identify appropriate nutritional therapies.
- ✔ Evaluate the effectiveness of nutritional support.

Use the guidelines in the following sections to do a baseline nutritional assessment so that the nutrition team can formulate a customized nutritional support plan that fits the needs of your patient.

Obtaining your patient's weight

In assessing your patient's nutritional status, you can use several different methods to measure his body weight, but the most common methods involve relationships between height and weight and comparisons between actual weight and usual weight. Whichever method you use, obtaining an accurate baseline body weight is critical in establishing your nutritional support plan, evaluating the results of the plan, and adjusting the nutritional support components as the patient progresses through the plan.

Body mass index

One of the most frequently used methods of assessing weight is the *body mass index* (BMI). BMI uses the relationship between body weight and height to measure overall lean or fat body mass. In other words, it measures a person's underweight or overweight status. A high BMI indicates obesity, whereas a low BMI suggests inadequate nutritional intake.

BMI is easy to calculate, especially if you use one of several online BMI calculators (check out www.nhlbisupport.com/bmi/). But if you like doing math, you can calculate BMI the old-fashioned way with one of two equations. Which equation you use depends on whether you're using metric units (meters, m, and kilograms, kg) or standard American units (inches, in, and pounds, lb). Here's a quick example of the BMI equation, using metric units:

$$BMI = weight\ (kg) \div (height \times height)\ (m^2)$$

$$BMI = 60\ kg \div (1.7\ m \times 1.7\ m)$$

$$BMI = 60\ kg \div 2.89\ m^2 = 20.8$$

Here's an example of the BMI equation, using standard American units:

$$BMI = weight\ (lb) \div (height \times height)\ (in^2) \times 703$$

$$BMI = 160\ lb \div (66\ in \times 66\ in) \times 703$$

$$BMI = 160\ lb \div 4{,}356\ in^2 \times 703 = 25.8$$

After you have your patient's BMI, use Table 18-1 to identify his weight status.

Table 18-1	BMI Weight Status
BMI	*Weight Status*
Below 18.5	Underweight
18.5–24.9	Normal weight
25.0–29.9	Overweight
30.0 and above	Obese

BMI uses the same standard weight status for both men and women over the age of 20. But infants and children have weight status categories that are specific for both age and gender (check out www.cdc.gov/healthyweight/assessing/bmi/childrens_bmi/about_childrens_bmi.html for details).

When used with clinical evaluation and weight loss history, BMI is one of the best methods for weight assessment because it's easy to use and accessible to all clinicians.

Actual weight as a percentage of usual weight

Another method of assessing patient weight is by comparing the percentage of usual body weight (UBW) to actual body weight (ABW). In fact, actual weight as a percentage of usual weight is one of the most accurate and reliable methods of determining weight loss. To calculate actual weight this way, you must know the patient's usual body weight, which you can usually get from the history and physical or by asking a family member.

To calculate the actual weight percentage of usual weight, multiply actual weight in pounds by 100 and divide by usual body weight in pounds. The minimum actual weight percentage for survival is 48 to 55 percent of usual weight. Here's a simple example for a patient who actually weighs 150 pounds with a usual weight of 180 pounds:

% of UBW = (actual weight × 100) ÷ usual body weight

% of UBW = 150 lb × 100 ÷ 180 lb

% of UBW = 15,000 ÷ 180 = 83.3%

Reviewing your patient's blood work

In addition to measuring a patient's weight, a thorough nutritional assessment involves reviewing the patient's laboratory results, especially results that measure visceral proteins and complete blood counts. These two particular lab tests can help evaluate whether the patient is suffering from malnutrition and how well his immune system is functioning.

Visceral proteins

The most common type of malnutrition in hospitalized patients is *protein malnutrition,* in which visceral proteins are significantly depleted. *Visceral proteins* are synthesized in the liver and are considered to be some of the most accurate indicators of a patient's protein stores.

The patient's initial chemical profile should screen for the following visceral proteins:

- **Albumin and prealbumin:** Albumin creates an osmotic force that maintains fluid volume within the vascular space (normal values are between 3.2 and 5 grams per deciliter, or g/dL). Prealbumin provides a general idea of a person's nutrition (normal values are between 18 and 36 milligrams per deciliter, or mg/dL).

- **Transferrin and retinol-binding proteins:** Transferrin is a plasma protein that transports iron through the blood to the liver, spleen, and bone marrow (normal reference ranges are 204–360 mg/dL). Retinol-binding proteins are carrier proteins that bind retinol (normal reference ranges are 65–276 international units per deciliter, or IU/dL).

Serum albumin decreases in malnourished patients as the body breaks down protein to create energy. Although it takes several days or sometimes weeks before a patient's protein stores are depleted enough to show a decrease in albumin, the initial lab screening of albumin provides a baseline for later comparison.

When a patient's albumin levels start decreasing, the patient is at high risk for complications of malnutrition. Albumin values that drop below 3.2 g/dL are associated with increased morbidity and mortality in hospitalized patients.

Levels of prealbumin, another visceral protein measured in the initial blood work, indicate a depletion of protein stores earlier than albumin. It takes only a few days from the onset of protein breakdown for lab work to show a decrease in prealbumin. For this reason, prealbumin is considered to reflect an accurate picture of the patient's current nutritional status. It's also a specific indicator of the effectiveness of nutritional therapy and is used to evaluate and direct ongoing nutritional support.

The other visceral proteins, such as transferrin and retinol-binding proteins, are helpful in evaluating baseline nutritional status, but they aren't responsive enough to be useful in acutely ill patients.

Complete blood count

Another set of blood work measurements used to assess your patient's nutritional status is the *complete blood count* (CBC). It provides a comprehensive look at the patient's blood components. You can then use the patient's CBC to do a comparison between the patient's lab values and normal values. Here's what the CBC measures:

- ✔ **Red blood cells (RBCs):** RBCs transport oxygen from the lungs to the rest of the body by means of an oxygen-binding, iron-rich protein called *hemoglobin.* When RBCs and hemoglobin values are low, the patient is clinically *anemic,* and anemia is one of the earliest laboratory indicators of protein depletion associated with malnutrition.

- ✔ **White blood cells (WBCs):** WBCs reflect the status of a patient's immune system. High levels of WBCs may indicate infection or inflammation, and low levels may suggest impaired immune function. Low measurements of a specific type of WBC, the *lymphocyte,* have been linked to malnutrition.

- ✔ **Blood platelets:** Although blood platelets are the smallest blood cells in the body, they, too, provide information about a patient's nutritional status. After all, malnutrition frequently alters the size, shape, and number of platelets in the blood.

Assessing your patient physically

Assessing a patient's physical appearance is an important component of any nutritional screening. Changes in hair, eyes, skin, and mucous membranes are frequent markers for nutritional deficits. Table 18-2 lists the main physical characteristics you need to look for in your patient and the nutritional deficits they may indicate.

Table 18-2   Physical Assessments and Nutritional Deficits

Focus of Assessment	Findings	Nutritional Deficit
Hair	Hair loss, change in pigment, dry hair	Protein, calories, zinc, linoleic acid
Mouth	Inflammation of mucous membranes, oral lesions, sores	Vitamin B
Tongue	Purplish, red, or beefy color	Vitamin B
	Varicose vein beneath the tongue	Vitamin C
Skin	Dry, flaky skin	Vitamin A, fatty acids
	Hemorrhagic spots, easy bruising	Vitamins C and K
Musculoskeletal	Muscle wasting, atrophy	Protein, calories
	Kyphosis, osteoporosis	Calcium, vitamin D
Neurologic	Confusion, listlessness	Protein
	Sensory or motor impairment	Thiamine, vitamin B12

Besides just physically observing the characteristics listed in Table 18-2, you can also do a series of measurements called *anthropometric measurements* as part of the physical assessment. Anthropometric measurements are noninvasive, inexpensive techniques used to measure body dimensions to identify obesity and malnutrition.

Asking questions about dietary history

Obtaining a dietary history from your patient is another important element in nutritional assessment. A dietary history not only evaluates adequate intake of all macro- and micronutrients needed for proper nutrition but also provides insight into the impact of physical, psychosocial, and cultural factors on the patient's attitudes about food intake and nutrition. In doing so, it aids in the early detection, prevention, and treatment of malnutrition in hospitalized patients.

A thorough dietary history asks questions about the following potential problems:

- Altered taste or smell
- Breathing, chewing, or swallowing difficulties
- Dental cavities, missing teeth, or ill-fitting dentures
- Ethnic and cultural preferences
- Fad diets and diet modifications, such as low fat or low sodium
- Food allergies, aversions, or intolerances
- Frequent fasting, NPO (nothing by mouth), or clear liquid status
- Inability to prepare food or feed self

By obtaining a thorough dietary history of your patient, you can determine the duration and amount of recent or past weight loss and identify food allergies.

Using a clinical scoring system

To speed up the process of identifying nutritional deficiencies in patients, scientists have developed more than 50 clinical scoring systems for use as hospital admission screening tools. Of the many scoring systems available today, however, only a few have been tested and proven to accurately identify nutritional deficiencies and predict clinical outcomes.

The most common and widely used scoring system is the *Subjective Global Assessment* (SGA). The SGA, an in-hospital screening tool, is considered the gold standard for nutritional assessment, especially when used with gastrointestinal (GI) surgical patients.

The SGA takes into account the following five factors of patient history:

- ✔ Dietary intake change
- ✔ Functional capacity
- ✔ GI symptoms
- ✔ Relationship of disease to nutritional requirements
- ✔ Weight change

In addition, the SGA considers the following five features of the physical examination:

- ✔ Ankle edema
- ✔ Ascites (peritoneal fluid)
- ✔ Loss of subcutaneous fat in the triceps
- ✔ Muscle wasting in the quadriceps and deltoids
- ✔ Sacral edema

Based on these ten criteria, the SGA ranks the patient's nutritional status as one of the following:

- ✔ Well nourished
- ✔ Mild/moderate or suspected malnutrition
- ✔ Severe malnutrition

Figure 18-1 shows the basic elements needed for the SGA clinical scoring system and includes an overall rating that quickly identifies the degree of risk for malnutrition.

In addition to the more than 50 clinical scoring systems readily available to clinicians (see the nearby sidebar for a quick look at a few of these), many hospitals have developed their own nutritional-assessment systems. Check your facility's guidelines for details. Incorporating a clinical scoring system into your baseline nutritional screening routine enables you to provide early detection and intervention for patients at risk for malnutrition.

Patient Name: _____ ID #: _____ Date: _____

WEIGHT

Baseline Weight: _____ (Dry weight from 6 months ago)
Current Weight: _____ (Dry weight today)
Actual Wt loss/past 6 mo. _____ % wt loss _____ (actual loss from baseline/last SGA)
Wt change over past two weeks _____ No change _____ Increase _____ Decrease
RATING: 1 2 3 4 5 6 7

DIETARY INTAKE

_____ No change (Adequate)   _____ No change (Inadequate)
Change:
Sub optimal Intake _____ Protein _____ Kcal _____ Duration _____
Full Liquid _____ Hypocaloric Liquid_____ Starvation _____
RATING: 1 2 3 4 5 6 7

DIETARY INTAKE

(*Frequency: Never, daily, 2-3 times/wk, 1-2 times/wk, >2 weeks, <2 weeks)

Symptom:	Frequency: *	Duration:
_____ None	_____	_____
_____ Anorexia	_____	_____
_____ Nausea	_____	_____
_____ Vomiting	_____	_____
_____ Diarrhea	_____	_____

RATING: 1 2 3 4 5 6 7

FUNCTIONAL CAPACITY

Description:	Duration:
_____ No Dysfunction	_____
_____ Change in Function	_____
_____ Difficulty with ambulation	_____
_____ Difficulty with activity (patient specific "normal")	_____
_____ Light activity	_____
_____ Bed/chair ridden with little or no activity	_____
_____ Improvement in function	_____

RATING: 1 2 3 4 5 6 7

DIAGNOSIS/CO-MORBIDITIES RELATED TO NUTRITIONAL NEEDS

Primary diagnosis _____ Comorbidities_____
_____ Normal requirements   _____ Increased requirements
_____ Decreased requirements
Acute Metabolic Stress: _____ None _____ Low _____ Moderate _____ High
RATING: 1 2 3 4 5 6 7

PHYSICAL EXAM

_____ Loss of subcutaneous fat   _____ Some areas _____ All areas
    (below eye, triceps, biceps, chest)
_____ Muscle wasting   _____ Some areas _____ All areas
    (temple, clavicle, scapula, ribs quadriceps, calf, knee, interosseous)
_____ Edema (related to undernutrition/use to evaluate weight change)
RATING: 1 2 3 4 5 6 7

OVERALL RATING

_____ 6-7=Very Mild risk to well nourished; most categories or significant/continued improvement
_____ 3-4-5=Mild/Moderate; No clear sign of normal status or severe malnutrition
_____ 1-2=Severely Malnourished; most categories/significant physical signs of malnutrition

Figure 18-1:
Sample SGA
clinical
scoring
form.

Illustration courtesy of ESRD Network 13

Scoring nutrition status with a few other clinical scoring systems

Here's a quick peek at some of the most common clinical scoring systems in addition to the SGA:

✔ **Mini-Nutritional Assessment (MNA):** This widely used screening tool is similar to the SGA and consists of 18 questions that assess the patient's dietary history and subjective evaluation of nutritional status.

✔ **Council on Nutrition Appetite Questionnaire (CNAQ):** This eight-item self-assessment questionnaire is designed for older and high-risk patient populations. The CNAQ deals with quantity and quality of food intake, appetite, and eating patterns and asks patients to rate themselves on a scale of 1 to 5, with low scores indicating high risk for nutritional deficiencies.

✔ **Simplified Nutritional Appetite Questionnaire (SNAQ):** The SNAQ is a shorter version of CNAQ; it asks only four questions about food intake, appetite, and eating patterns. The SNAQ is tailored for hospitalized patients and is highly sensitive and specific in identifying patients at risk for weight loss during hospitalization.

✔ **Malnutrition Universal Screening Test (MUST):** This screening test was developed by the British Association for Parenteral and Enteral Nutrition and is used more commonly in Europe. It uses BMI, unintentional weight loss, and acute disease effect to assess nutritional status. This test has been shown to predict length of hospital stay, discharge destination, and mortality. One advantage of the MUST system is that it offers treatment options based on test scores. The major disadvantage is that it's more difficult to use because it requires calculating BMI.

Calculating your patient's energy requirements

After determining that the patient needs nutritional support to promote healing and enhance recovery, the next step is to calculate the patient's energy requirements in order to identify what kind of nutrients the patient needs. Calculating energy requirements in hospitalized patients usually requires the use of an energy equation, and many equations use kilocalories, body weight, and activity levels as a starting point.

We show you how to calculate energy requirements in the following sections. Flip to Chapter 8 for details on how to identify the kinds and amounts of nutrients you need to meet those energy requirements.

Focusing on kilocalories

A *kilocalorie* (kcal) is a unit measurement of 1,000 energy calories. In technical terms, 1 kcal is the amount of energy needed to raise the temperature of 1 kg of water by 1 degree Celsius. In food calorie terms, 1 kcal is equal to 1 food calorie, and the calories on food labels and calorie calculators are interchangeable with kilocalories.

Most average adults need between 1,800 and 2,500 kcal per day to meet their energy needs. Of these kilocalories, approximately 1,000 kcal come from carbohydrates in the form of glucose, 525 to 550 come from lipids, and 350 to 375 come from proteins.

One of the most common ways to use kilocalories to calculate energy requirements is to estimate the number of kilocalories needed per kilogram of body weight per day. Critically ill, nonobese patients need about 25 to 30 kcal per kg of body weight. Critically ill, obese patients need only about 21 kcal per kg of body weight.

Other common methods of calculating energy requirements based on calories and kilocalories include the following:

- ✔ **Harris-Benedict equation:** This equation uses weight, height, age, sex, and body weight to estimate *basal energy expenditure* (BEE) in kilocalories. Basal energy expenditure calculates daily energy expenditure based on gender, age (in years), height (in centimeters, cm), and weight (in kg) for caloric requirements. Here's what the Harris-Benedict equation looks like for males and females:

    Male BEE = 66.5 + (13.75 × weight in kg) + (5.003 × height in cm) − (6.775 × age in years)

    Female BEE = 655.1 + (9.563 × weight in kg) + (1.850 × height in cm) − (4.676 × age in years)

    Check out this website for a handy online BEE calculator: `www-users.med.cornell.edu/~spon/picu/calc/beecalc.htm`

- ✔ **Indirect calorimetry:** This widely used method for calculating energy expenditures and requirements uses metabolic measurements of the body's oxygen consumption and carbon dioxide production over a period of time. It also measures loss of nitrogen through the urine. Although indirect calorimetry is considered to be one of the most accurate ways of determining a patient's energy needs, it requires expensive monitoring equipment and isn't available in all facilities.

Including basal energy expenditure and activity levels in the energy equation

Another way to calculate energy requirements is to use basal energy expenditure in conjunction with activity levels (labeled *activity factors* and *injury factors*). This method is especially common in predicting energy expenditures of critically ill patients because stress, activity, illness, trauma, burns, and cancers can increase daily caloric requirements.

Additional energy equations are available online to calculate energy requirements, but no matter which equation you use, you must remember not to exceed recommended nutrient levels. Exceeding recommended daily maximums can result in hyperglycemia and impairment of hepatic, respiratory, and kidney function. (Flip to Chapter 8 for the skinny on recommended nutrient levels.)

Concentrating on concentrations

Getting the right nutrients in the right amounts to supply a patient's energy needs is only one step in the creation of a successful nutritional support plan. Getting the right concentrations of nutrients is another.

Table 18-3 provides guidelines for the most common nutrient concentrations used in PN support regimens. Turn to Chapter 8 for all the details on creating a balanced, effective PN solution with all the right macronutrients, micronutrients, and trace elements.

Table 18-3	Standard Macronutrient Concentrations in Parenteral Nutrition			
Macro-nutrient	**Normal Range**	**Usual Dose**	**Maximum Dose**	**Considerations**
Protein	0.8–2 g/kg/day	1.1–1.5 g/kg/day	2.0 g/kg/day	Should have high concentrations of amino acids; must be specifically dosed in renal and liver disease
Calories	20–35 kcal/kg/day	20–30 kcal/kg/day	Determined by patient status	Not to exceed 25 kcal/kg/day in critically ill patients

Macro-nutrient	Normal Range	Usual Dose	Maximum Dose	Considerations
Glucose	70–80% of nonprotein calories	Determined by patient status	7g/kg/day or 4–5 mg/kg/min	Improved outcomes noted when blood glucose maintained at < 110 mg/dL in critical patients and > 150 mg/dL in stable patients
Lipids	15–30% of nonprotein calories	Determined by patient status	2.5 g/kg/day	Limited benefit noted when > 30% of nonprotein calories; must be slowly infused; not indicated in patients with pancreatitis or hyperlipidemia

Note: g/kg/day = grams per kilogram of body weight per day; kcal/kg/day = kilocalories per kilogram of body weight per day; mg/kg/min = milligrams per kilogram of body weight per minute; mg/dL = milligrams per deciliter

Administering Parenteral Nutrition Products through a CVAD

PN comes in two types, both of which can be infused through a vascular access device (VAD):

✔ *Peripheral parenteral nutrition* (PPN) has a smaller concentration of nutrients and less than 10 percent dextrose, making its osmolarity low enough to give through a peripheral IV. PPN is usually given for a short period, usually no longer than a couple of weeks.

✔ *Total parenteral nutrition* (TPN) has a higher nutrient concentration, making its osmolarity caustic to peripheral veins, and is usually given for an extended period of time for acutely and chronically ill patients who need PN infusions for weeks, months, or even longer. Therefore, TPN has to be given centrally through a central vascular access device (CVAD). CVADs are the best option here because they provide safer long-term access for continuous, repeated infusions associated with nutritional support therapy.

For more on the differences between PPN and TPN, turn to Chapter 8. Because infusing PPN through a peripheral IV is so similar to infusing any other medication, we don't cover that topic in detail here; flip to Chapter 12 for details. Here, we focus on safely administering PN products through a CVAD. (Refer to Chapter 13 for a lot more info on administering through CVADs.)

CVADs are catheters that are placed in large veins of the neck, chest, arm or groin for long-term, repeated infusions. Central catheters allow large amounts of medications, including chemotherapy drugs and nutritional support products, to rapidly dilute and move into the patient's bloodstream.

Getting started

When administering PN, the first things you need to do are check the physician's order and verify that the pharmacy's admixture matches the physician's order. Next, you have to inform the patient about the anticipated treatment, explain the benefits of PN, and answer any questions she may have. After doing so, you're ready to verify the CVAD's tip placement.

Obtaining an order for a chest X-ray and confirming placement

Before using a CVAD to administer TPN, verify the location of the catheter tip either by using an existing chest X-ray or by obtaining an order for a new chest X-ray. Verifying the tip's location ensures that the catheter is in the right place and that the fluids and medications will flow freely into the central venous system.

Because TPN products may be caustic, never administer them through a newly placed CVAD. Always confirm that the catheter tip is in a large, free-flowing vein, typically the superior vena cava or the inferior vena cava (for femoral placement), before you start TPN therapy.

Filtering the line

TPN solutions are infused through a filtered line and infusion control pump. Frequently, these solutions arrive from the pharmacy stamped with the type of filter required for infusion.

Typical nutritional solution filters include 1.2 micron, 24-hour filters for TPN mixed with lipids and 0.2 micron, 72-hour filters for TPN without lipids. Refer to your facility's protocol for filter recommendations to make sure you use the correct filter.

Starting the infusion gradually

Gather all the supplies needed to administer IV infusions. (Remember that PN solutions are usually refrigerated and you need to remove them from the refrigerator at least an hour prior to infusion.) Before starting any infusion, especially PN infusions, wash your hands thoroughly with soap and water. When initiating therapy, start slowly at 50 percent of the calculated requirements. Progress should be followed on a flowchart. (Refer to Chapter 13 for more on administering central IV infusions.)

Cycling the administration

When administering PN, you do so either continuously over 24 hours or cyclically in shorter periods of time, usually 12 to 14 hours through a CVAD. You usually administer PN continuously in acutely ill patients and those requiring only short-term PN. You usually give cycled administrations to stable patients who require long-term PN or patients who require PN after being discharged from the hospital.

Considering hang time

Sky divers think of *hang time* as a glorious free fall before they deploy their parachutes. Parenteral nutritionists, on the other hand, refer to *hang time* as the length of time that's considered safe for PN administration before bacterial counts start to grow.

According to the American Society of Parenteral and Enteral Nutrition (A.S.P.E.N.) and the Centers for Disease Control and Prevention (CDC), the maximum hang time for a total nutrient admixture is 24 hours, and the maximum time for a lipid solution is 12 hours.

Hang time begins from the time the formulation is compounded, reconstituted, or warmed or the original seal is broken. Extending hang time beyond the A.S.P.E.N. and CDC recommendations places the patient at risk for sepsis and other complications caused by bacterial contamination.

Maintaining the administration set and tubing

Guidelines for changing IV sets and tubing for PN are often based on the manufacturer's guidelines for the IV sets, filters, or admixtures you're using. For example, some filters specify changing them every 24 hours. Refer to your facility's protocol or pharmacy for specifics on changing and maintaining PN IV sets.

Monitoring the infusion

You must closely monitor PN IVs to ensure accurate infusion rates, compliance with hang times, and central line patency. Of course, you have to closely monitor the patients, too, to prevent overloading the metabolic system with a barrage of concentrated nutrients. The following sections provide guidelines for monitoring patients who are receiving PN.

Testing 1-2-3: The importance of blood glucose monitoring

Hyperglycemia (or high blood sugar) is the most common complication of PN, so insulin is frequently added to PN solutions to prevent hyperglycemia and to maintain glucose control. For example:

- ✔ For patients with diabetes who require insulin before PN, 1 unit of regular insulin for every 10 g of dextrose is added.

- ✔ When blood glucose levels are consistently above 200 mg/dL, more insulin needs to be added.

- ✔ To provide even greater glucose control, the doctor may order sliding-scale coverage with regular insulin.

Be sure to consult your physician, nutritional team, or pharmacy if you have any issues with glucose control.

Rapid-acting insulin analogs help control glucose, but they're incompatible with PN solutions. Regular insulin is the only insulin you can safely add directly into a PN formulation.

Tight glucose control is essential in nutritional support because hyperglycemia prevents the metabolism of nutrients in PN, placing the patient at greater risk for infection and delayed healing. Daily reformulations based on laboratory values are frequently necessary to prevent hyperglycemia from overfeeding. Preventing hyperglycemia results in better patient outcomes and shorter hospital stays.

Evaluating your patient and monitoring progress

When you're working with patients on PN, you need to monitor them for clinical symptoms, biochemical findings, and nutritional status:

- ✔ Clinically, you need to monitor patients for vital signs, weight, intake and output, and a host of routine physical assessments, such as CVAD site inspection, dressing condition, and adverse reactions to PN. (See Chapter 13 for details on inspecting the CVAD site and dressing condition, and check out the next section for info on how to manage adverse reactions.)

✔ Biochemically, you need to monitor your patient's lab values for glucose levels, liver function, blood count, acid-base balance, electrolytes, and a host of other lab tests to monitor kidney, gallbladder, and pancreatic function.

✔ Nutritionally, you need to use clinical assessments and biochemical values to monitor your patient's nutritional progress so nutritional components and medications can be added or deleted and the doctor can generally direct the course of treatment.

Many institutions use flowcharts and an interdisciplinary nutrition team to monitor the patient throughout PN therapy. The team members check the patient's weight, CBC, electrolytes, and blood urea nitrogen (BUN) often (daily for inpatients). They monitor plasma glucose every six hours until the patient's glucose levels become stable. They monitor fluid intake and output continuously and assess liver function tests prior to and periodically during PN infusion. Other assessments, measured twice a week, include plasma proteins, prothrombin time, urine osmolality, and calcium, magnesium, and phosphate levels. A full nutritional assessment (including BMI calculation and anthropometric measurements) should be repeated at two-week intervals. Consult your facility's protocol for patients on nutritional support regimens so you know how to best monitor them.

Managing Common PN Complications

PN is a complex form of IV therapy that saves lives, but it also carries risks for life-threatening complications. As a medical professional, your job is to minimize and manage the many metabolic, technical, and systemic complications of PN therapy.

To help manage the following metabolic complications, carefully check the patient's lab results and use the monitoring techniques we describe in the earlier section "Monitoring the infusion":

✔ **Fluid and electrolyte balance:** Monitor electrolytes daily and adjust electrolyte dosing frequently to match the patient's changing needs for replacement due to disease and stress.

✔ **Glucose imbalance:** Monitor glucose levels closely to prevent hyperglycemia, which places the patient at risk for life-threatening complications such as bloodstream infection. Report blood glucose levels consistently above 200 mg/dL to the physician.

✓ **Nutritional imbalance:** Monitor the patient's liver, kidney, and other organ functions through lab values. Correct imbalances by notifying the physician to add or delete nutritional supplements to the PN mix.

Here are some of the most common technical complications of PN, along with ways to minimize or manage them:

✓ **Air embolism:** Ensure that all ports are closed before changing IV sets.

✓ **Embolism or occlusion:** Monitor for slow infusions or no blood return.

✓ **Venous thrombosis:** Check for sluggish infusions, paleness, or soreness or swelling of the extremity.

Bloodstream infection, or *sepsis,* is the most common systemic infection associated with PN, and it's usually caused by microorganisms introduced into the bloodstream through a central line. Fever is the hallmark symptom of sepsis, so any time you notice a fever in your patient, be sure to investigate to find the source. If you can't find a source and fever persists for 24 to 48 hours, the physician may order the catheter to be removed. Before the removal of the catheter, draw a blood culture specimen from the catheter, as ordered by the physician or directed by facility protocol. After the catheter is removed, cut 2 to 3 inches off the catheter tip with sterile scissors and place it in a sterile culture tube, according to facility protocol. For additional tips on preventing and managing sepsis, follow the infection management techniques we cover in Chapter 13.

Another complication of PN, *refeeding syndrome,* occurs when a malnourished body is flooded with nutrients, resulting in a metabolic overload of systems and organs. You can help minimize refeeding syndrome by starting PN slowly and gradually increasing it to the desired amount.

Discontinuing Parenteral Therapy

A physician's order is required to discontinue PN because it's a medication. But a general rule of thumb for when to discontinue PN therapy is when enteral or oral feedings supply more than 50 percent of the daily estimated kilocalories required to meet the patient's energy needs. However, you may need to start PN again within two to three days after discontinuance if the patient's intake drops below 50 percent of her daily requirements for energy calories. The following sections cover a few things you need to keep in mind when discontinuing PN.

Tapering off versus stopping abruptly

Many IV therapists and physicians *taper off* (or decrease gradually) PN infusions to prevent *rebound hypoglycemia,* a significant decrease in blood glucose levels that patients can experience when PN is discontinued. Those in favor of tapering off recommend a 50 percent reduction of the infusion rate for the first hour of discontinuation, followed by an additional 50 percent reduction in the second hour.

Other clinicians feel that tapering off is unnecessary. They say that the risk for rebound hypoglycemia is extremely low, especially in patients with stable glucose levels, and studies support their position. Check the physician's orders and your facility's protocol for details on how you should approach PN discontinuation.

Although experts continue to debate the tapering off controversy, most agree that patients prone to hypoglycemia may benefit from a short one- to two-hour tapering off period before a complete discontinuation of PN.

Considering when to withhold or withdraw

In critically ill patients, PN is a life-sustaining treatment, which means that deciding whether to withhold or withdraw PN is equivalent to deciding whether to remove a patient from a respirator or heart pump.

Much of the discussion about withholding or withdrawing PN revolves around the same medical, legal, and ethical issues related to removing other life-support measures. Because most critical patients die after being removed from life support, the decision to discontinue PN ultimately rests with the healthcare team, the patient, and the patient's family. Your contributions during this dark period are reassurance, concern, and support for the decision made by the patient and the patient's loved ones.

Disposing of Parenteral Nutrition Products

Nutritional waste products contain high concentrations of nutrients and may be hazardous when handled without proper protective equipment. So be sure to follow institutional guidelines or established policies and procedure protocols when disposing of all nutritional waste products. Usually the disposal process involves the following:

✔ Discard any unused medications in specific unused medication receptacles.

✔ Discard nutrient waste products, infusion bags, and tubings in specified biohazardous containers.

✔ Discard needles, ampules, and other sharps into designated sharps containers.

✔ Wear protective gloves and clothing when appropriate and discard them in designated containers when you're finished with them.

Part V
Considering Unique Populations

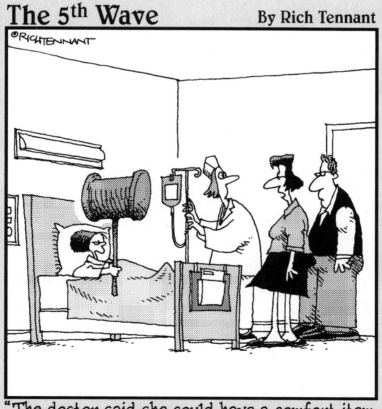

The 5th Wave   By Rich Tennant

"The doctor said she could have a comfort item during the IV insertion."

In this part . . .

Part V explores the special needs of different patient populations. It offers several insider secrets on meeting the challenges and special needs of pediatric IV patients and geriatric IV patients. It also identifies the special skills and experience you need to provide IV therapy to patients at home.

Chapter 19

A Little Dab'll Do Ya: IV Therapy for Infants and Children

....

In This Chapter

▶ Identifying the differences between pediatric and adult IV therapy

▶ Calculating pediatric dosages

▶ Delivering peripheral and central IV therapy in infants and children

....

*I*n many ways, IV therapy in children is very different from IV therapy in adults. As a result, even experienced IV nurses have to relearn certain administration techniques and develop new ways of thinking to make a successful transition from adult to pediatric IV therapy.

Dealing with squirming infants, initiating therapy in smaller veins, and calming anxious parents are just a few of the difficulties pediatric IV nurses face on a daily basis. In addition, they have to be aware of the different types of equipment needed for children and the different types of calculations used in pediatric dosing. Lucky for you, this chapter takes you on a how-to journey of all this and more, including how to start IVs, administer IV therapy, and manage central lines in kids.

In short, this chapter explains how to deliver safe IV therapy to children and how to guide them through one of the scariest times in their lives.

Understanding How Pediatric IV Therapy Is Different

Children respond to IV therapy based largely on their age, previous experiences, education, and family. Hence, administering IV therapy in children is a daunting task for pediatric nurses because it requires a different manner of communication, a different level of monitoring, and a different set of tools and techniques. From using fiber-optic lights to identify small veins in chubby arms to starting IVs in the scalp, IV therapy in children is miles apart from IV therapy in adults. In contrast to their adult counterparts, children require

- ✔ Distractions, such as pacifiers and sucrose bottles, during the procedure
- ✔ Lower and slower infusion rates (as a rule of thumb, hang only one 500 mL bag at a time; 100 mL/hour, or 2,400 mL/day, is the normal maximum amount)
- ✔ Smaller equipment (see the section "Making equipment modifications")
- ✔ Specific insertion sites based on age and type of therapy (see the later sections "Selecting the best venous access site" and "CVAD IV Therapy for Kids")

IV therapy in children also differs from that in adults on the following levels:

- ✔ **Anatomical:** Infants and children have approximately half the number of accessible veins as adults, and their veins are smaller, deeper, and more difficult to visualize than adults'. Plus, when you're working with infants in the early stages of development, you have to take special age-appropriate insertion precautions, such as avoiding IVs in the thumb-sucking extremity. As you can see in Figure 19-1, nurses frequently use scalp veins and lower extremities for IVs in pediatric patients, while they rarely use those sites for IV placement in adults.

- ✔ **Emotional:** During hospitalization, children tend to regress to an earlier age, causing them to exhibit developmental behavior younger than their actual chronological age. For example, even older children may cry more frequently and more loudly and express hostile emotions more openly than they normally would. Pediatric IV nurses must remember to provide care for the children's developmental age, not their chronological age.

- ✔ **Epidemiological:** Unlike adults, who are frequently hospitalized for chronic conditions, children are usually hospitalized for episodic care of acute conditions. Thus, pediatric IV therapy requires developing techniques to deliver safe therapy within a wellness framework. Most pediatric patients are normal, otherwise healthy children whose childhoods have been interrupted by acute disease or traumatic events. Pediatric patients still enjoy and want to participate in regular activities of childhood, and IV nurses are in an optimal position to help children receive the care they need while providing a safe yet playful hospital environment.

- ✔ **Physiological:** The physiological body composition of infants and children is approximately 70 to 90 percent water, compared with 60 percent in adults, which places children at greater risk for fluid deficit and/or fluid overload than adults.

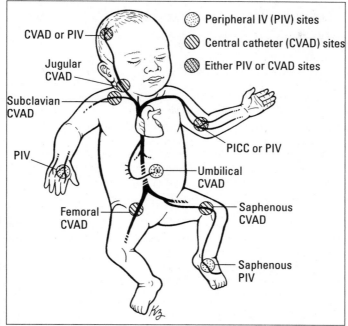

Peripheral IV (PIV) sites

Central catheter (CVAD) sites

Either PIV or CVAD sites

CVAD or PIV

Jugular CVAD

Subclavian CVAD

PIV

PICC or PIV

Umbilical CVAD

Femoral CVAD

Saphenous CVAD

Saphenous PIV

Figure 19-1: Anatomic placement of IVs in pediatric patients.

Illustration by Kathryn Born

Making equipment modifications

To prevent IV complications, such as fluid overload and inaccurate dosing, most healthcare facilities use specialized child-sized equipment for pediatric administration. Here's some of the most commonly used equipment:

✔ Ambulatory infusion pumps for active, older children

✔ Low-pressure infusion pumps and smaller IV fluid bags

✔ Low-volume IV tubing to reduce flushing volumes

✔ Micro IV tubing that delivers 60 drops/milliliter (drops/mL) rather than the 10 to 15 drops/mL delivered in adults

✔ Pediatric arm boards, stabilization devices, and flexible net tubing

✔ Syringe pumps for accurate delivery of small infusion volumes

Dealing with fear and establishing a positive relationship

Pediatric IV therapy involves creating a protected environment for children (and their families) to recover, regroup, and rehabilitate while receiving IV treatment. Ask a child and her family about their greatest fear in the hospital, and most will say *needles!* Pediatric IV nurses enter a child's hospital room with the fear factor looming large in everyone's mind, and creating a positive relationship with the child and her family is central to alleviating this fear and setting the stage for a successful IV outcome. Through entertaining teaching techniques, alleviation of pain with topical anesthetics, and creation of innovative distractions during IV insertion, nurses can transform a scary procedure into a show-and-tell event.

To establish rapport early in the child-family-nurse relationship and to make the whole therapy process as smooth as possible, follow these tips:

- ✔ Include the child and her parents in patient education to prepare them for what will take place during the IV procedure.

- ✔ Use hands-on teaching tools that show the steps of starting an IV, and encourage the child to feel the soft catheter that remains inside the vein.

- ✔ Be honest and tell the child that the insertion procedure will hurt for a short time, about the time it takes to count to 50, and encourage the parents and child to count to 50 during the insertion. Also let her know that IV fluids may feel cold or that medications may sting but only for a few seconds.

- ✔ Ask parents to stay during the procedure to distract their child with videos or games, such as blowing bubbles through a straw, and encourage the child to hold a comfort item, such as a favorite toy or stuffed animal.

- ✔ When appropriate, enlist the child's help in the process by having her tear tape, open alcohol pads, or choose her favorite bandage color.

- ✔ If possible, keep the child's room a *safe room* by administering medications and performing procedures in an adjacent treatment room.

Involving the child and her family in the process early and frequently lessens anxiety, inspires courage, and encourages compliance.

Child life specialists, when available as a resource, are invaluable in creating activities that help children and families deal with the fears of IV therapy. See the nearby sidebar for details on what to do if a child life specialist isn't available.

Taking the fear out of IV therapy

Here are a few tips you can use to help make the infusion process less scary for children and their families, particularly if a child life specialist isn't available to help before and during the procedure:

✔ Perform venipuncture in a neutral place, such as a treatment room.

✔ Avoid applying restraints as much as possible and allow parents to hold and hug the child.

✔ Use creative forms of distraction by having the patient sing, blow bubbles, play with toys, or watch a movie.

✔ Use a tourniquet appropriate for the size of your patient by cutting a typical tourniquet down to fit the patient's extremity.

✔ Let the parents be with their child, especially with patients under 7 years old, because parents can help reduce anxiety.

Avoiding complications: Keeping a watchful eye

Some of the most common complications in adults, such as infiltration, phlebitis, and displacement, also occur in pediatric patients, and they're frequently associated with a child's activity and restlessness. Frequent IV restarts, which are the result of these complications, place children at a higher risk for hematomas and infection than adults.

To help prevent infiltrations, phlebitis, and displacements in your pediatric patients, do the following:

✔ **Be sure to perform hourly site assessments.** Hourly site assessment is typically the policy for infusing IVs in infants and allows for early detection of warning signs.

✔ **Use age-appropriate arm boards for splinting.** These arm boards allow for maximum mobility and easy viewing of the IV site.

✔ **Secure the site with a stabilization device.** Doing so limits catheter micro-motion associated with tape securement, reduces catheter-associated complications and unscheduled restarts, lengthens IV dwell time, and increases patient comfort.

From Preemies to Teens: Dosing for Peds

Most pediatric medications have recommended safe-dosing ranges based on the child's weight or age. Some medications have small, specific ranges, while others, such as broad-spectrum antibiotics, have wider safe-dosing ranges.

When calculating pediatric doses, check a pediatric handbook and have another nurse check to ensure that the dosage you calculated is in the safe-dosing range. If the dosage is out of range, check with the physician or pharmacist before administering the medication.

Understanding the importance of age and weight

A child's age group and weight are key considerations in determining pediatric dosages. Children's age groups are important because they affect how a child's body reacts to medications. From preemies to adolescents, the main age groups are

- ✔ **Preemie:** *Preemie* is short for *premature infant,* born before the 38th week of pregnancy.
- ✔ **Newborn:** Also called *neonates, newborns* are 1 month old or less.
- ✔ **Infant:** An *infant* is between 1 month and 1 year of age.
- ✔ **Child:** A *child* is in the broadest age group, from age 1 to age 12.
- ✔ **Adolescent:** An *adolescent* is in the teen years, from age 13 to age 18.

Because children vary so much in weight, size, and tolerance, using weight in your dosage calculations gives you a more accurate dose than using age alone. After all, the size of a 6-year-old pediatric patient may vary significantly from one child to another, depending on genetics, chronic disease, nutrition, and other independent factors.

For this reason, using weight to calculate pediatric dosing is the most common and accurate method. Fortunately for you, it's also the easiest. Most medications are dispensed and labeled as milligrams (mg), making it simple for IV nurses to weigh a child, convert the weight from pounds (lb) to kilograms (kg), and calculate the dosage based on mg of medication per kg of body weight.

Practicing your dosage calculating skills

To use the weight method to calculate pediatric dosages, the first step is to convert a child's weight from pounds (lb) to kilograms (kg). To convert weight from lb to kg, multiply the child's weight in lb by the conversion factor of 1 kg equals 2.2 lb (in other words, divide the child's weight by 2.2). Here's an example for a child who weighs 44 lb:

44 lb ÷ 2.2 = 20 kg

After you have the child's weight in kg, you calculate the total daily dose in mg and then the dose of each administration. Finally, you convert that dose to milliliters (mL). Here's an example that can help you practice your dosage calculating skills:

The physician's order calls for IV administration of ceftriaxone in mL to treat meningitis in a 5-year-old who weighs 40 lb. The ordered dose is 100 mg/kg, administered once per day, and the drug comes pre-diluted in the concentration of 40 mg/mL. How much medication, in mL, do you give in each dose?

To answer this question, use the following steps:

1. **Convert the child's weight from lb to kg by using the conversion factor 1 kg equals 2.2 lb.**

    40 lb ÷ 2.2 = 18.2 kg

    The patient weighs 18.2 kg. Round down to 18, or as directed by facility protocol.

2. **Calculate the daily dose in mg.**

    18 kg × 100 mg/kg/day = 1,800 mg/day

    The daily dose is 1,800 mg/day.

3. **Divide the daily dose by the frequency of administration.**

    1,800 mg/day ÷ 1 dose/day = 1,800 mg/day

    The once daily dose is 1,800 mg.

4. **Convert the once daily dose to mL.**

    1,800 mg/dose ÷ 40 mg/mL = 45 mL/dose

    The correct dose is 45 mL once daily.

Considering alternative methods for calculating dosing

Although most pediatric dosing is based on mg of medication per kg of body weight, dosages for certain medications, such as chemotherapy and critical-care drugs, are sometimes determined by body surface area and other alternative methods. Being familiar with one or two additional methods of calculating pediatric dosages is useful because it allows you to verify dosages you calculated based on the weight method (see the previous sections). Alternative calculating methods that nurses sometimes use include

- **Body surface area:** Body surface area (BSA) is a method of calculating dosing based on square meters of body surface. It requires using a relationship table known as a *nomogram* to determine dosing. To use the nomogram, you simply find the child's weight and height on the table and then find the corresponding BSA. You then divide the child's BSA by the average adult BSA and multiply by the normal adult dose of the medication.

- **Clark's rule:** Clark's rule is a rarely used rule that uses a combination of weight and adult dose to calculate dosing. You simply divide the child's weight by 150 and multiply that number by the adult dose.

- **Young's rule:** This rule uses a combination of age and adult dose to calculate dosing. You just add 12 to the child's age, divide the sum by the child's age, and divide the adult dose by the number you get after dividing by the child's age.

Peds-Specific Peripheral IV Considerations

Healthcare professionals perform more than 18 million peripheral venous access procedures on children each year in U.S. hospitals. Unfortunately, children and families report these IV procedures as being the most feared and most painful procedures associated with hospitalization. In fact, studies indicate that only half of IV starts are successful on the first try, and on average, it takes 2.2 attempts before venous access is successful.

The good news: Nurses are in a central position to reverse this attitude of fear by making the IV procedure as successful and painless as possible — on the first attempt. The following sections offer guidance on how to do so.

Selecting the best venous access site

To improve your chances of having a successful IV start and a successful procedure altogether, you need to know which sites are best for venous access in which children. Desirable sites in children and infants include

- ✔ Scalp veins in babies who are less than about 12 months of age

- ✔ Saphenous veins in babies who require larger vascular access device (VAD) lumens

- ✔ Feet and leg veins in children who are not yet standing or walking

- ✔ Hands and forearms in ambulatory, active children

Less desirable sites include the antecubital fossa and the palmar aspect of the wrist. The Infusion Nurses Society (INS) doesn't recommend using them due to an increase in complications at these sites.

Choosing the most appropriate peripheral IV

Which vascular access device (VAD) you use also impacts how successful your IV procedure will be. To select the best VAD with the right peripheral IV gauge for your pediatric patient, you need to know the child's age and weight. Table 19-1 presents general guidelines for selecting the right peripheral IV gauge for your pediatric patient.

Table 19-1   Guidelines for Peripheral IV Gauge Selection

Patient's Age	Patient's Weight in Kilograms (kg)	Peripheral IV Gauge
Premature infant	3 or less	26–22
Newborn (neonate)	3–4	26–22
Infant (1 month to 1 year)	4–10	24–20
Toddler (1 to 2 years)	10–13	24–20
Preschool (3 to 5 years)	13–18	24–20
School age (6 to 12 years)	18–40	24–18
Adolescent (13 to 18 years)	40–75	24–18

Using special techniques in venipuncture

Nurses at the forefront of pediatric IV therapy use special venipuncture techniques to provide the greatest opportunity for successful IV starts on their first attempt. Here are a few techniques you can try:

- Illuminate veins with approved fiber-optic or infrared light sources.

- Always insert the peripheral IV with the bevel up.

- Use anesthetic creams, such as EMLA, or a freezing spray, such as Pain Eze, to reduce pain and a warm compress to promote local vasodilation.

- Use warming packs and dangle the extremity to enhance circulation.

- Use pediatric blood pressure cuffs to provide vein distention.

To further increase your number of successful IV starts, we recommend that you also take part in the following educational and skill-building exercises:

- Observe multiple IV insertions and learn from your fellow nurses.

- Practice on mannequins, virtual programs, and IV access simulators.

Knowing what to do after a successful IV start

When your IV start is successful, quickly secure the site with a stabilization device, transparent dressing, flexible net tubular wrap, and age-appropriate arm board (see Chapter 3 for details on this and other IV equipment). *Note:* If you have an unsuccessful IV start, you can try again, but be sure to quit after two attempts and call the IV team.

After you stabilize the VAD and dress the site, you have to determine the IV fluid requirements for your pediatric patient. You do that by following your facility's protocol. Policies on pediatric fluid requirements vary from hospital to hospital, but Table 19-2 lists some commonly used guidelines for fluid requirements.

Table 19-2	Guidelines for Pediatric Fluid Requirements
Weight Range	*Daily Fluid Requirements*
0–10 kg	100 mL per kg of body weight
10–20 kg	1,000 mL + 50 mL per kg over 10 kg
20–70 kg	1,500 mL + 20 mL per kg over 20 kg
More than 70 kg	2,500 mL (same as adult requirement)

CVAD IV Therapy for Kids

Central vascular access devices (CVADs) are IV catheters with tips that are located in the superior vena cava near its junction at the right atrium or in the inferior vena cava if inserted through a lower extremity. You use central lines for vesicant agents, such as chemotherapy, and for long-term therapies that require frequent administrations. (Find details about adult CVADs in Chapters 3 and 13.)

Pediatric CVADs are similar to their adult counterparts, except that they have smaller lumen sizes and shorter lengths. Plus, with pediatric catheters, the patient's age, weight, and height are decisive factors in determining which type of pediatric CVAD to use. Table 19-3 shows CVAD sizes commonly used in pediatric central venous therapy.

Table 19-3	Recommended Pediatric CVADs Based on Age and Weight		
Age in Years	*Weight in Kilograms (kg)*	*Gauge*	*Length in Centimeters (cm)*
< 1, newborn	4–8	24	5–12
< 1	5–10	22	5–12
1–3	10–15	20	5–15
3–8	15–30	18–20	5–25
> 8	30–70	16–20	5–30

The following sections outline the four major types of CVADs and explain what you need to know when using them with children.

The non-tunneled percutaneous CVAD

Non-tunneled percutaneous CVADs are inserted by a physician often via the neck, chest, or groin and threaded through the vein to the superior vena cava (the same process as in adults). Another option, used mainly for pediatrics, is to insert the CVAD into the saphenous vein of the leg; in this case, the catheter tip ends up in the inferior vena cava. Non-tunneled central lines are used for short to intermediate dwelling times to provide frequent access for fluid or medication administration. Pediatric CVADs may require insertion under general anesthesia and typically require more vigilant monitoring for occlusion due to smaller catheter sizes.

The biggest problem with non-tunneled catheters is that they have a section of catheter that's exposed above the skin's surface, making them easier to displace in active children. For this reason, most doctors recommend tunneled catheters for active children who need longer-term therapy.

The tunneled catheter

As in adults, *tunneled catheters* are usually inserted in the chest and tunneled beneath the skin to enter via the subclavian or jugular vein; the tip ends up in the superior vena cava. Physicians typically insert tunneled catheters in children for long-term IV therapy.

The PICC line

Peripherally inserted central catheters, also called *PICC lines,* are inserted peripherally, usually through the arm, and threaded to the superior vena cava. In pediatric patients, doctors have other options for the placement of PICC lines, including the scalp vein, umbilicus, and saphenous veins. Qualified nurses usually insert PICC lines for use in long-term therapies. PICC lines stay in place for months and are used for treatment of children with serious disorders such cancer, leukemia, or hemophilia.

The implanted port

Implanted ports are central lines that are surgically implanted under the skin by a physician. The catheter is tunneled under the skin and enters via the subclavian or jugular; the tip ends up in the superior vena cava. Ports have a reservoir with a self-sealing septum that you access through the skin with a special non-coring needle. Ports are used for long-term therapy such as chemotherapy, antibiotics, or parenteral nutrition. Accessing a port, especially in children, may require using topical anesthetic, such as EMLA cream, or a freezing spray, such as Pain Eze, to decrease the pain. Always use sterile technique when you access an implanted port.

Chapter 20

When Aging Is an Issue: IV Therapy for the Elderly

. . . .

In This Chapter

▶ Considering the effects age has on IV therapy

▶ Dealing with common issues when working with older patients

▶ Following a few important insertion guidelines

▶ Knowing what to look for when monitoring infusions in elderly patients

. . . .

*I*n 2001, the American Nurses Association (ANA) estimated that likely more than 8.5 million people will be over the age of 85 in the United States by the year 2030. This figure represents a significant amount of the population that may be hospitalized and need IV therapy. As people get older, their body organs age with the rest of their bodies. These physiological changes affect the way the elderly body deals with medications. As a result, older adults are generally more sensitive to IV therapy than their younger counterparts due to decreased drug absorption, binding, distribution, and excretion.

In this chapter, you find out about the specific risks facing elderly IV patients and the special precautions you must take when medicating and monitoring them. You get some insider tips on starting IVs in thin, fragile veins, and you discover how to recognize and manage complications that are specific to the elderly.

Understanding How Advanced Age Impacts IV Therapy

When administering IV therapy in elderly patients, you have to consider all the effects aging has on their bodies. Specifically, you need to consider how aging affects the body on the following three levels:

✔ **Cellular:** At the cellular level, age-related changes in cell structure impair the immune system, lessening the body's ability to fight infection.

✔ **Organic:** On an organic level, aging causes diminished function of body organs, such as the liver and kidney, which leads to a reduced ability to absorb, metabolize, and excrete medications.

✔ **Systemic:** Systemically, aging results in the body's decreased ability to repair itself, leading to impairment of major systems, such as the immune, respiratory, and circulatory systems.

As the human body ages, body composition changes: Lean muscle mass decreases, fat increases, and the basal metabolic rate (BMR) slows down. Every ten years after age 45, the average person loses approximately 10 percent of his lean muscle mass and gains the same amount in body fat. As the body mass shifts from less muscle to more fat, the body's ability to absorb, metabolize, and excrete medications slows down.

The same metabolic changes that cause decreased muscle mass and increased fat deposits also cause metabolic diseases, such as diabetes and hypertension. These metabolic changes are associated with decreasing levels of hormones and antibodies and increasing levels of insulin resistance. They also cause a decrease in the regenerative capacity of stem cells, hampering the body's ability to repair itself and maintain health. Age-related metabolic changes decrease the body's ability to metabolize amino acids and store protein and decrease glandular activity, impairing thyroid and adrenal function.

With all these changes taking place in your elderly patient's body, it's no wonder that he's at greater risk for the following complications during IV therapy:

✔ **Adverse drug reactions (ADRs):** Older patients typically have one or more chronic, coexisting diseases. As a result, they're usually on multiple prescription medications, making them more vulnerable than younger patients to ADRs during IV therapy. As a healthcare professional administering IV therapy, you're at the forefront of preventing and managing these ADRs. (We explain how to prevent ADRs in the later section "Identifying adverse drug reactions.")

✔ **Dehydration:** Older patients are at greater risk for dehydration because they're frequently undernourished and are more vulnerable to age-related shifts in water balance. Older patients also typically take multiple medications, such as diuretics, that deplete body fluids, and they have medical conditions, such as diabetes, that cause excessive urination, placing them at even greater risk for dehydration. Therefore, you have to be especially vigilant about looking for signs of dehydration in your elderly IV patients. (We tell you how to deal with dehydration in the later section "Managing dehydration.")

✔ **Infections:** Because elderly patients often have impaired immune systems, they're at greater risk for infections, particularly when they're in the hospital. And their risk rises even more if they have frequent, extended stays at the hospital.

Pneumonia and influenza are two of the most common infections in elderly patients. In fact, pneumonia results in the death of more than half of all hospitalized patients 65 years and older, and influenza accounts for more than 15,000 deaths in the elderly each year. Another common infection is *hospital-acquired infection* (HAI), a healthcare-related infection that usually occurs within three days of admission and is frequently related to a medical procedure or treatment (in this case, IV therapy). (We explain how to prevent these infections later in the section "Preventing infection.")

Optimizing Therapy for the Older Adult

To meet the specific challenges of IV therapy in the elderly, you must give special consideration to the age-related issues we outline in the preceding section that impact every aspect of IV therapy. This section covers the problems and solutions most frequently associated with IV therapy in the elderly, from starting an IV in thin, fragile veins to obtaining informed consent from a cognitively impaired senior.

Be patient with your patient. More than 40 percent of all hospital patients are 65 years and older, meaning that you'll certainly be caring for elderly patients during your healthcare career. Using patience to explain procedures and outline treatment plans helps build relationships and promote patient compliance. Educating patients about self-care procedures maximizes independence and prevents recurrence of symptoms. Discussing the importance of proper nutrition, compliance with medication schedules, and well-patient checkups also improves patient outcomes.

Assessing the elderly patient

Before you start an IV in an elderly patient, you need to perform a basic patient assessment that focuses on the following factors:

✔ **Chronic, coexisting medical conditions:** Elderly patients may be admitted to the hospital for treatment of an acute condition like pneumonia, but they may also have a chronic existing medical problem, such as diabetes, that impacts their ability to tolerate dextrose in IV fluids.

✔ **Cognitive status, current medical problems, and health history:** A thorough patient assessment must evaluate an elderly patient's current and past health conditions, as well as her ability to comprehend her medical treatment and communicate effectively with the healthcare team.

✓ **Loss of functionality, vision, or hearing:** Assessment must also include an evaluation of physical function to determine the patient's ability to ambulate safely, evaluate the patient's risk for falling, and determine the need for any special provisions.

✓ **Medications, allergies, and drug interactions:** Patient assessment must also include a thorough medication evaluation because many elderly patients take multiple medications and are at greater risk for adverse drug reactions — a risk that's identified at the time of the initial assessment and communicated to coworkers throughout therapy via proper documentation.

Use your assessment results to develop a nursing care plan that focuses on any complex problems your patient has, the multiple medications she's taking, and the associated need for a multidisciplinary team of healthcare providers. Be sure to document your findings to inform other healthcare team members.

Obtaining informed consent

As with the general population, doctors must obtain informed consent (as determined by the facility's policies and local, state, and federal regulations) before performing a defined procedure or therapy. The healthcare provider who's performing the procedure or treatment needs to obtain the consent. The Infusion Nurses Society (INS) recommends that the informed consent include full details of the procedure, its risks and benefits, any alternatives, and all complications associated with the treatment or therapy in a manner that the patient or their legal representative can understand. The nurse should advocate for the patient's (or the patient's legal rep's) right to accept or refuse treatment.

Obtaining informed consent from cognitively impaired older adults presents a whole different challenge for IV therapists. Informed consent makes sense only for people who can make informed decisions, and nurses are frequently in the difficult position of helping doctors decide who can and can't make informed decisions.

Of course, deciding that an unconscious or severely mentally impaired patient is incapable of making an informed decision is easy to do, but deciding whether patients with mild cognitive impairment are capable is more difficult. In patients with questionable cognitive ability, the physician must decide whether the patient is capable or incapable of making an informed decision. To help you and the physician decide whether a patient truly understands the concept of informed consent, assess the patient's ability to understand relevant information, consequences of a decision, and communication of a decision. For example, ask the patient her name, birth date, current year, and current president and ask her if she knows where she is and why she's in the hospital.

Some older patients elect to take a formal test to gauge mental status, while others choose to appoint a surrogate decision maker through legal documents, such as advance directives or durable power of attorney for healthcare.

Considering the dose

When calculating the IV dose for an older patient, the optimum dose is the smallest dose that can achieve the desired effect. After all, older patients have age-related changes that impair the body's ability to circulate, metabolize, and excrete drugs, leading to a slower response to IV medications (see the earlier section "Understanding How Advanced Age Impacts IV Therapy" for details).

If a patient can't metabolize and excrete a medication quickly enough, the drug circulates in the bloodstream for a much longer period of time than it does for the average person. As a result, you need to take the following dosing considerations into account when you're working with elderly patients:

- Lower doses to accommodate the slower metabolism
- Longer time intervals between infusions
- Microdrips and slower infusion rates to prevent overhydration

Turn to Chapter 10 for a ton more details on IV dosing.

Selecting the best venipuncture site

Selecting the best injection site in elderly patients can be a challenge. Older veins are thinner, less elastic, more superficial, and less stationary. The subcutaneous tissue that anchors veins in younger people is diminished in older patients, making veins more likely to roll and more prone to punctures in the vein's back wall.

Use the following tips to help you select the best veins to use in older patients:

- Select a vein that enables you to pull the skin taut toward you to anchor the vein and prevent it from rolling.
- Choose a vein that lets you reduce the angle of insertion to prevent puncturing the back wall. Your goal is to reduce the angle to almost flat when penetrating the vein and then to reduce the angle even more when you obtain flashback.

✔ When possible, select a vein that you can clearly feel and see by occluding the vein with finger pressure above the insertion site so you don't have to use a tourniquet. Older veins and skin are more vulnerable to damage from tourniquets.

Check out the later section "Gentleness Is Key: Following Some Basic Insertion Guidelines" for details on how to successfully start an IV after you've selected the best insertion site.

Choosing the most effective equipment

In addition to the standard IV therapy equipment (such as infusion bags, IV tubings, and IV poles), other supplies you may need for geriatric patients include nonirritating paper tape for applying dressings to fragile skin, antiseptic solutions, and a wide variety of small-gauge vascular access devices (VADs).

Selecting the right VAD is important in IV therapy, but it's even more critical when you're dealing with elderly patients. The most ideal VAD for the older patient includes the following features:

✔ Smallest catheter gauge and shortest catheter length possible for the infusate

✔ Least invasive device and least number of lumens

Other factors to consider when choosing the VAD include the type of infusate, the catheter dwell time, and the frequency of IV additive administrations (see Chapter 3 for details on which VADs to use when).

A general rule of thumb is that therapies lasting longer than 96 hours or containing vesicant medications require a central vascular access device (CVAD) (see Chapter 13 for details).

When administering to older patients, you also need to use the following two pieces of equipment to control infusion volume and prevent fluid overload (see Chapter 3 for more details on each one):

✔ **IV infusion pump:** Set the infusion pump at the slowest possible infusion rate to prevent rupturing or damaging your older patient's fragile veins.

✔ **Microdrip IV tubing:** This tubing works great for elderly patients because it allows you to infuse smaller amounts of medication with greater accuracy and control.

Gentleness Is Key: Following Some Basic Insertion Guidelines

Inserting IVs in older patients can be an intimidating task. After all, older veins roll, are less elastic, and move during insertion. They're easily blown (ruptured) during IV insertion and may be flattened by dehydration. Plus, older skin bleeds and bruises when you apply tourniquets too tightly.

But don't worry! This section offers some basic tips and guidelines to help you insert IVs in elderly patients with confidence every time.

Prepping your elderly patient's skin

When prepping your elderly patient's skin for IV insertion, follow the instructions on the prepping solution. Be gentle so you don't damage your patient's thin, fragile, easily torn skin.

If you use alcohol pads, cleanse the skin with short, gentle strokes that disinfect the minimum area needed for the insertion and dressing. Make sure that the prepped area is dry before you or the doctor inserts the catheter.

Inserting the VAD

To maximize success when inserting the VAD in an elderly patient, keep in mind the following guidelines:

- Use a soft, lightly applied tourniquet or a slightly inflated blood pressure cuff.
- Stabilize the vein for the insertion by applying traction below the insertion site.
- Use the smallest catheter possible and a flat angle of insertion.
- Insert the catheter directly on top of the vein and avoid side entry.

Stabilizing the device

The INS recommends using catheter stabilization devices rather than tape to secure VADs in elderly patients. Stabilization devices protect the integrity of the insertion site and prevent the VAD from loosening when patients try to adjust the dressing. Improved stabilization with manufactured devices also restricts micromovements that can lead to infiltration, leakage, and IV restarts.

When prepping your patient's skin for a stabilization device, use the prepping solution that accompanies the device. The solution provides a thin coat of protection that allows the device to stick to the prep rather than to the patient's skin.

When removing the stabilizer, use an alcohol pad to easily release the device without tearing or bruising your patient's skin.

Monitoring the Infusion to Prevent Complications

You have to monitor VADs in elderly patients more frequently than in younger patients because the risk for infiltration, drug interaction, and other complications is greater in older patients. In fact, in hospitalized patients 65 years and older, medication reactions occur 2.5 times more frequently, and treatment mishaps occur 4 times more frequently than in younger patients. Part of the reason for these healthcare-related complications is that older patients are frequently more acutely ill and require longer hospital stays than their younger counterparts (see the earlier section "Understanding How Advanced Age Impacts IV Therapy" for more on why older patients are more prone to IV-related complications).

To minimize risk for your elderly patient, take the following precautions:

- ✔ Closely monitor patients with cognitive impairment for possible drug reactions.
- ✔ Identify patients who experience an onset of confusion or sedation, discontinue the infusion, and give appropriate reversal agents (antagonists) according to the doctor's order.
- ✔ Monitor patients frequently when they're frail or lack family support.
- ✔ Obtain orders for nutritional support when applicable.
- ✔ Obtain orders to stop a drug when symptoms subside.
- ✔ Start IV drugs *low and slow* (that is, slowly give the lowest possible dose when starting a medication) and titrate dosages up to the desired rate.

The following sections provide more advice for guarding against some of the most common IV complications in the elderly.

Preventing infection

Unfortunately, the typical signs and symptoms of infection, such as fever or increased white blood cell count, are often absent in the elderly because of impaired immune function. In fact, in some cases, the only symptom that signifies infection is altered mental status or impaired cognitive function. For this reason, you need to be especially vigilant in preventing hospital-acquired infections (HAIs) from spreading and checking your elderly patients for infection. As part of your regular monitoring, be sure to do the following:

✔ Inspect the dressing for dampness and the insertion site for swelling.

✔ Maintain strict adherence to aseptic technique.

✔ Wash your hands frequently with antibacterial soaps.

✔ Prevent cross-contamination among patients.

✔ Disinfect the catheter hub by vigorously scrubbing it for at least 15 seconds with an appropriate antiseptic.

✔ Use a needless system (specifically a split-septum system) to access the IV tubing.

✔ Change the needleless connection every 72 hours or according to your facility's policy and procedure.

Two of the most common infections that elderly patients suffer from are pneumonia and influenza. The most successful way to prevent these respiratory infections is by vaccination. The pneumococcal vaccine decreases risk for pneumonia by 75 percent, and influenza vaccines reduce risk for infection by 30 to 70 percent in elderly populations.

Other general factors that help prevent infection in the elderly include the following:

✔ Decreased hospital stays

✔ Less invasive surgery and strict infection control

✔ Less frequent use of urinary catheters

✔ Nutritional assessment and intervention

Dealing with equipment issues

The normal aging process causes many physiological changes in the skin and veins of geriatric patients, requiring you to pay special attention to the equipment you use during IV administration. Small equipment failures that occur from the time of IV insertion to IV discontinuation may result in serious complications for older patients. To minimize the risk for these complications in older patients, use the following guidelines to double-check equipment and supplies:

- ✔ Visually inspect IV bags and bottles for contamination through damage or cracks, which lead to a serious risk for phlebitis and other complications.
- ✔ Check IV solutions for precipitates that may cause additional problems in older, sclerosed veins.
- ✔ Verify that the medication labels on infusion bags are the correct medication and dosage as ordered by the physician.
- ✔ Inspect IV tubing for kinks, closed clamps, or damage and change macrotubing to microtubing.
- ✔ Ensure that infusion pumps are working properly and set up for accurate infusion volumes and drip rates to prevent fluid overload.
- ✔ Use lightly inflated blood pressure cuffs rather than tourniquets to insert IVs with less damage to fragile skin.

Identifying adverse drug reactions

Adverse drug reactions (ADRs) from treatment with IV antibiotics are one of the most common problems associated with geriatric IV therapy. To identify suspected ADRs, monitor patients for the following adverse symptoms, which are frequently associated with IV antibiotic therapy:

- ✔ Respiratory distress
- ✔ Skin rash or hives
- ✔ Swelling, particularly in the hands and face

Sometimes ADRs manifest themselves in older patients in atypical ways, such as the following:

- ✔ Confusion, hallucinations, or delirium
- ✔ Falls or slipping injuries
- ✔ Gastrointestinal problems such as diarrhea, constipation, or abdominal pain
- ✔ Kidney problems such as flank pain or dehydration

Prevention is the first step in avoiding IV complications in elderly patients. To prevent ADRs from occurring, follow these guidelines every time you administer IV therapy to elderly patients:

✔ **Conduct a thorough patient assessment of your patient's prescription and over-the-counter medication history.** Elderly patients are twice as likely as their younger counterparts to self-medicate for common ailments. Finding out about all medications your patients are taking at the initial assessment enables the healthcare team to avoid duplication and potential overmedication.

✔ **Closely monitor and observe your elderly patients throughout therapy.** Any new symptom or exacerbation of an existing symptom may indicate an adverse reaction to a medication.

✔ **Consider those patients who are at higher risk for ADRs.** Patients taking more than five medications and patients taking high-risk medications, such as the following, are inherently at greater risk for adverse reactions:

- Antibiotics

- Anticoagulants

- Antipsychotics

- Antiseizure meds

- Diuretics

Managing dehydration

When monitoring your elderly patients before, during, and after their infusions, be sure to assess them for dehydration. As part of this assessment, do the following:

✔ Evaluate the patient's health history, particularly for patients with a history of dehydration and an increased risk for recurrence.

✔ Assess the patient's physical, nutritional, and hydration status by assessing the patient's health history, physical assessment, laboratory tests, functional assessments, fluid intake behaviors, and risk identification.

✔ Review any and all laboratory findings, including the following:

- **Blood chemistries:** These can help you detect electrolyte imbalances that are frequently associated with dehydration.

- **Complete blood count (CBC):** CBC measures the number of red blood cells (RBCs), number of white blood cells (WBCs), total amount of hemoglobin in the blood, and the fraction of the blood composed of RBCs (hematocrit). Increased RBCs or high hematocrit may indicate dehydration (possibly from severe diarrhea).

- **Blood urea nitrogen (BUN) and creatinine:** BUN measures the amount of urea nitrogen in the blood (normal results are 6–20 mg/ dL). Creatinine is a breakdown product of creatine, which is an important part of muscles (normal values are 0.7–1.3 mg/dL for men and 0.6–1.1 mg/dL for women). Higher values indicate dehydration.

- **Urine specific gravity:** This measures the kidney's ability to concentrate or dilute urine in relation to plasma (normal values are 1.002–1.030). Higher levels indicate dehydration.

If you identify dehydration in one of your elderly patients, notify the physician immediately and implement the following hydration management therapy:

- ✔ Calculate a daily fluid goal and monitor intake and output.
- ✔ Minimize fasting times for tests or surgery.
- ✔ Provide the patient with a variety of fluids to drink.
- ✔ Teach the patient to use a urine color chart to monitor his own hydration status.

Replacing and Discontinuing Peripheral IVs

As in younger patients, peripheral IVs in the elderly must be replaced at the first sign of phlebitis or when clinically indicated, as recommended by the INS. However, you may be reluctant to replace a noninfected, working IV in an elderly patient who has no suitable veins for replacement. In these situations, notify the physician for an order to preserve the existing IV or to replace it with a midline or central venous catheter.

When peripheral lines are left in longer than recommended, the infection rate rises significantly. Closely monitor the insertion site for infection and carefully document the reasons for not replacing the catheter.

When discontinuing peripheral IVs in the elderly, prepare to work in slow motion and keep the following guidelines in mind:

- ✔ Remove the tape and dressing slowly to prevent tearing the skin.
- ✔ Remove the catheter gently and slowly to prevent damaging the vein.
- ✔ Because elderly patients are more prone to hematoma, apply pressure to the insertion site more gently and for a longer period of time than you do in younger patients.
- ✔ For seniors on aspirin or anticoagulant therapy, monitor the insertion site and reapply gentle pressure if needed to stop bleeding.

Check out Chapter 12 for more details on replacing and discontinuing peripheral IVs.

Chapter 21

There's No Place Like Home: IV Therapy for the Homebound Patient

. . . .

In This Chapter

▶ Assessing the neighborhood, home, and patient

▶ Creating a care plan for your homebound patient and choosing the right infusion equipment

▶ Practicing safe IV therapy in the home

▶ Preparing your patients and their families for self-care

. . . .

*H*ome healthcare is the fastest growing sector in the multibillion-dollar healthcare industry, and it's growing larger every day. In fact, home healthcare anticipates a 66 percent increase over the next ten years and expects to be servicing more than 7 million patients per year. With rising hospital costs and shrinking healthcare dollars, a growing number of patients are taking their central lines and catheter bags home with them to complete treatment and recovery.

In this chapter, we take a look at the unique safety issues you face in home healthcare, and we explain how to make the home environment as safe as possible for you and your patient. We introduce you to ambulatory home infusion pumps and the increasingly sophisticated types of infusions you may administer to homebound patients. We explain how to manage home IV therapy, including complications that may arise during a home visit, and we offer some tips to help a patient and family become self-sufficient in administering IVs at home.

Ensuring Safety: Assessing the Home Environment

Hospital and home therapy are a lot alike for the provider in terms of the equipment, treatments, and medications used; however, one major difference is the unregulated environment. In hospital environments, the patient is the primary variable needing assessment, but in home healthcare you also have to assess the overall environment, including both the neighborhood and the home itself.

Checking out the neighborhood

Home healthcare workers have no control over their patient's neighborhood location, but they do have control over how they assess the neighborhood and implement precautions to ensure their safety and that of their patient. Because most reports of violence or threats of violence to home healthcare workers come from high-crime areas, home healthcare workers must thoroughly assess their patient's neighborhood to identify high-risk times and areas and come up with a safety plan to deal with them.

To assess the neighborhood, research the area for factors associated with location, such as crime rate, police presence, and population demographics. Your research can consist of doing Internet searches to check demographics or driving through the area to assess it visually. Here are a couple of great online resources to check out: `http://quickfacts.census.gov/qfd/index.html` and `www.brookings.edu/about/projects/state-metro-innovation/resources`.

If your neighborhood assessment shows that your patient's home is located in a high-crime area, take the following precautions to ensure your safety during each home visit:

- ✔ Call your patient ahead of time to confirm the appointment and get detailed directions.
- ✔ Keep your car's gas tank full.
- ✔ Keep the home's doors locked and windows closed.
- ✔ Post and update your schedule with your facility or a coworker and request daytime assignments when scheduling with your facility or the patient.
- ✔ Trust your instincts and leave the area if it feels unsafe.

Dealing with safety issues in the home

Managing health and safety hazards in the home is one of the greatest challenges facing home healthcare workers. After all, residential settings are plagued with problems that can place the patient and the healthcare provider at risk.

Patient safety

Homebound patients face a number of safety risks that hospital patients don't have to worry as much about, including the following:

- **Unsanitary conditions in the home:** Exposure to raw meats, pets, and unsanitary conditions poses a significant risk for patient infection, especially for patients with central line catheters, who are already at higher risk for bloodstream infections and sepsis.

- **Cross-contamination from blood-borne pathogens, such as HIV/AIDS, Hepatitis, and methicillin-resistant Staphylococcus aureaus (MRSA):** This risk can lead to infection and usually involves mismanagement of central line dressings, discarded IV sets, and other medical waste.

- **Environmental factors:** Tripping falls are the most common cause of injury in the home; they frequently involve cluttered pathways, poor lighting, rugs, stairs, small pets, and inadequate access for wheelchairs and walkers.

To minimize risks for home patients, home healthcare workers must employ the following safety measures:

- Ensure that the patient and family adhere to strict *aseptic technique* (a set of specific practices performed under carefully controlled conditions with the goal of minimizing contamination by pathogens). The goal of aseptic technique is to protect the patient from infection.

- Ensure that you and your patient properly manage all dressings, sharps, and medical waste (see the later section "Properly discarding hazardous waste in the home" for details).

- Ensure that walkways are clear and free of all tripping hazards.

Healthcare worker safety

Homebound patients aren't the only ones at risk in home-care settings. Rates of injury to home healthcare workers are 50 percent higher than the rates for their hospital counterparts.

According to the U.S. Bureau of Labor Statistics, home healthcare workers face multiple safety risks, ranging from falls over tripping hazards to hostile animal bites. Exposure to hazardous substances in the home, such as asbestos insulation and lead paint, and unexpected factors, such as illegal weapons or illicit drugs, also increase risk for home healthcare workers.

To minimize risk when you're working in a home setting, use the following guidelines to tip the scale in favor of your own personal health and safety:

- ✔ **Expect the unexpected.** Be aware that homes, unlike acute-care settings, are constantly changing, unpredictable environments that you must monitor continuously.

- ✔ **Watch your step.** To avoid stepping on a nail, tack, or piece of glass, keep your shoes on when you're in a patient's home. Also pick up any tripping hazards you see as you walk through the home.

- ✔ **Protect yourself.** Identify any weapons or illegal drugs in the home and make sure they're removed before you initiate therapy.

- ✔ **Don't touch the animals.** Even when animals appear to be friendly, ask that animals be kept away during your visit. We recommend calling the patient ahead of time to discuss this issue.

Optimizing IV Therapy for a Homebound Patient

Home infusion therapy presents multiple challenges (besides just the safety issues we mention in the preceding section) to home healthcare workers. For one, home healthcare providers work alone, without the on-site support of coworkers or emergency response teams. They also have to depend on the patient or family members to carry out treatments and provide medications during the healthcare worker's absence. Plus, increasingly sophisticated infusions of parenteral nutrition, antibiotics, and immunoglobulin therapy are now being administered at home by using increasingly sophisticated equipment.

As a home healthcare nurse, you play a major role in optimizing therapy for homebound patients despite these challenges. The first two steps you take to get the most out of home IV therapy are completing a patient assessment and creating a comprehensive patient care plan.

Completing a patient assessment

Initial patient assessments for home infusion patients involve the same evaluation criteria you use for hospital patients, including medical history, medications, allergies, and a review of body systems (see Chapter 14 for details).

If you're dealing with elderly homebound patients with multiple medical conditions, you also have to assess the following:

✔ **Available support systems and functional limitations:** These support systems may include family members, caregivers, or neighbors who can assist the patient when they have limitations, such as being nonambulatory, bedbound, or wheelchair bound.

✔ **Cognitive and psychosocial status:** Cognitive impairments associated with delirium, dementia, and depression place patients at greater risk for injury due to short attention spans, impaired memory, disorientation, and confusion. Psychological and social aspects of your patient's life can contribute to both positive and negative overall outcomes, so you need to make sure you evaluate them early on.

✔ **Need for physical, occupational, or speech therapy:** These therapies can increase your patient's long-term quality of life and positively impact treatment outcomes by restoring strength and mobility, reducing pain, and increasing the patient's ability to communicate effectively and manage everyday tasks such as bathing, eating, and dressing.

✔ **Technical skills or need for a social worker or nurse aid:** Some patients need help performing tasks related to their medical equipment or regular daily activities, such as getting in and out of bed, moving around, and using the toilet. That's where a nurse aid comes into play. For other patients, a social worker can help them and their families find community resources, get counseling, and coordinate a variety of available services.

Taking care of the multiple needs of homebound elderly patients frequently requires a team approach to provide the services described in the preceding list. Identifying the patient's needs early in patient assessment helps you establish a team of healthcare professionals that can address all the patient's needs and achieve a better outcome.

After you complete your patient assessment, a detailed plan of care needs to be prepared (see the next section) and then coordinated with all members of the healthcare team to organize the delivery of services needed by the patient.

Developing a patient care plan

Developing a complete, detailed patient care plan, as with inpatient IV therapy, is central to the success of home infusion therapy and does the following:

- Summarizes the initial patient assessment
- Identifies the patient's needs
- Establishes a plan to meet those needs
- Outlines which home healthcare team member is best equipped to address the patient's specific problem
- Determines a time line for intervention and resolution of the problem

When developing your care plan, be sure to include these details:

- Types of services, equipment, and supplies required
- Frequency of visits and activities planned
- Functional limitations, rehabilitation potential, and prognosis
- Medications, treatments, and physician orders
- Mental status and nutritional requirements
- Environmental circumstances and safety measures
- Evaluation of progress and time line for discharge or referral

After you create your patient's care plan, you have to ensure that the patient understands the differences between hospital and home IV therapy as well as the role the he has to play in self-administered therapy at home. See the later section "Teaching Your Patients (And Their Families) How to Care for Themselves" for details.

Getting Comfortable with Home Infusion Equipment

Today's home infusion equipment employs technology that permits self-administration and automated drug delivery outside the hospital and that has become more sophisticated and adaptable. The shift in healthcare delivery from the inpatient setting to the outpatient and home settings makes selecting reliable, effective infusion equipment a critical part of safely delivering medications.

Even though most home IV equipment is similar to acute-care IV equipment, one exception is the infusion pump. The infusion pumps typically used in homecare are called *ambulatory pumps.* These pumps are smaller, hand-held versions of their hospital, pole-mounted counterparts. They often perform the same functions as larger devices, but they're designed specifically for use in home settings with ambulatory patients and can be carried in backpacks and fanny packs during infusions.

Which ambulatory infusion pump is best for home infusion depends on several factors, including the therapy, the patient's disease state, possible financial reimbursement, and the patient's ability to operate the equipment and troubleshoot complications. Here are some of the ambulatory pump functions most frequently used in home infusions:

- ✔ **Continuous flow delivery:** The continuous flow setting infuses a specific volume of fluid over a specific time. You typically use this setting for medications that must be closely monitored, such as pain medications and potassium, but you can also use it for 24-hour infusions of antibiotics and parenteral nutrition.

- ✔ **Continuous flow with bolus:** This setting allows the patient to press a button to receive a bolus or extra dose of medication; you use it exclusively for pain control. Also known as *patient-controlled analgesia* (PCA), this type of IV therapy requires the physician to prescribe the medication, the bolus dose, and specific time intervals between dosings.

- ✔ **Intermittent therapy:** You use the intermittent setting to give several medication doses throughout the day. For example, on this setting, you can program the pump to give one dose of medication, such as an antibiotic, every four hours and to run at very slow drip rates between doses.

- ✔ **Escalating rates:** The escalating rate setting starts medications slowly and escalates the flow to a certain target rate, enabling you to monitor for drug reactions during early periods of infusion. This setting comes in handy when you need to monitor first dosings of new medications.

- ✔ **Ramping rates:** The ramping setting starts at a very slow rate, increases to a target rate over a specific period of time, and slowly tapers off to zero. You use this setting to administer parenteral nutrition overnight.

Many homebound patients are discharged from the hospital with existing peripheral or central lines, but occasionally, you may have to start a peripheral IV in a home patient. Before you do so, you have to choose the right vascular access device (VAD).

When selecting a peripheral VAD, ensure the proposed therapy lasts for less than a week or is being administered infrequently. Longer therapy durations or more frequent administrations require central lines. After determining that the infusion is appropriate for a peripheral VAD, select the smallest gauge and shortest needle length adequate for delivering the intended therapy.

The most common VAD used in home IV therapy is the short, 3-inch-or-less, over-the-needle catheter that leaves a polyurethane catheter in place in the vein. You have to replace the catheter and rotate the site when clinically indicated, in accordance with the *Infusion Nursing Standards of Practice*.

See Chapter 3 for more on IV equipment and Chapter 12 for more on peripheral lines.

Managing Your Home Patient's Therapy

Working with homebound patients, you're an autonomous healthcare provider without the comfort and resources of on-site personnel and emergency response teams. You have less direction from supervisors and physicians and more direction from the patient and family members. The following sections provide guidelines on how to safely manage IV therapy outside the safety net of a hospital setting.

Having an emergency plan in place

When you're administering IV therapy in your patient's home, one of the most important things you must do is have an emergency plan prepared in the event of an anaphylactic reaction to medication. Unlike the hospital setting, where you can call a code blue and get emergency assistance, you're on your own in the patient's home.

As part of your preparation for an emergency situation, you first obtain a physician's order to initiate treatment and implement emergency orders. Then you put together an anaphylactic kit to take with you whenever you go to your patient's home. Anaphylactic kits usually contain the following items:

- Acetaminophen
- Epinephrine
- Diphenhydramine
- Hydrocortisone
- Needles and syringes
- Administration sets
- Sodium chloride IV solutions

Fortunately, anaphylactic reactions are relatively rare because most patients start therapy in the hospital and continue the same therapy at home. Some patients, however, receive their first dose of a new medication at home, and these situations raise the risk for anaphylactic reaction.

To minimize risk for first-dosing reactions to new medications, start the infusion low and slow and closely monitor the patient's vital signs. When vital signs are stable and you notice no evidence of adverse reaction, advance the infusion to the desired rate.

Monitoring IV therapy in the home

Monitoring home infusions requires all the same processes you use in acute-care settings, plus a few others that pertain specifically to homebound patients. (See Chapters 12, 13, and 14 for details on monitoring IV therapy in the hospital.)

Because most home patients are ambulatory, you have to be aware of several mobility factors that can cause infiltration or accidental removal of the IV catheter when you're monitoring home infusion patients. Pay attention to the usual problem suspects, including the insertion site, dressing, administration set, and patient. In addition, be sure to monitor the following factors that can be impacted by mobility:

- ✔ Secure ambulatory pump (should be secured to the patient by pump sash, backpack, or fanny pack)
- ✔ Availability of unobstructed ambulatory pathways
- ✔ Secure insertion site thanks to a stabilization device
- ✔ Secure IV tubing and infusion bag to prevent tripping or inadvertent catheter removal

Home patients who are receiving the following types of infusions require especially close monitoring:

- ✔ **Blood and blood component transfusions:** These may be administered at home when procedures required by the American Association of Blood Banks are followed. The home-care nurse arranges for an on-call physician and paramedic to stand by for emergencies. The nurse monitors the entire transfusion procedure and then monitors the patient for 90 minutes following the transfusion (or according to the nurse's facility protocol).

✔ **Chemotherapy agents:** A home-care nurse monitors these infusions throughout the course of administration and then discontinues the infusion, changes the tubing, and removes biohazardous waste. Refer to Chapters 6 and 16 for more details on chemo infusions and check out the Oncology Nurses Society website (www.ons.org) for particular guidelines.

Avoiding complications

Whenever potent medications and IV lines are involved, home patients are at risk for a host of IV-associated adverse reactions, such as infection, infiltration, extravasation, and embolus. In fact, the same complications associated with IV therapy in acute-care settings (see Part IV) are possible in home-care settings, plus the following additional complications:

✔ Ambulatory complications, such as accidental catheter removal

✔ Patient-administered medication errors

To prevent medication errors at home, clearly label and store medications in a designated section of the refrigerator, away from food items and out of the reach of children.

Documenting your actions

Home healthcare is a team effort that involves practitioners from various healthcare specialties. This team approach requires communication and coordination among multiple agencies and relies heavily on accurate, complete documentation in the patient's medical record. Hence, documentation is just as important in home-care settings as it is in acute-care settings.

The members of any home health team use documentation as the primary communication tool to inform each other about the patient's problems, treatments, and progress. Home-health agencies use that same documentation to evaluate and optimize risk management, to measure compliance with accreditation standards, and to get reimbursement from third-party payers such as insurance companies, government agencies, and assistance programs.

As part of your home-care documentation, be sure to include the following details:

✔ Nursing assessments and care plans

✔ Coordination and communication with other service providers

✔ Reports of incidents, interventions, treatment, and outcomes

✔ Evaluation of progress and assessment for discharge or referral

✔ Patient and family teaching, including the materials and methods used, the subjects taught, and the comprehension by the patient and family (see the later section for more details)

Properly discarding hazardous waste in the home

Managing home-generated hazardous waste became safer in 1988, when Congress directed the Environmental Protection Agency (EPA) to provide guidelines and protocols for safe handling, but although each state now regulates the transportation, storage, and disposal of medical hazardous waste, the home-care setting isn't easy to regulate. Home healthcare workers still report that patients and their caretakers frequently discard sharps in used food cans and dressing bandages with food and plastic refuse.

A major task facing home healthcare workers is teaching patients and their families to use designated sharps containers and biohazardous plastic bags to discard medical waste. An even more daunting task is getting a sick patient to properly discard a bandage when throwing it away in the regular trash is so much easier.

Fortunately, in recent years, specialized infusion companies have begun to provide licensed personnel to pick up biohazardous, infectious waste from the home and transport it to designated medical waste facilities for safe disposal.

Teaching Your Patients (And Their Families) How to Care for Themselves

Home infusion nurses face the multifaceted task of performing healthcare, teaching patients to care for themselves, and assessing the patients' competence at self-directed care. For example, home IV nurses have to teach their patients and their families everything about IV infusions, from drug preparation to infusion pump operation. Without the nurse's diligence in education, homebound patients would never experience the convenience and other benefits of home therapy.

Figuring out how to self-administer IV infusions is a strange (and potentially dangerous) new process that can overwhelm newly discharged patients. Thus, as an IV nurse, you need to break down the education into bite-sized pieces, omitting background information, and insist on return demonstrations to help patients learn and gain confidence.

Here are some of the most important things you need to teach your patients and their families:

- ✔ **How to recognize complications:** Common complications include redness, swelling, or pain at the insertion site; these can be signs of infiltration (see Chapter 12 for details).

- ✔ **When to call the physician versus when to call 911:** Common complications, such as hives or rashes, for example, require a call to the physician. More serious complications, such as respiratory distress or loss of a level of consciousness, demand a call to 911.

- ✔ **How to prevent medication errors:** Teach your patient to match the medication label with the dosage, drip rate, and frequency of administration on the prescription. Explain how to check the medication's expiration date, storage instructions, and possible side effects.

- ✔ **How to use the infusion equipment:** Ensure that your patient knows how to program the infusion pump, read the display screen, and respond to messages and alarms.

- ✔ **How to flush and maintain patency:** Discuss and explain to your patient how to properly flush peripheral and central lines to maintain a viable catheter.

Part VI
The Part of Tens

The 5th Wave
By Rich Tennant

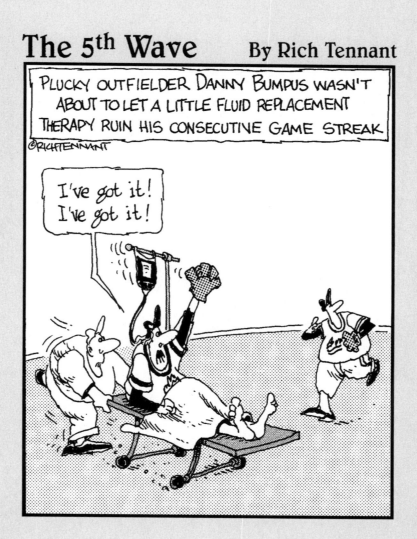

In this part . . .

Part VI is a handy reference that highlights some helpful tips and tricks you need to know as an IV nurse. First, it identifies ten important rules of thumb that every practitioner needs to remember about IV therapy. Then it reveals ten important tricks of the trade for successfully starting IVs.

Chapter 22

Ten Things You Need to Know in IV Therapy

In This Chapter

▶ Choosing the right site for IV placement

▶ Choosing the right catheter for the job

▶ Starting IVs the safe way (and knowing when to hand over the job to someone else)

▶ Monitoring your patients throughout the infusion

*I*f you're like most healthcare students and professionals, you probably have a million things on your mind every day. Having so many things competing for your attention can make remembering the nitty-gritty of IV therapy a little difficult. That's where this chapter comes into play. It contains ten things you need to know— from finding the right insertion site to monitoring the site during administration — before you begin IV therapy. So make sure you don't skip this chapter!

Start Your Site Search Distally

Vein preservation is one of the keys to successful IV therapy. When you're starting IV therapy on a new patient, begin your insertion site search low on the distal part of the extremity to preserve veins on the proximal part. Even if the patient's hospital stay is only short-term and you don't expect to administer multiple IVs, the best practice is to start the first IV distally so you can preserve veins in the proximal forearm for unexpected emergencies. (Turn to Chapter 12 for more on choosing the right insertion site.)

Avoid Starting IVs in Areas of Joint Flexion

If you place a peripheral IV in a joint area like the wrist or elbow, the flexible plastic catheter can collapse or crimp every time the patient bends her arm to eat or drink. To avoid sluggish IV flow rates and an increased potential for clots from crimped catheters, select veins in the hand, forearm, or other areas without joint movement. (Check out Chapter 12 for more on choosing the best veins for IVs.)

The Infusion Nurses Society (INS) recommends not starting IVs in the lateral surface of the wrist from the base of the palm where the wrist starts to approximately 4 to 5 inches up the arm due to the risk of pain and nerve damage.

Use Your Sense of Touch to Find a Vein

Finding a vein for IV therapy requires a combination of visual inspection and physical palpation. In many cases, the best veins for infusions are frequently difficult to see but easy to feel at first. If you're having trouble finding a vein, press your fingers to your patient's forearm or hand in common locations for veins and palpate for the spongy, bounce-back feel of a vein. When you can trace a spongy, spring-back channel between the soft-tissue areas of the forearm, place a tourniquet above the area and watch as the vein becomes more noticeable. When you see a tubular distention, you've found a vein.

Avoid Inserting IVs into Vein Valves

All veins have *valves,* which help with cardiac function by allowing the blood to flow in only one direction. When you start an IV, avoid choosing an insertion site that goes directly into a valve; instead, insert it above or below the valve.

To locate the valves in a vein, place a tourniquet above your intended insertion site and watch as the valves distend and protrude slightly from the vein. A distended valve appears as a small, round outcropping from the main shaft of the vein. You know you've found a valve if the small outcropping disappears when you release the tourniquet.

Clip Excess Hair That Interferes with the IV Area

If you have to start an IV in an area where excess hair may interfere with cleansing, inserting, or stabilizing the IV, remove the excess hair before you start the procedure. Many professional standards and protocols recommend clipping excess hair rather than shaving it because shaving causes microscopic cuts and abrasions that may potentially cause infection.

Choose the Right Gauge Based on the Patient's Situation

In most cases, the type of IV therapy you're administering, the condition of your patient, and the duration of therapy help determine the required catheter *gauge,* or size. For example, high-volume infusions during an emergency may require 14- to 18-gauge catheters, whereas most other situations require 20- to 27-gauge catheters. ***Note:*** INS recommends using a 14- to 24-gauge catheter for adults and a 22- to 24-gauge catheter for pediatrics and neonates to administer blood or blood product transfusions. See Chapter 12 for more information on selecting the correct catheter gauge.

Rely on a Blood Flashback

A *blood flashback* is a flash of blood either in the catheter or flashback chamber of an over-the-needle peripheral IV. Blood flashbacks allow you to confirm that the needle is entering the vein correctly. Outside factors such as low blood pressure, low fluid volume, and vein valves frequently decrease the presence of blood flashbacks.

If you don't observe a flashback or blood return after inserting an IV, the catheter tip may be resting near a valve. One way to assess for blood return is to apply the extension set and syringe and slowly pull back the plunger of the syringe while slowly pulling back the catheter. If you still don't see a blood return, you can attempt a gentle saline flush. If you don't see any sign of *infiltration* (pain, redness, or swelling at the needle insertion site), you can try to start the infusion slowly and monitor it closely. If you see any sign of infiltration, remove the IV, apply pressure to the insertion site, and start the IV in a different location.

Follow the Two Strikes, You're Out! Rule

If you encounter difficulty starting an IV, particularly when you're just beginning your IV career, make two attempts and then turn to an experienced IV therapist for help. Doing so isn't an admission of defeat; it's an admission of concern for your patient. Use the situation as a learning experience, and identify at least two things you'll do differently on your next attempt.

Never Push or Pull against Resistance

If you encounter resistance when starting, flushing, or withdrawing an IV, whatever you do, *don't* push or pull or try to force it. Here's what the resistance could mean:

- Resistance when starting an IV may indicate that you've encountered a valve or missed the vein and need to reposition the needle. If repositioning doesn't work, discontinue the attempt and try a vein in a different area. Never forcefully push the catheter off the needle. Doing so can cause trauma to the vein and pain for the patient.

- Resistance when flushing or withdrawing a catheter may indicate that the catheter is crimped and the patient needs to reposition his extremity to release the catheter. If resistance to flushing persists after repositioning, you may be dealing with a more serious complication, such as a blockage or occlusion from a clot. If you suspect a clot, notify the physician and follow orders or facility protocol for managing possible occlusion by clot or thrombus. Never push or pull against resistance.

Don't Rely on an Alarm to Alert You

Infusion pumps are wonderful assistants, but they can't replace the watchful eye of a vigilant IV nurse. Make sure you monitor your patient's IV at least twice during every eight-hour shift. When you add medications to the mix, be sure to monitor the IV immediately after medication injection, at least once during administration, and at the completion of administration.

Chapter 23

Ten Tricks of the Trade for Starting IVs

Gone are the days of trying over and over again to start an IV on your patient. In the *Infusion Nursing Standards of Practice,* the Infusion Nurses Society (INS) recommends that you make only two attempts to start an IV before you call in someone else. Because starting an IV can be tricky, we dedicate this chapter to giving you ten tricks of the trade to help you get it right the first time, saving your patient (and you) the anxiety and discomfort caused by multiple sticks.

Turn Up the Heat

Heat dilates blood vessels and increases blood flow and blood volume in distal veins. So you can use approved heating packets or warm, moistened towels to heat the extremity where you want to start the IV to help distend the veins. Apply the packets or towels approximately five to ten minutes before IV insertion and remove them immediately before prepping the site.

Pump Up the Volume

If you're dealing with dehydrated or critically ill patients, you can increase venous dilation (and, in turn, distend their veins) by doing one of two things:

✔ Apply a lightly inflated blood pressure cuff, no more than 60 millimeters of mercury (mmHg) of pressure, rather than a tourniquet and maintain inflation until venipuncture is complete. ***Note:*** Using a tourniquet with fragile or underdeveloped veins can cause the veins to blow when the needle is inserted.

✔ Ask the patient to pump his fist several times after you apply the tourniquet.

If neither of these tricks works and you've tried the other methods we cover in this chapter, ask another nurse to try. If another nurse can't do it either, talk to the patient's physician to see whether you can obtain an order for a midline or central line placement.

Make Gravity Your Best Friend

Use gravity to help distend veins by dangling the patient's hand and arm below heart level. As the hand dangles, gravity distends the veins in the hand and distal forearm, providing easier IV access and less risk for penetration of the back wall of the vein.

Don't Slap the Vein Silly, but Do Gently Tap It

To increase distention of the vein, you can gently tap, rub, or thump the vein after you apply a tourniquet. Tapping the vein with two to three fingers increases dilation of the vein with blood and facilitates easier insertion.

Use an Alcohol Pad to Help with Visualization

Not only do alcohol pads disinfect the IV insertion area, but they can also help you visualize veins. The friction you create by rubbing the patient's skin with alcohol pads aids in distending the vein, and the alcohol's presence on the skin highlights the vein and provides a three-dimensional appearance to the vein structure.

Disinfect the insertion site in the direction of the venous flow. Doing so improves the filling of the vein by pushing the blood past the one-way valves.

Get Cozy with Your VAD

Not all peripheral vascular access devices (VADs) are created equal! Although many VADs do share some common features, such as universal colors to designate the gauge, universal lengths, and some form of safety mechanism, they also come with a wide variety of options:

- ✔ **Safety features:** Some VADs have an *active safety feature* in the form of either a push button that retracts the needle into a plastic sheath when you press it or a push-pull system that retracts the needle within a plastic sheath as you push the catheter in and pull the needle back. Other VADs have a *passive safety feature* in the form of a small metal shield that either covers the needle tip as you pull the needle through the catheter or automatically sheaths the needle in plastic housing as you remove it from the catheter. ***Note:*** INS standards recommend a VAD with some form of safety feature to reduce the incidence of needle-stick injuries. Find out more information on sharps and sharps injury prevention at the International Sharps Injury Prevention Society's website: www.isips.org/index.php.

- ✔ **Flashback options:** Most VADs have flashback options, such as a flash chamber or a notched needle. The flash chamber allows blood to flow up the needle into a chamber so you can confirm that the needle tip is in the vein. The notched needle has a small hole in the needle a couple millimeters up the shaft, which allows a flash of blood into the catheter, so you can confirm that the needle tip is in the vein.

- ✔ **Closed versus open systems:** Some VADs are *closed systems,* meaning the extension tubing is attached to the catheter as an integrated system. The system is considered *closed* because it creates a closed fluid path, which has been proven to significantly reduce blood exposure during insertion. Others are *open systems,* meaning the extension set is attached to the hub of the catheter after the catheter is inserted into the vein. Open systems are the most common.

Familiarize yourself with the VADs you use. Read the manufacturer's directions, and when possible, watch a nursing associate insert the different types of VAD or ask her if she has any insider secrets to successful insertion. Turn to Chapters 3 and 12 for more on the different types of VADs.

Use an Anesthetic

If a physician order or your facility's protocol approves the use of topical or local anesthetics when starting IVs, you can use them to promote patient comfort and compliance. One of the most commonly used topical anesthetics, *EMLA,* is a cream mixture of two local anesthetics: lidocaine 2.5 percent and prilocaine 2.5 percent.

As an alternate to cream, some IV therapists inject a local anesthetic of 1 percent lidocaine, 0.1 to 0.2 mL, with a tuberculin syringe prior to venipuncture.

Anchors Away! Provide Vein Stability

Before you insert the VAD, anchor the vein by gently applying traction, or pulling the skin tightly, below the insertion site. Pulling the skin taut below the insertion site anchors the vein, prevents it from rolling, and provides vein stability as you insert the needle and advance the catheter. For more on stabilizing veins during IV insertion, check out Chapter 12.

Consider Using an Indirect Insertion

Inserting a VAD directly into the vein is the most common method of insertion, but in some cases, you may want to insert a VAD by the indirect method. In other words, you pierce the skin alongside the vein and enter the vein's sidewall. Nurses sometimes use indirect insertions to access elderly fragile veins because the indirect method allows them to place the VAD into the vein's sidewall, increasing success. For more details on indirect vein insertions, see Chapter 12.

Never Let 'Em See You Sweat

When a patient fears a procedure, that fear triggers an autonomic nervous system reaction, known as *vasovagal response,* where the patient becomes sweaty and nauseated and can have blurred vision and hearing loss. Vasovagal response can elicit a drop in blood pressure and heart rate and may even cause the patient to faint.

To prevent this response, enter your patient's room with confidence and do everything you can to alleviate his fears. Remember your countless hours practicing on IV mannequins, your knowledge about the IV procedure, your familiarity with the VAD you're using, and the insider secrets you've learned from experts. Take a moment to establish rapport, alleviate your patient's fears, and instill confidence. When your confidence is high and your patient is emotionally prepared for IV insertion, you've set the stage for a successful procedure.

Index

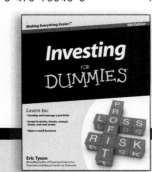

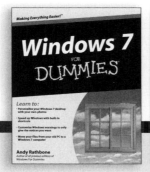

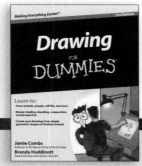

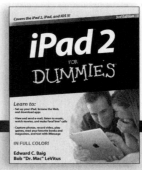

ailable wherever books are sold. For more information or to order direct: U.S. customers visit www.dummies.com or call 1-877-762-2974.
U.K. customers visit www.wileyeurope.com or call (0) 1243 843291. Canadian customers visit www.wiley.ca or call 1-800-567-4797.

Connect with us online at www.facebook.com/fordummies or @fordummies

Math & Science

Algebra I For Dummies,
2nd Edition
978-0-470-55964-2

Biology For Dummies,
2nd Edition
978-0-470-59875-7

Chemistry For Dummies,
2nd Edition
978-1-1180-0730-3

Geometry For Dummies,
2nd Edition
978-0-470-08946-0

Pre-Algebra Essentials
For Dummies
978-0-470-61838-7

Microsoft Office

Excel 2010 For Dummies
978-0-470-48953-6

Office 2010 All-in-One
For Dummies
978-0-470-49748-7

Office 2011 for Mac
For Dummies
978-0-470-87869-9

Word 2010
For Dummies
978-0-470-48772-3

Music

Guitar For Dummies,
2nd Edition
978-0-7645-9904-0

Clarinet For Dummies
978-0-470-58477-4

iPod & iTunes
For Dummies,
9th Edition
978-1-118-13060-5

Pets

Cats For Dummies,
2nd Edition
978-0-7645-5275-5

Dogs All-in One
For Dummies
978-0470-52978-2

Saltwater Aquariums
For Dummies
978-0-470-06805-2

Religion & Inspiration

The Bible For Dummies
978-0-7645-5296-0

Catholicism For Dummies,
2nd Edition
978-1-118-07778-8

Spirituality For Dummies,
2nd Edition
978-0-470-19142-2

Self-Help & Relationships

Happiness For Dummies
978-0-470-28171-0

Overcoming Anxiety
For Dummies,
2nd Edition
978-0-470-57441-6

Seniors

Crosswords For Seniors
For Dummies
978-0-470-49157-7

iPad 2 For Seniors
For Dummies, 3rd Edition
978-1-118-17678-8

Laptops & Tablets
For Seniors For Dummies,
2nd Edition
978-1-118-09596-6

Smartphones & Tablets

BlackBerry For Dummies,
5th Edition
978-1-118-10035-6

Droid X2 For Dummies
978-1-118-14864-8

HTC ThunderBolt
For Dummies
978-1-118-07601-9

MOTOROLA XOOM
For Dummies
978-1-118-08835-7

Sports

Basketball For Dummies,
3rd Edition
978-1-118-07374-2

Football For Dummies,
2nd Edition
978-1-118-01261-1

Golf For Dummies,
4th Edition
978-0-470-88279-5

Test Prep

ACT For Dummies,
5th Edition
978-1-118-01259-8

ASVAB For Dummies,
3rd Edition
978-0-470-63760-9

The GRE Test For
Dummies, 7th Edition
978-0-470-00919-2

Police Officer Exam
For Dummies
978-0-470-88724-0

Series 7 Exam
For Dummies
978-0-470-09932-2

Web Development

HTML, CSS, & XHTML
For Dummies, 7th Edition
978-0-470-91659-9

Drupal For Dummies,
2nd Edition
978-1-118-08348-2

Windows 7

Windows 7
For Dummies
978-0-470-49743-2

Windows 7
For Dummies,
Book + DVD Bundle
978-0-470-52398-8

Windows 7 All-in-One
For Dummies
978-0-470-48763-1

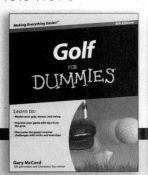

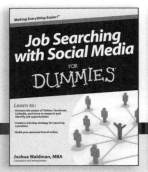

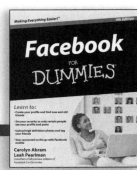

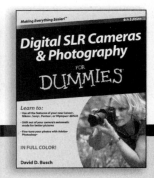